DISCLAIMERS

I have tried to recreate events, locales, and conversations from my memories of them. In order to maintain their anonymity **in all instances**, I have changed the names of individuals and at times places, I may have changed some identifying characteristics and details such as physical properties, occupations and places of residence.

This book is not intended as a substitute for the medical advice of physicians. The reader should regularly consult a physician in matters relating to his/her health, particularly with respect to any symptoms that may require diagnosis or medical attention.

Statements in the book have not been evaluated by the FDA.

Spare Changing For Trauma:

A memoir of pain and healing

By

April .L. Graham

Self Published via Docucopies 636 Commerce Dr, Hudson, WI, 54016
1-877-222-4842

Dedicated to some girl out there on a forgotten highway

Her pack is too full

Her stomach too empty

Feet stained with dirt

Eyes full of held back tears

Heart full of cynicism

Though she knows what's likely coming

She keeps walking anyways

Contents

4

I can't imagine that anyone really wants to read about the things I will be talking on here, maybe because I can't fathom living them again and, in a way, it feels like putting these words to paper is doing just that. But I know that it will also be a release for me, and maybe give some insight for those who care to know a bit more about the things that have shaped me as a person. In that, I would like to call bullshit to the folks who like to sing about how our traumas do not define us. I find this to be a deep form of self denial. Are we only our traumas? No, but do they play a pivotal role in who we are as people? Of course, they do. We can be so much more than just in a perpetual state of hurt from these things - our things - that have happened to us. They can be empowering, they can be crippling, and all of the states found in between. Today, as I type these words, I am both empowered and fucking crippled from the fear of it.

I want to talk on how my mind works for a moment here, just to brace you for what may be chaotic to read. Time for me during this particular chunk of my life - shit, life in general - is seemingly interchangeable. I mean, I know which scenario led to the next but that's not how the story always flows in my head, so this will not be chronological. At times I don't even know how old I was. Sometimes I wonder if this was all even my life. It just seems like so much to have happened in such a small time frame.

I know many want to hear it all, every phase and every tidbit, but there is just so much that I can't. I can't relive it all at once. So here in this space with you, I will be meandering through the highways, interstates, piss smelling camps, and the hunger that defined a chunk of my life between the approximate ages of 13 and 18, and we will see what comes of it. If it doesn't break me, if it helps others in some way, if it helps me, well, I can keep going.

Some asked for an herbal book. Some asked for a book about my traumas. Honestly, I don't know how to write about one and not the other, so I won't.

I don't suspect this will be an easy read, and that's about the only warning I'm gana give.

.1.

Swallowing Trauma

I just wanted out. Away. Gone. Fuck this place and everyone in it. Fuck your faces, your voices, your kind words that echoed with emptiness. They didn't take away the hurt that led me to run. And damn, did I run. I stole your rig at twelve and got them girls who knew how to drive to join me. We made it all the way to Portland before the cops found us. They screamed 'kidnap' and my face hit the pavement with a knee to my spine. They drug me back.

I cut the screws out of the window frame meant to keep me in with a dremel tool and ran down to the carnival that comes every year. They were happy to let me join them. I mean, I had enough tits to make them happy and there was lots of dope to go around. They drug me back.

I ran in the dead of winter, up under that bridge where people went to have life damaging experiences. I was skinny enough to get through that rebar and away from that man - hanging, dangling above the sub-zero raging water of the mighty Umatilla. The other girl was not so lucky. Her screams still haunt me, though there was nothing I could do. They drug me back.

I met those men in town, working on the new road that benefited no one. I talked that one girl into picking me up. I hitchhiked for the first time on the highway. There are so many truckers who really don't care. They drug me back. Again and again, they drug me back.

Then I met a boy much older than me, as usual, who said "wanna robo fry?"

Of course, I did. Why not? By that time I had eaten plenty of mushrooms and even some shitty brown acid. "What could cough syrup really do to me?" I asked.

He quickly replied, "This is the pure stuff in the cough syrup that fucks you up. My mom works at the psych ward and they give it to the crazy fucks to make them normal, but it will get us high!!"

I am crying as I write this. If there was ever a time I wish my folks had rolled up and drug me into their rig it was this time. I'd choose this time. Instead, this guy, easily eight years older than me, would hand me three huge pills and I would swallow them with such confidence, not noticing the very evil smile on his face. I know where your mind went, but the pills were what he said they were.

"Have fun with that!" he said and went on his way.

I decided to head home. It was only four small town blocks away, but by the time I was no more than fifty steps away from my window I was having a hard time moving my legs. I took the screen off the window and made it back into my room undetected. I remember clear as day thinking "I don't wanna do this. I'm just going to go to sleep instead." So that's what I did. Only those pills had a different plan for my seventy pound at best on a well fed day body.

I was screaming in my sleep. Jezus Christ, I remember in my dream it was solid black fear. I was just dreaming the feeling. But our house was old and had shifted, so sometimes when my bedroom door opened it made an extremely loud POP sound as the door broke free from the pressure of the frame. This, of course, was the sound of my parents running to their child's room that was screaming at the top of her lungs like she was being murdered. But to me, it was the sound of hell breaking through. It awoke me to the visions of the fear I was feeling. It awoke me to full on DXM overdose induced hallucinations.

The pills were 800 milligrams. Each.

As my parents saw their half naked daughter flailing in fear, I saw robotic Hellraiser type demons that were trying to get cold metal into my veins so they could encase my heart. I kicked my mother in her jaw as slices of darkness went across my vision, like shards of glass that could somehow rip new layers. These slices, these new voids, somehow allowed something beyond darkness to creep in. The screams of a million, the smell of cold, stainless steel that had somehow rusted. I am not entirely sure that I didn't actually slip this reality so close to death and see Hell. I am sure I kicked my poor mother in the jaw. I have never fought so hard in my life.

I remember the sidewalk that leads to the front door and dragging my nails across it trying to stop them from taking me deeper into the darkness. Of course, this was my father trying to get me to the rig. Trying to save his daughter. I could smell blood, It was blood from my nails ripping back against the pavement. As my mother held me in her lap the best she could with the help of the seatbelt, I underwent the sensation of those needles filling my veins and finally reaching my heart. I could feel the cold metal tighten with each fading beat.

As we went flying down the overpass that led to the hospital I suddenly had a completely sober moment. Anyone who has eaten acid knows what I'm speaking on here. I remember seeing the terror in my dad's face and saying, "I'm fine now we can go home."

and my mother saying "You're not fine!" before slipping back into that dank crushing darkness.

When we got to the hospital I was in and out of these reality slips. I remember this male nurse who kept screaming in my face "What are you on!?!?!" and I would scream back "ROBO FRY!!!"

But you have to understand at this time they had no clue that people could chug cough syrup to get high, let alone hallucinate. At least not in rural NE Oregon. They managed to hold me down to get a catheter in. They needed a urine sample to see what I was on. This entire time I was ravaged by creatures with metal shards that oozed out of their rotten skin. I got a hand loose. I was in survival mode. The rooms of the hospital were individual personal hell-like chambers, where I could see every undesirable experience each poor soul was undergoing. I ripped out my catheter as well as my IV. I'll never forget the sudden splatter of bright red as my blood painted that cheap cotton curtain.

One last needle came and I went to sleep, but what really happened is I was paralyzed from conscious movement for the comfort of those around me. I went deeper into this dark place. There are things I will never be able to put to words. Just feelings, images, smells. But what I do know is once I decided to just let the pain swallow me, to find peace in the death of it, I saw a light.

I saw a light in all of the screams. I smelled moss. That dank earthy scent was such a comfort compared to the smell of metal, sterilized blood, and fear. So I crawled as my flesh was torn away by what I do not know. As my muscles ripped away, my bones were becoming weak and I could feel them growing hollow. I was being eaten alive, stripped down like a deer hanging on a rusty triangle from the old locust tree in our yard.

As my hand reached for this light, that was not any color I can describe, I felt my bones turn to dust and I woke up...

The clock hands on the wall would move an hour at a time. My brain could not register the individual tick movement and they would all just happen at once. It's funny how sharply I remember all of this but nothing about the return trip home or what the following night was like, but the morning after I remembered something distinctly. Sitting out in that grass, it smelled so sweet. It was so vibrant that it and all of the other plants around me made feel safe. Not just feel safe, I was safe. I had never felt this in my life.

I also remember sitting with my sister's boyfriend at the time, who is still, to this day, a brother to me. He was smoking a joint - right there in front of my house - while he talked on someplace I can't recall he was going for a party or the like. My mom came out and I didn't hide the herb. I just asked if I could go and she said, 'I don't care."

Mom, if you are reading this I understand this was the moment I broke you. That it just didn't matter anymore. I don't think it could if you were going to survive. I don't blame you.

I know many are wanting to get through this story and find me an awoken or more enlightened individual, or that maybe seeing these Hells would get me closer to my Creator, but in my ignorance of youth it was nothing more than a story to tell. I am still processing the trauma of it at 34. So instead I talked that guy from far away into getting me a bus ticket to Eugene. Mom, I will never forget that night as I sat on the greyhound bus waiting for it to leave. When you walked on and I cried and said "let me go", not in the way that meant I wanted you to let me go to Eugene, but you know...to let me go.

And you did.

Just like that at the age of 13, I was on my own.

I understand Mom, but I wish you would have drug me out by my hair and beat the ever loving shit out of me right then and there. That would have been kinder than the next six years or so of my life.

For those still reading, welcome to a split second glimpse into my teenage years.

Yarrow Stops the Bleeding, but Not the Trauma of the Wound.

I could start a million chapters with 'I stepped off that bus in Eugene', or 'I hopped out of that van/truck/car/train' and tell any of a million tales. At the time, Eugene Oregon was the place to be homeless. Long before they tore out the strip and chased the street kids away it was a Mecca of sorts.

I stepped off of that bus and walked as quickly as I could towards the bustling strip before night fell in the hopes of finding a group of street kids to camp with. As a young girl sleeping was a dangerous affair, and while much pain came from within these hodgepodged groups, at least I had a better chance of knowing the name of who was possibly going to rape me. I quickly met an older man, probably in his twenties, that went by Mellow. He was fucking skeezy, to say the least, but he was talking of a place that grabbed my interest. An Intentional Community is what folks like to label them these days, but it was your run of the mill, in the woods homeless commune. They preached love, kindness, and a wide open view of the world, all while turning a blind eye to rampant sexual assault, abuse, poverty, and dirty half-starved, underdressed children that were being taught less than the family dog on a daily basis.

The reality is I had been running with, and to, the "Rainbow Family" since I was about nine. I just knew how and where to find these people, in the national forest squatting fourteen days at a time, fourteen days at a time starting AFTER the ranger has given notice. Then we would just move the mandated five miles and start the clock again. But this camp was different. It was isolated. The homeless population was at an all time high within the city, so a huge amount of us being out in the woods subsisting off of food stamps, food boxes and the occasional full grocery cart of food blatantly stolen, was preferred to the lot of us aggressively flying signs and spare-changing. That shit's for sure no good for tourism! They left this commune alone, and in doing so it's numbers swelled to a shocking amount as word spread. At one point there were easily 300 or more people there, just fucking up the land and making the found natural hot springs a cesspool for staph infections of all kinds.

When humans live like this on the streets and form groups we revert back into something more primal, a pack. There are pecking orders. Alphas, Omegas - there are just these unspoken things that I always thrived on quietly observing. It's not something you really see in a more "civilized" setting. After about a week securing my spot with an all male group of "kids", I talked a doe-eyed, fresh to the dorms college kid into paying $40 for a

$10 bag of weed that was probably worth $5. You had to have some sort of worth and for me, no matter what impression you glean from these pages, I strived for that worth to be greater than the young vagina between my legs.

I'm not going to lie, being fuckable was a factor. However, I tried very hard to make my worth be what my hustle could supply.

Time went by in a blur of flying signs and soup kitchens, bottles of liquor for breakfast and bags of dope for dinner because sometimes it was safer to stay awake all night than sleep. Suddenly it was the 4th of July and the whole strip all the way to the courthouse was packed with booths, bands, protests of things I don't recall giving a fuck about if I'm being honest. But as evening fell and I assumed we would head up to the bluff where we had been camping, Mellow said, "Let's camp on the courthouse lawn as a form of protest!"

There was more to his rant and reasoning, but I wasn't listening because the only thing that was ever on my mind as the sun went down was, "Where can I sleep tonight?" or "How do I stay awake?" Back then the courthouse had a large unfenced yard that kids always hung out on during the day beating their drums, playing hacky sack and straight-up smoking herb, but apparently no one until us we're stupid enough to sleep there. I mean, the police station was on the backside of the building, after all.

When you read 'camp' I am guessing you picture tents and other common camping comforts you may be accustomed to. Allow me to set your mind right. Our 'camps' were what we carried on our backs, and what we carried on our backs were packs with very little space. Most of us only had a blanket or a very thin sleeping bag. I knew several kids, especially those who were along the lines of the gutter punk persuasion, that didn't even have a pack, let alone a blanket. I had a paper thin sleeping bag and most of the synthetic filling had settled to the bottom. We passed out on that lawn behind a big ol' oak tree near the building, hoping that car lights would not hit us as they passed for fear one would be a cop.

I drifted off to sleep and began to dream. In it, I was drowning while on dry land. I woke up gasping, and in that deep breath, I damn near filled my lungs with water! I was so baffled in those split seconds of first waking up. How was it raining in July? How was the rain getting under my sleeping bag? But it wasn't raining. It wasn't raining at all. Some courthouse maintenance man likely decided to deal with the homeless problem on the lawn by turning the sprinklers on full blast and my lucky fucking head just happened to be resting on one.

By the time we got off the grass, we and all of our packs were soaking wet. Some may be thinking, "At least it's a warm July night", but a 50*F night quickly turns deadly when you are soaking wet. By that time in my life, I already had a full head of dreadlocks, so my hair was not drying anytime soon and we had nowhere dry to be, let alone anywhere we could start a fire. We sat there on those concrete blocks for what seemed like an eternity until I realized I had stopped shivering and began feeling sleepy.

I told this to a kid named Hank who had been in the national guard and served overseas. He screamed at me "GET UP AND MOVE!" At first, I didn't understand I was already pretty out of it from the early stages of hypothermia. He grabbed me by the arm and made me walk.

Soon we had walked to the backside of the police station where a vent was blowing warm air from the underground parking garage. We laid on that vent soaking the warmth up like it was mother's milk, eventually falling asleep. I woke up feeling the first rays of warmth from the dawns sun, and in an instant, I realized not only was Hank gone, I had not grabbed my pack when he dragged me away. Utter panic gripped me and I could not catch my breath. My mind went a million miles an hour.

I ran back to the courthouse lawn but they were long gone. I checked the bluffs. I checked the soup kitchens. I checked the corners we liked to fly signs on. By mid morning I had spiraled into full disparity. I may as well just die, not because I had lost my group, but I had lost my pack. It was my life in every literal sense. That evening I curled up under the stairwell of some apartment complex that was out of easy sight, trying to sleep on the concrete with nothing more than two scratchy welcome mats that I had stolen underneath me. The next morning my throat was becoming sore and my bones were aching deeply. I got up and started walking towards a bakery that always tossed their day olds out by the dumpster in a plastic bag, hoping to get them before anyone else.

Afterward, I was walking down some random road that was supposed to take me to a youth outreach center. I was hoping they would have a spare backpack and blanket, or maybe some food, as I ate nothing but a tub of pure sugar icing found in the dumpster. Suddenly a car pulled up screeching its tires. It startled the hell out of me. This short dude with a bull ring in his nose said "Hey, you're that April chick who almost froze to death right? Get in the car!"

I said, "I don't have time to get raped today. I need to find a new backpack…"

He replied, "I know where your pack is and the kids who lost you too!" Hopping in his car I muttered something about guessing I do have time, and he just smiled and said, "My name's Blue. I'm from Nebraska and were headed to the woods!"

Just like that, I was finally on my way to the commune, and I was fucking livid. I had been telling these guys for weeks that we needed to go there and was always met with almost hostile resistance. Now I'm in some fancy car with a guy from Nebraska who's fucking blaring Moby because that's where they went in the night. It was a long drive and I tried desperately to avoid the thoughts in my mind that were screaming I was actually headed to some remote place where no one would hear me scream. Sometimes you just had to ignore those thoughts and hope for the best because a situation you were escaping was worse.

When the last turn onto a remote logging road came, almost bottoming out his car before leading to a field of tents, RVs and slapped together shacks next to the river, I don't think I have ever been more relieved in my life. I b-lined to the half-assed A Camp section where alcohol was openly allowed knowing that's where I would find them. Sure enough, I did, every one of them shit faced and Mellow using my pack as a fucking chair, smashing the few valuable to me things I had. I yanked my pack out from under him and they all erupted in laughter. I walked away without saying a word. You can't trust people who will leave without waking you to keep you safe, and the reality is in settings like this with a lot of new people around group structures get shook up, usually ending with a violent explosion.

I was so tired. Just utterly drained from being bone cold and eating nothing but sugar. I wanted to sleep, and I can't stress enough that I did not feel well. I ended up on the outskirts. This is usually where people are calmest, mostly because they are older or have kids. I took out my mildew smelling sleeping bag and found a thick bedding of moss under some alders growing a few hundred yards away from the river and passed out. I didn't fall asleep. I passed the fuck out.

When I woke up the next afternoon I was once again soaking wet, but I was not freezing. Instead, I was burning up with fever, and in an instant realized I could barely take a breath because my throat was so swollen. I tried to stand, but my leg muscles where jelly and I felt like I was dying of thirst. The sound of the river running was the only thing that gave me motivation to not lay there and die. My fevered brain thought to itself, "if I could just drink some of that cold water I would be okay." I crawled on my hands and knees the best I could. It was so far away. I lost control of my bladder and pissed myself. It took about an hour to get to the river, and once there I drank freely, not thinking or caring about the repercussions.

I curled up there next to the river and would wake in the night even iller. I began to shit myself from the Giardia or maybe Campylobacter I had likely contracted from drinking out of a river. Doing so wasn't safe in general, let alone next to that many people camped out. Honestly, I feel like this was an exit point my soul could have chosen to take. I clearly had pneumonia or something and now was losing what little bodily fluids I had. The people that had come across me quickly decided to avoid me. I was too ill to speak, and I remember thinking this must have been what it felt like when the first person in a camp got smallpox and was left in the woods to die. My Grandma used to tell me stories about things like that.

As night began to set in, my breaths were shallow and I could no longer feel much of a heartbeat in my chest. I did not have the ability to cry. I'm not sure if it was because I was too dehydrated or if my body was too weak to pull up those emotions. Two men came across me and I laid there listening to them debate with one another if anyone knew I was over there or if they could catch what I had if they took turns raping me. I couldn't move. I couldn't cry out. I couldn't anything. When they finally walked away, I remember feeling a wave of relief hit my burning muscles that had been tensed, the only movement my body could afford. To my terror minutes later in my somewhat blurry, made worse by the darkness vision, I saw a mountain of a man walk up to me. He scooped me in his arms like a hawk takes a mouse from a field and I checked out of my body, sure I was being taken to be violently gang raped.

I came to but was afraid to open my eyes. I could hear the crackling and popping of a fire and what sounded like rocks bashing and scraping together. Soon the slight breeze shifted and the smell of smoke that was burning my chest with every labored breath gave way to the familiar pungent smell of Yarrow. I faded in and out of consciousness a lot, not sure if I had been raped. I couldn't really feel my body. Finally opening my eyes, I saw an old teapot stained black from many campfires being filled with water. I saw the man throw more wood into the flames. I heard those rocks smashing again. I smelled the Yarrow even stronger now. I had a conscious thought, "If they kill me maybe they will bury me in the Yarrow field." I oddly found comfort in that idea, and once again slipped out of consciousness.

I am not sure how long I was asleep, but suddenly this man was forcing me up and dumping a warm, pungent liquid down my throat - the first thing I had drank since the river. That smell of Yarrow had now turned into the bitter, astringent taste of earth and volatile oils. I felt every cell in my body scream out for it as I gasped for air between the forced drinks. It almost made me feel dizzy to realize this man, who had still not spoken a word, was helping and not harming me. All night he woke me up and made me drink cup after cup of that fresh Yarrow he had been smashing up between two rocks and boiling in that old teapot. I must have drunk a gallon's worth before I had to piss. That's how utterly dehydrated I was.

By the dawn, I was no longer burning up with fever, even though the Yarrow made me flush with heat. The man had fried up bread for me to eat and I had never been so grateful for greasy flour and salt, still not a word spoken. Come early morning he carried me to the river, fully undressed me, washed me, put me in new to me clothing, and carried me back to his fire. More Yarrow, more Yarrow, and more Yarrow. By the afternoon my breath came with much more ease and the muscles in my legs began to firm up. Still no words, but I could hear him humming quietly to himself as he worked, his melodies so familiar and reminding me of home. That evening he fed me potatoes and some kind of meat and it made me cry. The utter feeling of sustenance, of being truly nourished. To this day I still fight the urge to cry when I eat a good meal. I fell asleep and slept more deeply than I could ever recall. I dreamt of those Yarrow fields and the smell of hot fresh wild blood on a blade I'd never seen before. I think I may have dreamt of the summer lands.

I woke up to the birds. Listening to them sing a sincere feeling of contentment washed over me. I could smell that early morning dew mixed with the scent of a fire that had burned itself to ash. I sat up and he was gone. The camp was gone, that fire stained teapot was gone, but one thing remained. That knife I had never seen in waking life but had in my dreams was stabbed into a note.

"You don't die here. You have too much work to do."

I stood up, legs shaky but firm enough, head woozy from laying down so long, blood running down my legs as my moon came early, and I was determined to live. I had it in my head that this was the moment that all things would change because it could not possibly get any worse. I set out to find that field of Yarrow. I just needed to see her.

There was no Yarrow to be found in any of the barren trampled down fields. Sometimes I'm not sure there was ever really a man, either.

The only thing I can say for certain is that for many years that blade was never far out of my reach.

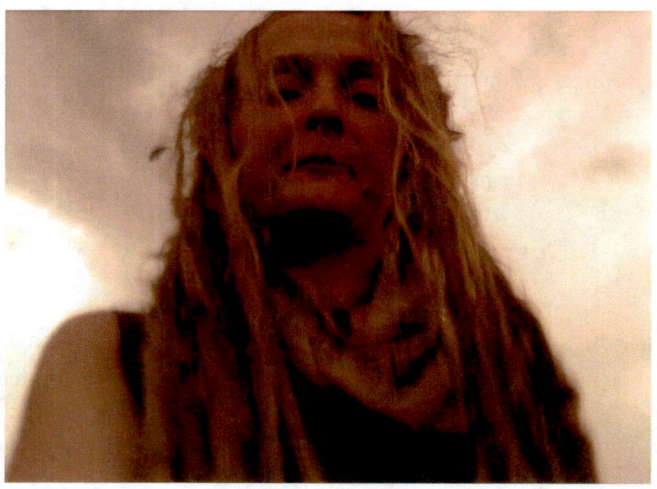

·3·
Yarrow

Achillea millefolium

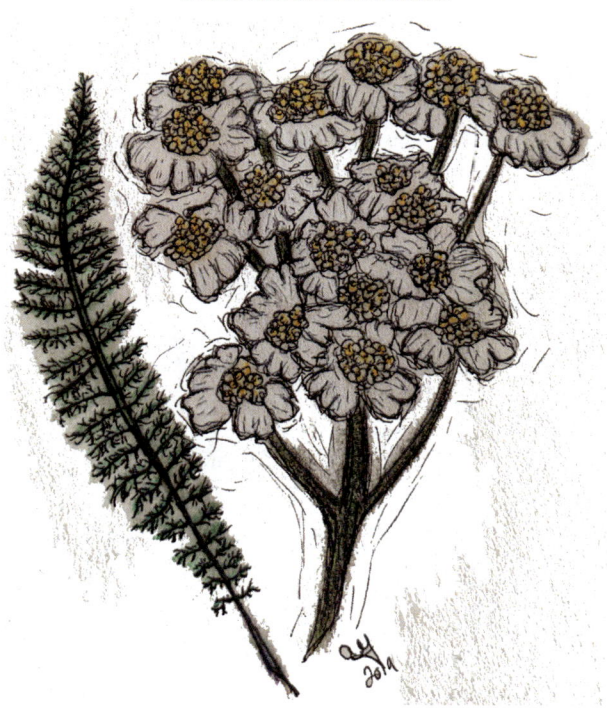

There's something about Yarrow and her affinity for blood that makes me see her as a true warrior, and it's not because she stops the bleeding. I'd say, for me, it has more to do with her ability to help us persist through the blood that is going to fall whether we like it or not. I suppose that's what I consider a warrior - not the person who walks through life with an unscathed appearance, but someone who can be openly bleeding from trauma and keep walking any damn how.

The truth? I don't know. I don't know if those men truly walked away. I don't know if that man who scooped me up prevented a violent rape or took pity for me in the aftermath. I do know that sometimes knowing won't do much for the healing, and I trust my mind's decision in that.

Regardless, I'm going to choose to keep walking even though the blood keeps falling. It's either that or give up and, though at times I wish it was, it simply isn't in my nature to do so.

The History of Yarrow:

A thing - in written history terms, anyhow - can not exist without a name. In so many ways the name of a thing is usually the key to remembering the stories that occurred that wrote this name into the history books of humanity in the first place. When we name something we give it the ability to live on, for others to imagine alongside us, even if they were not by our side at the time, even if it happened so long ago that it is now considered a fairy tale.

You see, the history I love is not all rigid facts, but rich with story.

She was so afraid of her child being wounded as he grew and faced the terrors of the world that she dangled her infant by nothing more than his heel and submerged him in that bath of simmering Yarrow - all so no hurt may ever befall him. But - as it often happens when we attempt to overprotect our children, to shield them from their hurts, to shield them from the harsh reality we live in at any given moment in history - there will always be a weak spot. This weak spot is almost always their sheer inability to see themselves as a humble human, to see that wounds bleed, to process the horrors we have been shielded from.

So when that arrow struck Achilles' heel, the one spot his mother did not dip into that water thick with Yarrow's protection, he quickly met his death. His mortality was realized. This is the ancient Greek tale of Achilles, a Yarrow blessed soldier who died in the Trojan war.

Yarrow's Latin name is Achillea millefolium. Achillea is a reference to the story of Achilles' heel. In this story that we have barely touched on above, our fierce lady Yarrow was also used to heal the many wounded soldiers and to stop the bleeding of spear wounds, as well as to prevent festering. She is the very definition of a warrior's plant ally, having been regularly used well into the Civil War.

Now it would be easy to take the image of a warrior and cast them into the role of rugged, harsh, dangerous, and only needed when the going gets tough, but she has a gentle side too should she been seen in a calm breezy meadow before the bloodshed ensued. Her beautiful lace like leaves unfurling into almost dainty like ferns granted her the second half of her Latin name *millefolium*, which is an adaptation from the french word 'millesfeuilles', describing her lacy, feathery, fern-like leaves. She is, in reality, a very gentle lady, so long as she is shown the respect she is deserving of. She holds the power to stop our bleeding, but she also has the power to start it. This is the case for any warrior if we really think about it.

Let's step off of mythical tales and into some reality though, because I find that just as exciting!

She is such an ancient ally that her pollen was found in the Shanidar burial caves near Iraq dating as far back as 65,000 years ago and, seeing how humans did not (as far as we can tell) bury their dead with flowers until after the Cro-Magnon era. The popular theory is that Yarrow's pollen was present as a result of medicinal use before they died, possibly in a shamanic sense as well.

Neanderthals from El Sidron, Spain that date to about 50,000 years ago have also been found with Yarrow residue in their teeth. Seeing how Yarrow is a very bitter, some would say a pungent, lady from her high volatile oil levels it is not very likely that these ancestors were eating her as a regular food source so much as they were likely eating her for her many healing abilities! Many have a false notion that Neanderthals were unintelligent humans just barely surviving the elements, but the truth is these humans had a deeper relationship to the land and the plant allies it held, more than we could ever fathom. Quite simply put, they damn well knew what plants were good medicine!

So there is a bit more to her name we can talk about. There is a bit of a debate as to if she was named after Achilles of Troy, or perhaps was she named after Achillo, an ancient Greek doctor who used her to cure wounded warriors.

Today we call her Yarrow, but this word comes from the Old High German name 'Garawa', a word that to date has no pre-existing origin known. To me that is powerful. Think about that for just a moment. A word, a name, the magic of speaking something into existence for the very first time, proclaiming her as Garawa. Doesn't seem all that magical, eh? Well, what if you consider that, if you speak English, almost all the words that come out of your mouth are not original words, but a language based off of the evolution of a language that adapts and steals from others, such as the word Yarrow from the word Garawa.

When Garawa fell into the mouths of the Anglo-Saxons the word is adapted to 'Gearwe', and became the common synonym for 'mirifillo' in many books of the 725 A.D. era. This name continued on until about 1503 when the word 'Yarrow' was born.

She has many names across many lands though, such as staunch grass, bloodwort, knight's milfoil, sanguinary, soldier's woundwort, carpenter's grass, gordaldo, nosebleed plant, old man's pepper, devil's nettle, thousand-leaf, and thousand-seal.

These names and the many others she knows often speak on her blood influencing abilities, but so many differing names (no way is above a complete list) means that mankind of all walks around this vast earth has valued her enough to speak her into humanity's history.

I am grateful they did.

The many uses of Yarrow:

Struggling with oral health issues? Gum disease? Receding gum lines? Excessive bleeding when brushing? Canker sores? Abscesses? Swelling? Is your breath just straight up nasty, and it's not gut health related?

Prone to sore throats? Sinus infections? Struggle with bacterial infections in general?

Pretty sure you're gana up and die from a fever?

Is your body a never ending fountain of too many fluids? I mean is your nose chronically running?

Bloody noses?

Intestinal tract kinda sorta got you bleeding internally? Bleeding stomach ulcer? Maybe you can't stop taking loose shits? Is your digestive health a nightmare?

Need to slow down your moon time bloods? Maybe you need to make them come if it's not a pregnancy that has them late?

Is your skin waging war against you? Acne? Psoriasis? Eczema? Rosacea? Some sort of stubborn fungus?

Super nasty cut? A really stubborn wound that won't heal? Did your cat lose its mind and shred your legs all up?

Are you suffering from hemorrhoids? Constantly dealing with UTIs? Need some help pissing?

Do bugs find your blood delicious and you'd like to keep them the hell off of you?

Since I know you are a human reading these pages I'd be willing to bet at least a few of these issues hit the nail on the head!

How can Yarrow do so much for us?

I wanna take a second or two to talk about how I'll be breaking this all down for you in each herb chapter. Bear with me.

In every plant, there are chemical compounds of all varieties. these are how any given plant does any given thing to our body.

Talking about said chemical compounds can for sure get super dry, scientific, and leave us feeling not only confused but overwhelmed, which usually shuts the average person down to learning. This is no big surprise, as not many people like this kind of drudgery and it sure as hell does not make for easy learning.

At the same time when I read most herbal books geared towards the average human I am more often than not let down with the shocking lack of 'why'. I mean, the 'why' should not be the most important thing in our relationship with plants, but it's still for sure a thing that should be a part of it to an extent.

So my aim in these chapters is to the best of my ability explain the why in such a way that just about anyone reading will understand it.

I'm not saying I won't utterly fail at this, but I'm gonna give it a good go and see what happens!

So back to how Yarrow can do so many amazing things for us! The first thing to know is that she has well over 100 unique compounds in her, but let's just focus on the ones I feel inclined to talk about and how they help us.

Like some pretty powerful compounds such as achilleine, sesquiterpene lactones, azulene, menthol, cineole, camphor, camphene, limonene, sabinene, and eugenol.

Even looking at that small example of her compounds it's probably easy to see why when we dive into this side of the pool it can leave us feeling like we're gonna drown in the depth of it all. I kinda sorta half ass promise to not let that happen. Let's talk about how Yarrow and bleeding wounds go together like bees and honey.

It's all about her Achilleine content which makes her a legit hemostatic/styptic, which basically means she is able to make our blood clot as well as shrink up blood vessels to help reduce bleeding. That may not sound like much of a magic trick when it's put so simply, but let's break the impact of this down section by section.

For the sake of humoring me I want you to imagine you just cut the ever loving shit out of yourself with something less than clean. Let's also picture it was not a super sharp thing, so we don't have the luck of an easily healable cut. Like, oh I dunno, an old, rusty, serrated knife that spends as much time in the garden as it does in a chicken coop. Now, as a person who was once hacking through a summer's worth of inch thick tomato vines with said style of rusty knife, slipped and cut well into my knee cap's membrane. I can tell you these wounds are fucking impossible to heal well and excessively prone to infection because each step we take basically opens the wound again.

So there I am, feeling less than sharp myself, half limp, running through my teaming with microbes garden, just bleeding out like a stuck pig. I make it to the yarrow patch (it was a BIG garden so it took a moment) and chewed up wads of very bitter leaves that I could spit (yes, spit) directly onto my serrated knife to the bone wound. I wanted to really get that visual across.

It was clear I had nicked a little vein or something as, well, let's just say the blood with each heartbeat was doing a little more than running down my leg! Within no more than two minutes this wound that likely needed medical attention (cough cough, no insurance) had FULLY stopped bleeding. Now don't get me wrong here. I don't mean pressure and allowing my heart rate to drop made the flow slow down. I'm straight up saying I was able to, after only two minutes, take off the yarrow poultice and walk to the house with no new blood running anywhere.

When I chewed her up it made her super high levels of volatile oils available, and when that wad of spit went from my mouth to my wound it quickly made my blood cells shrink up (open your hand fully and then quickly make a fist to imagine what she does to blood cells). Instead of waiting on my immune system to respond and begin creating blood clots the Achilleine took care of it!

I'm gana branch off here a moment to talk about why beyond her ability to stop my bleeding she's the top ally I choose when I cut myself in really dirty places, which I am honestly prone to doing in life.

A few compounds that make her pretty pungent in smell and taste alike are menthol, camphor, cineole, camphene, sabinene, and limonene. Yeah, these things are why she smells and tastes the way she does, but they are also the main how, what, and why to her ability to kill all gram positive bacteria on contact, attack and/or outright prevent infections from happening, and even take on some serious fungal issues.

Hmm, that's cool. Let's sink this in a bit deeper with one little example of gram positive bacteria.

MRSA is a gram positive bacteria (although it's also capable of being gram negative). What's MRSA? Oh, ya know, just the type of staph infection that will no joke eat your body alive from the outside in and has become resistant to practically all antibiotics. The antibiotics that are still kinda sorta killing it are so strong that they can kill you too. When I sliced my knee with a knife that had all sorts of fecal matter on it from the life of gardening with livestock I was at real risk of, at the very least, getting a basic non MRSA staph infection.

That's a pretty broad stroke of a few of the vast array of compounds that make her smell, so let's keep on getting off track here while I also oddly narrow in on a few of these things because, eh...that's just how my brain works!

Are you SUPER into smoking herb (Marijuana) and really pay attention to the terpenes?

If so, I'm guessing you noticed a few of those names associated with Yarrows scent, namely camphene, limonene, menthol, and sabinene. Maybe you don't recognize any of these things, but they are all indeed terpenes with some pretty awesome abilities when it comes to healing up wounds.

Camphine is how Yarrow acts as a gentle analgesic, which is just a fancy word for pain relief, and you'd better believe that gash on my knee was sending some pain signals to my brain. These terpenes are pretty well studied for medicinal values, and not simply because the marijuana industry is booming at the moment. These terpenes are found in a lot of plants that have been used in varying folk medicine for thousands of years.

Scientists usually deeply want to know the 'why', and sadly the why is usually discovered via animal testing. Camphine is a perfect example, as it was some little lab mice that were put into a state of pain and inflammation in one way or another that showed it was able to gently relieve the pain response by pulling down inflammation again and again. You're going to see me talking on animal studies often in these pages, I don't condone them but I also acknowledge this is how we know the 'why' of many things that truly end up saving lives.

So what about limonene? This is something that the average human is encountering on more than likely a daily basis. This terpene is HOW lemons smell like lemons. It's a vastly extracted "VOC" which means volatile organic compounds, and in large amounts can really fuck our health up. But in small **naturally occurring levels** it can act as a powerful antifungal and antimicrobial. There is a big difference between antimicrobial and bacterial, just to put that out there. An antibacterial can only kill, you guessed it - bacteria. An antimicrobial kills not just bacteria, but viruses and funguses as well.

Then sabinene and azuline come dancing in and while both are great antibacterial/antimicrobial/antifungals, they also have some pretty amazing anti-inflammatory properties. In fact, it's pretty critical for sabinene to be present alongside CBD if we expect to see any real inflammatory relief, and she can be detected in most "full spectrum" oils.

I'm sure we all recognize menthol from varying reasons in life (Have you smoked menthol top tobacco? That shit will be why I one day die of cancer, hah!), but as a terpene she's pretty legit at also relieving pain, although it is usually more related to muscle and skeletal pain. Beyond that, she's the main 'Who's Who' of annihilating staph infections. Of course, once again we owe this knowledge to some mice who were given a raging staph infection and then treated with isolated menthol, with decent success.

I mean, the ability to simply chew up some leaves and have so much amazing support for a nasty wound in one single place sure seems like magic to me!

Of course a lot of these terpenes that helped my wound heal up to completion in under a week when it should have taken two (even if I got the stitches I legit needed) are how we can also rely on yarrow to attack fungal infection, acne, stubborn wounds, or even rosacea (if you, like me, stand on the side of the fence that believes that issue is caused from a bacterial infection of the skin).

What about internally though? I mean, what was going on in my body as I drank way too much hot yarrow brew so many years ago? Internally there was a serious cascade of reactions going down, but we'll start off with the fact that while there were many things I could have died from, fever was likely a top contender!

Yarrow's ability to influence our entire vascular system (how blood moves through your body) truly astonishes me, and I just want to take a moment to say I find her affinity for my blood, any blood, a beautiful thing. Maybe because blood is the ultimate life source for all animals on this planet. It's just...magical to me in some way that I'll likely never be able to fully put words to.

Most are going to tell you that Yarrow will only cure a dry fever - this is a fever where you are not sweating. The idea is Yarrow drank as a warm tea will induce sweating, and that's for sure what will happen. Her achilleine we already jabbered on a bit when ingested will raise our body temp, but she also encourages all of our pores to open wide. So as we sweat bullets our pores open up, allowing heat to escape and our temperature drops.

But here's the funny thing - I have never been able to get a cold or even lukewarm cup of yarrow tea to make me sweat out, so, and I'm just sharing my thoughts here, while we know thanks to some test rats and rabbits that achilleine can induce sweating, it seems that it does not increase our body temperature high enough for sweat without the extra kick of heat. I'd even dare to say it might have something to do with the fact that our body processes warm water more slowly compared to cold water, so that warm tea is setting in your "core", heating you from the inside out.

When it comes to a wet fever - which means we are covered in sweat already from our body attempting to kill some thing or another that is invading us - yarrow is still worth reaching for! She has such extensive control over not just our vascular systems but our neurovascular systems (your veins + nerves) that she can outright control blood pressure, both clot and un-clot, move blood to the surface and away from it.

So that last bit, where she can cause our body to pull blood inward or push it up near the surface of the skin is important. I want you to imagine that it's really cold outside and you heat your home with a woodstove - an old wood stove in an old house with shitty insulation. The kinda situation that you have to keep the fire blazing and the house hot as hell since it loses heat so fast and you will be just as cold as if you were outside. Now imagine you have to go out into the, I dunno, sub freaking arctic temperatures compared to your really hot house. You put a ton of layers on and went outside where you're not cold but also not hot and you go about, let's say sledding.

So your joyous afternoon of sledding is over and you head back into your super hot house. Suddenly the many thermal long johns under your already insulated pants, a long sleeve shirt, a wool sweater, undercoat, then a thick winter coat are making you feel like you're gana have a fucking heat stroke. With each layer removed you get a smidgen of relief. You snap at a kid or your partner about how damn hot it always is in the house, but about 10 mins after you have stripped down to your underwear you realize that you were a bit of an asshole since it's nowhere near as hot in the house as it was when you first came in.

I may have gone too deep there, but this scenario is meant to paint a picture of how Yarrow can help with even a wet fever. You underneath all of those layers were the "core" of the heat being generated and the only way you were gonna find relief while still in the house is to allow your heat to NOT be the core, but move to the surface by stripping off all of your layers. So when Yarrow enters a hot body and moves your hot blood from your "core" to skin level it's the same thing as taking off all of those layers, there's nothing in the way of your heat escaping your body from your wide open pores.

Her blood influencing abilities go so much further though. With her natural tannins that make her a powerful astringent combined with her ability to tighten, tone, and sooth blood vessels, she's gonna be your new best friend when it comes to getting those hemorrhoids to shrink up and your moon blood to stop flowing so heavily. Let me break these out into sections. I mean, they are kinda sorta in the same area but nowhere near the same "thing" in our bodies.

So hemorrhoids really suck, There might we one random human in the world that really loves hemorrhoids and may read this then send me a nasty letter but I can't please em all! For those of us who are not in love with our busted ass veins (pun intended) you're probably gana rejoice in yarrow's ability to shrink 'em back up! The thing is that the uncomfortable situation you've got going on down there is caused by enlarged and swollen blood vessels, and if you remember from a ways back Yarrow's achilleine content makes her a styptic, which is something that tightens up and tones our blood vessels.

In other words, I want you to put Yarrow on your ass.

Now, I know that sometimes these blood vessels that are acting like real assholes (I can't stop myself) get to stinging, burning, and of course, bleeding. We already know that she will stop the bleeding, but let's not forget she can also help with the pain due to her camphine bits sprayed on our bits.

Let's talk about the blood that comes from somewhere else and how when we are flooding during our moon time we can get our body to slow it's horses some. This really does come down to, you guessed it, her achilleine as well as her tannins. With her affinity for blood, she's amazing at tightening and toning the uterus, which also helps to staunch that heavy flow!

But how then can she also be a blood thinner?

Well, there are a few ways. The first is her eugenol content which is actually the main thing in Yarrow that gives her smell, and while anything with smell tends to have antibacterial/microbial/fungal abilities, another action she has is being a straight up blood thinner. Isn't that kinda interesting? Think about the fact that Yarrow contains compounds that not only can stop us from bleeding but cause us to bleed.

This is why some folks feel really intimidated to use her and while she for sure needs our deep respect, there's no need to fear something that is simply showing us how a well balanced regulator of our body works. That is in truth what she is, a legit blood regulator.

So when our wombs are having a hard time releasing the uterine wall and its **not due to a pregnancy,** her astringent abilities that tighten, tone and stimulate our uterine muscles (which encourages our body to release our endometrium - the lining of our womb and what's mainly coming out of us when we bleed) pair up with her eugenol content that thins out our blood, making it even easier for our wombs to do what they do best, sloth off their lining once monthly. This is how we can use her to both start a late period but slow down a heavy flow if it really gets to going like crazy!

Wanna hear another kinda crazy example that really illustrates her ability to both stop our bleeding and start it depending on how we use her? Okay, so if you smash up a fresh yarrow leaf and stick it up your nose the odds are damn good that you'll end up with a nose bleed, BUT if you have a nose bleed and you take some yarrow tincture every 5-10 mins she will stop the bleeding! Wana know something even crazier? Years ago when I was stepping back onto the path of friendship with plant allies when my life kinda sorta stabilized I, for the sake of truly understanding Yarrow, stuck her leaves in my nose and made myself have a nose bleed, then stopped said gushing nose with a tincture of yarrow I had on hand! I am not saying you should do this by any means, just felt like giving you another glimpse into my mind.

Maybe you don't have a womb or it's other areas of your body that seem to persistently explode bodily fluids. How can Yarrow help us out with these leaks we keep springing? It's all about her astringent nature which, just as a refresher, means she "dries things up". But with so many other aspects to her, it's usually because "x" compound is teaming up with her ability to dry us up.

When I was a kid I was a walking, barely breathing sinus infection. At one point I thought it was just something that happened every fall. Like a natural thing that heralded in the changing color of the leaves all around. Nope, it was just me getting chronic sinus infections and no one really cared to do anything about them. I guess in hindsight I'm grateful I didn't have copious amounts of antibiotics thrown in my little gut, but still. They suck, and no one wanted to be friends with the weird overtalkative girl, let alone when she could fill a fucking swimming pool with the volume of infection coming out of her nose.

This all stopped one day when my Grandmother Ruby said to my mother, "Oh Jezuz Judy, give her some Yarrow already!" After that I had a seasonal on again off again relationship with Yarrow, as she not only tacked the upper respiratory bacterial infections but dried up my snot and made coughing up thick phlegm (just made the gag sound) an easier task.

We already know that all of her badass terpenes are what made it a breeze for her to knock out my bacterial infections and it's her ability to dry out that slowed the snot down, but it's a little compound called cineole, also a terpene, that acts as an expectorant. This just means she helps us have a productive cough by thinning out the mucus in our chest. Cineole is actually found in a good amount of plants, but one you'll probably associate with easy breathing or using in the shower is Eucalyptus. Well, Yarrow has you covered here too!

But cineole goes well above and beyond simply helping us hack shit out of our lungs. In clinical trials she was also proven as an extremely effective anti-inflammatory agent (reduces swelling) that directly affects inflammatory related mucus. In other words, if you have a sinus infection or something respiratory related that your immune system is responding to with mucus, Yarrow steps in and not only slaughters the bacteria that's causing the issue, but also reduces the at times damaging effects of our own immune system. like making a little girl produce said swimming pools worth of snot.

Of course when we have infections another side effect is often fever, although that can be more typical of a viral infection. Either way, the compounds found in Yarrow's beautifully magical body make her ideal for dealing with bacterial based infections. Case in point, I was given the gift of strep throat from my teenage son's girlfriend and felt it set in yesterday morning when I woke with a throat on fire. After 12 hours of compulsively spraying Yarrow tincture directly into the back of my throat - which not only killed all of that gram positive bacteria on contact but also took away the horrendous sore throat with her awesome pain killing abilities - I woke up today and don't even feel the slightest tickle or burn!

Now just to be clear, I think an unused immune system leads to more serious lifelong chronic conditions, but I wasn't trying to use my immune system by battling a horrendous case of strep throat right now!

If the time ever comes that you need to chew up a Yarrow leaf for whatever reason you will quickly notice she is a pungently bitter ally. Of course, most of this comes from her varying terpenes, but this means she has the ability to stimulate your saliva production which triggers your digestive tract. That plus her bitterness makes her a pretty great digestive aid and carminative, which means if you are farting horribly from oh, I dunno, ingesting a bunch of infected snot, she is going to get rid of the gas in your digestive system. So that's for sure a great thing, especially for the human who has to be around us. Her very drying tannin levels will also give us the gift of helping us slow down diarrhea if it hits.

Her ability to do this paired with the fact that she can also help slow down internal bleeding of the intestinal tract means you should always have a bottle of Yarrow tincture in your cupboard as well as some dry leaves for making tea, especially if you have Crohn's or any other autoimmune issue or disease that makes you prone to bleeding in these areas .

Speaking of stomach issues, ulcers are another area where she really can give us a helping hand. Of course she can only help us out with the bleeding if that aspect is involved. There are a lot of different kinds of ulcers that have many different causes, and while some ulcers really benefit from improved digestion, Yarrow has a handful of compounds called sesquiterpene lactones that we're gana touch base on.

Where these compounds really shine is in their ability to reduce oxidative stress, encourage cell recovery to heal the wound, and if you suffer from Helicobacter pylori - which is a real jerk of a bacteria that causes ulcers and hides low enough in your stomach lining to not get wiped out by stomach acid - Yarrow is gana wage war on your behalf as soon as she hits your gut.

You're gonna see me talk a lot about oxidative stress in many different sections of this book like a broken record, but oxidative stress is such a HUGE cause of so many things in so many different parts of our body that it's pretty much just gata happen. There are these things most of us have heard of called antioxidants and there are these other things called free radicals. Your body is a war zone. That maybe doesn't seem like it fits, but hang with me for a moment. Every day you are breathing in air that has free radicals in it, eating food that has free radical in it, basking in the sun's that also delivers free radicals and as all of these free radicals enter your body antioxidants get busy slaughtering a good amount of them.

Also just to confuse you with the promise of explaining things later, free radicals can also be a good thing. This shit gets deep folks.

Okay back on track, oxidative stress happens when there are more free radicals in our bodies than there are antioxidants. While this imbalance causes all sorts of horrible health problems, in regards to stomach ulcers inflammation is the name of the game. Since sesquiterpene lactones specifically attack the inflammation caused by oxidative stress we now know (from inducing ulcers on poor lab rats) that they are actually really effective at healing them, but not just because of the oxidative stress link. Nope, let's keep diving.

Let's do a really quick guessing game. What do pharmaceutical medications meant to treat an array of ulcers and sesquiterpene lactones have in common? They're both cytoprotectants, which basically means something that protects the cells in our stomach from being damaged by upping our natural mucosal defense mechanisms, which is just super fancy talk for the mucus that protects your body from your own stomach acid amongst other things. It's the only reason you don't digest a hole through your stomach and when this mucus isn't doing so great an ulcer happens and your acids begin to digest your stomach lining.

These bits of Yarrow blow past pharmaceuticals though because when the scientists fed sesquiterpene lactones to their lab rats before making them ingest high proof alcohol to cause ulcers they discovered something pretty neat and I'm sure the rats were thankful for the small miracle - they acted as antiulcerogenics. This word that I will never pronounce correctly means something that protects against ulcers occurring in the first damn place!

So Yarrow can in one badass swoop stop internal bleeding, dry up diarrhea, improve digestion in multiple ways, heal and outright prevent ulcers? Yep yep!

Now I'm gonna jump back to how she improves digestion and then trail off a bit here. Do you recall how I said one of the ways she helps our digestion is by increasing the amount of saliva we produce? Did you know that one of the things good oral health relies on is ample spit?

Without spit our teeth straight up begin to rot out of their sockets, we are prone to all manner of infections, and even our immune system takes a hit, as a first line of defense in our main "opening" is shut down. So spit is like 90% water, but the rest is claimed by plasma B cells that reside in the salivary glands, and their main job is to produce antibodies that make up the rest of our spit.

Here's an odd thought. Every time you spit on the ground you're spitting out your immune system. There, now that's in your head.

I mean out teeth NEED a moist environment and they NEED these antibodies.

So when we brush daily with a bit of Yarrow on our toothbrush we are making sure we have spit to spare, but what else is going down? Tired of hearing about terpenes yet? Yep, all of those terpenes we've been talking about are going to kill off all of the nasty bacteria causing gum disease, cavities, abscesses, and horrendous breath that IS affecting your relationship even if they love you and say it's not. Let's not forget about her pain relieving abilities. Oh, or her anti-inflammatory ways! This means if you got yourself a toothache, swollen gums, or any other kinda jacked up thing going on in your mouth you need to get some yarrow in there.

A note about her ability to help with toothaches - remember she shares terpenes with clove, which is world renowned for helping us not kill ourselves from a toothache, a thing that used to legit be a common cause of suicide. So when I say yarrow can help with a toothache I don't say it lightly. Growing up one thing you'd always fine in my Grandma Audry's bathroom was this little brown jar filled with yarrow roots soaking in brandy and honey. Complain about a toothache at my Grandmas's house and you'd be chewing on a sweet and pungent yarrow root. In a few moments just about all of your mouth would be pretty close to numb!

After spending my youth as a dirty street kid I can tell you dental health was not on the top of my survival list. That life claimed a good amount of my teeth via no insurance, so pulling is all I could ever have done. But Yarrow IS the reason the teeth that survived that chapter of my life are alive and well in my head.

Sharp left turn - how often does it burn when you piss? Hot like fire? Damn, that's a urinary tract infection setting in! How many does that make for you this year? Wana make them a thing of the past? Yarrow can do that for ya! There's not really a place in our body that her terpenes can't tickle folks. I'm talking from your kidneys all the way to your urethra, she is going to wipe out the bacteria that are making situations a bit painful.

She does something else though because she's smart like that. Achilleine, the compound that never quits giving, acts as a natural diuretic, meaning you're gonna piss a bit more than usual. I don't overly notice this effect with a tincture honestly, but each body is different. Yarrow tea, however, will surely get you going, and this is a great thing. You see, the best way to flush the bacteria out of where it's crept into is to pee, and pee a lot. Yarrow is awesomely effective at dealing with UTIs because she not only makes you go more, she's also killing off the bacteria as she passes through.

There are a lot of stories from that camp that didn't make it into my shared traumas that are likely a traumatic tail another person cou;d write about. This camp happened to be right next to a group of hot springs that were a cesspool, and next to those we're kinda some marshy areas. Let's just say I'm pretty sure this is where the entire world's population of blood sucking mosquitoes originated. There was this guy who was getting targeted horribly by these diseases spreading little assholes, even when he stayed near the smoke of the fire. There was just something about his blood they got off on and one night a random drunk chick said "urine repels them!"

While that may be the case I don't think anyone fully expected this guy to spend all night pissing into a spray bottle and then joyfully walk around for the next few days he was in camp spritzing himself with it, and offering it to folks without telling them what was in the bottle.

I'm gonna go ahead and assume as much as you don't like mosquitos you probably don't feel like resorting to using your own urine. I mean, there's no real need to when you can keep mosquitos and ticks at bay with yarrow!

How she does this is how every highly scented plant does this. Her volatile oils. which are (wait for it) terpenes. I'll be going deeper into this further on in a chapter dedicated to rambling all about it, but let's just say we know that one of the primary reasons plants make these terpenes and other chemical scents is to **deter bugs and animals from eating them**, so we can tap into their **naturally occurring** levels of volatile oils to keep the bugs that want to eat us at bay too!

I feel the need to bring up the fact that every time someone mentions Yarrow can be used as an insect repellant they say "The US Army did a study and have shown it to be more effective than DEET!" With all due respect, go ahead and find that study, please. The only thing I have been able to find with my compulsive research ability is a single well known herbalist who claimed this study was conducted and said person is now quoted again and again as a source of the study.

So I'm not gonna say that Yarrow is more effective than a deadly chemical invented specifically so unfortunate men and women in the Vietnam war didn't have to die horrible mosquito disease related deaths. Is DEET safe? Hell no. If I was in the Vietnam jungle dealing with death-bringing mosquitoes swarming me in the BILLIONS would I choose yarrow over DEET? Hell no.

What I can say is that I, my Grandmothers, my Great Grandmothers, and beyond have used Yarrow tincture and oil to effectively keep an average load of mosquitos at bay.

What about ticks? In my area I solely use Yarrow to keep myself, kids, husband, and a pack of dogs free from ticks, but here's a moment of honesty. We are not outright infested here, and since I don't shave the hair off of my body if a tick does decide not to give a fuck that I smell like yarrow I can feel it the second it starts looking for a place to latch on.

In all honesty, I would not solely rely on Yarrow in deeply infested areas where tick borne diseases like Lyme are rampant and you can't even go into your well manicured yard without picking up a fucking tick (unless I was capable of not forgetting to spray it on every 15-20 mins and didn't shave my legs or anywhere else so I would have a better chance of feeling them on me).

This, and many other bits in this book, will likely get me some blowback. While there are many long standing traditional uses for plants that our ancestors didn't need a scientist to confirm, when it comes to saying something like Yarrow is more effective than DEET and that statement potentially leading to someone getting a life changing disease...well, I just can't comfortably spread that knowledge any further until I see actual proof of it.

Sincerely,
A woman who used to say Yarrow was more effective than DEET just because I read it in a book a long time ago that gives no cited sources.

That would have been a powerful place to end this section at, right? Ha, yeah but I AM a compulsive researcher! So while I have yet to find the mystical US army study on Yarrow that claims that she's more effective than DEET I did find this one:

Mosquito Repelling Activity of Compounds Occurring in Achillea millefolium L. (Asteraceae)
H. Tunón, W. Thorsell, and L. Bohlin
Economic Botany
Vol. 48, No. 2 (Apr. - Jun. 1994), pp. 111-120

You can use the internet to read the entire mind numbing article if you're into that kinda stuff, but if not I'm gonna take a sec to break down what they did.

They gathered Yarrow and decided to check out what compounds she had in her that would repel bugs. Tada - terpenes!

Then they dried a bunch of her in a 113*F oven for 24 hours so all of her volatile and other properties that only exist in the fresh plant matter would evaporate (more on this later), because these are the things that would not have very much staying power as a bug repellent. That is why you have to spray it on every 15-20 mins for it to be effective.

Then they ground up the Yarrow and dumped pure and poisonous ethyl alcohol (what most folks are told they have to make tinctures out of) over the top of the dried plant matter so they could rapidly extract her remaining compounds.

They then, after 48 hours of letting it steep, decided to "fractionate" it with some nasty petroleum and even harsher alcohol. This basically means they reached into what was present in the tincture and pulled out the differing compounds that had been extracted.

I swear this is leading somewhere.

Then they took all of these different compounds (there are A LOT) of varying kinds that they extracted from Yarrow and made up different test batches.

Of course, for this to work they also had to have a bunch of straight up pesticides to compare the follow human tests to.

They starved some mosquitoes for a few days making sure they would really zero in on an opportunity to eat. Then they talked some poor guys into slipping on gloves with a hole in them that exposed a small patch of skin. One patch of skin had the Yarrow extract on it. One patch didn't. They did this over and over again until they made their way through all of the batches of yarrow based repellent and the chemical ones.

With EACH test the hands remained in this box with bloodsuckers for 8 hours!

Over the hours another person was counting how many times they landed and fed.

Surprise surprise, the batches that were sky high in volatile oils helped keep mosquitoes from landing and or feeding as often.

But not as often as DEET did.

I will add they made a batch that had enough menthol in it to melt off the peoples skin that did keep pace with DEET, but it did not outpace it and there is the tricky issue of having to smear yourself with pure menthol volatile oil and at that point you're gonna end up with some legit chemical burns and a mosquito bite will be the least of your concerns.

So while I'd really love to see the study that the US Army supposedly did, I'm pretty sure that a Yarrow tincture sprayed on the skin is in no way, shape, or form as effective as DEET like the thousands of blog posts and books claim.

However, I still keep a bottle on me at all times in the summer!

Where does Yarrow grow?

While she's originally native to Europe, North America, and Asia, Yarrow can at this point basically be found worldwide as long as growing conditions are favorable, and they almost always are for this tough lady!

But here's an interesting thing to know - if you live in North America the Yarrow you know and love...well, there's a good chance she is not truly the Yarrow native to here!

In fact, our Yarrow is not the indigenous peoples' yarrow, nor is she the European peoples' Yarrow, not even Asians' Yarrow! She is someone "new", in the way that when the common Yarrow migrated here from Europe she got busy cross breeding with the Native Yarrow, and then the introduced Asian species joined in on the fun. A huge percentage of the time when you see Yarrow in North America you are seeing this melding.
We will never know the difference though, and neither would our ancestors, unless they somehow had the ability to look at her under a microscope.

She can be found in her favorite places - wide open sunny fields that don't hold onto water too late in the year. She's a master at tolerating droughts, which should probably be seen as a small miracle in our current climate crisis.

In the US you can find her atop my Subalpine forest range thousands of feet above sea level all the way down to below sea level, and you'd be pretty hard pressed to miss her between the months of April-October, assuming snow is no longer covering the ground. My main harvest time for her here at high elevation is July-August, but I can harvest her beautiful leaves before and after then too.

She really loves to creep into disturbed grounds, so expect to see her on overgrazed land - if you get there before the grazers do that is! I have also seen her take aggressive hold in old logged areas, but really you are almost guaranteed to find her in any open field that has been disturbed at all - 'disturbed' meaning the soil has been torn up in some way.

To get real specific, she prefers full sun locations with thin sandy soils, but I have seen her grow in part sun conditions too, the same way I have seen her grow well in beautifully rich soil. This is why she now grows all over the world. She is a master of adaptation.

Now please understand I am talking on wild white Yarrow here. I do not use the varieties that folks often grow in their garden, such as the pinks or yellows. There is some evidence that the compound levels I mentioned in the beginning tend to be much higher (on a problematic level) as a symptom of being cultivated for coloring. The same goes for the wild colored varieties.

When should we harvest Yarrow?

It is fine to harvest just her leaf in the spring, but when it comes to blooms I prefer to wait until all main blooms are in full bloom. A lot of this has to do with the belief that prior to that her volatile oil levels are too concentrated. I usually wait 2-4 days after she has bloomed before I harvest. Sound crazy? Well maybe, but go ahead and smell that bloom on the first day she opens and then smell it again 2-4 days later. The smell will have mellowed out noticeably. Do this sniff test long enough and you'll be able to walk up on a patch and tell just how long the majority have been in bloom by giving a few here and there a smell.

I'm thinking out loud here, but this makes me wonder if this is why I, nor anyone one I have ever gathered with, has ever experienced sun sensitivity or rashes when gathering Yarrow with bare hands. Is it possible that the higher oil levels are causing reactions because she was gathered right at the time of blooming?

I suppose it's a possibility. I like thinking about stuff like that, though.

I stop gathering her in mid summer, as deer in my area do depend on her for fall feeding and I don't want to be adding to that pressure on her.

What cautions should we take?

So there's one more compound we need to talk about and that's thujone. In small **naturally occurring** levels she can still fuck you up, people. She's bad for your kidneys, liver, brain, body, and is THE THING in absinthe that makes people absolutely lose their ever loving minds. Full blown hallucinations and murder suicide type shit, folks.

Freaked out? Let me bring ya back down a touch. So yeah Yarrow does have thujone in her in very, very, VERY small amounts. It's when we start messing around and using highly concentrated volatile oils (that the market calls for sales purposes "essential oils") that we are in real danger of thujone poisoning.

When it comes to a tincture made with fresh plant matter and 100 proof vodka we're golden, so long as we are not taking daily doses for longer than two weeks in a row.

Now I'm gana assume you brush your teeth for more than two weeks in a row (we all hope you do), so how can we use her safely for oral care then? Let's say you put 5 or so drops on your wet toothbrush and that you (like most humans) rinse and spit. The amount you will absorb through the membranes will be extremely negligible.

Keep in mind there are now a lot of botanical type drinks being sold in the stores for regular consumption. The companies that make these have to provide testing to show that the thujone is at an acceptable level, which is higher than what you'll find in a measly 5 drops of Yarrow tincture.

With that being said I'd not drink yarrow tea for weeks on end by any means, but would it use as needed for particular situations.

Okay, some more cautions - hey, these are not things to be afraid of, but simply what it looks like when a plant sets firm boundaries and asks us to respect them! Just thought I'd put that out there.

If you are allergic to plants in the aster family (chrysanthemums, daisies, safflower, ragweed, etc), there is a real possibility you may be allergic to Yarrow. This allergy may express itself internally, externally, or both. So, as always with any plant, proceed with caution. Rub some of the Yarrow oil, balm, or tincture on the inner elbow of your arm and wait a full 24 hours to see if you react. Didn't react? Cool, you can probably move forward with external use.

Internally if you have allergies so severe to the aster family that you go into anaphylactic shock don't fuck around with trying. If they just make your nose stuffed up and general seasonal allergy symptoms go ahead and try about 5 drops in a bit of water and see how that makes you feel over 24 hours. No bad reaction? Try 10 drops. Nothing? Good deal. You're allergies are probably not triggered by her. Oh, but if you're making tea out of her blooms the simmering will knock off pollen, so go easy there too until you know for sure.

Are you currently growing a kid in your belly? Yarrow needs to be hands off internally, although again I'd feel okay brushing my teeth with her still and using her externally, just not directly on my belly. Some poor pregnant rats took one for the team when we discovered that an extract of her volatile oils caused the rats placenta to get really big, but the babies' birth weight to be drastically reduced. Some of her terpenes and flavonoids I didn't touch on earlier do have a connection to our endocrine system (how we make hormones), and most things hormone influencing need to be hands off.

If that's not enough to keep you from using her while pregnant, please know that she can also cause your uterus to contract, so beyond a low birth weight, it's possible that she can make us miscarry. Don't take this to mean she can be used to give us an abortion. That is not what I am saying at all. Please don't try that with her. You'll hurt yourself.

Can we still utilize her during birth to stop ourselves from hemorrhaging out and heal ourselves up down there when our offspring has safely exited? Yep yep!

I also better tell you that Yarrow can increase sun sensitivity, though I have never experienced this and neither have my kids, partner, or any of my friends that join me when harvesting. I'm still thinking on this being due to us not harvesting same day opened blooms, not using tinctures made from dry plant matter, and never using her extracted volatile oils in any way shape or form. Does this mean that if you follow these things that you won't have a reaction to the sun or get contact dermatitis from her? I'll not make that guarantee, but this summer do a test patch after you've exposed your winter skin to the sun for a while and see how your body individually responds to her. This is important to know, especially if you plan to use her all summer as a bug spray!

What about medications?

She does not play well with lithium, and prevents it from exiting your body. If you're on lithium you already know it's a really dangerous medication that can kill your liver and such so a build up can be life threatening.

Taking medication to reduce stomach acid? She'd not be a great choice since she improves digestion via being bitter, which stimulates the production of stomach acid really efficiently.

Are you taking blood thinning or clotting medication or have a disease that makes you need these things? Yarrow is a powerful influencer of the blood, so don't mess around with her without hardcore supervision from your doctor and a very well studied clinical herbalist who holds a real medical degree (Since herbalists can't actually be "certified" in the USA, please be sure not to confuse fake certifications with medical degrees).

Some folks will say she should not be taken with sedating medications like benzos or opiates because they feel she has a sedating effect. While she does have the terpenes present to make this possible for certain bodies, I have never met anyone that feels sedated after taking yarrow as a tincture or even tea. I will say that there's a good bit of folklore I grew up with that said if we smoked her we'd get altered and since terpenes like heat that may be true. My own gut feeling always said she didn't want us to smoke her so I listened.

The main risk is that if she does have sedating effects you may become even more sedated and it may affect your breathing. So just proceed with caution, and take a small amount to see how she makes you feel before jumping in full on.

How much is too much?

So this section is kinda not really needed after the above info but, I know people like to skip from section to section in these kinda books so I'll repeat myself.

It's important that we don't take Yarrow tincture for more than 14 days in a row, and honestly if I am so sick with some issue that I need to be taking her in doses for that long...well, I pray to God by then I have health insurance! That is to say, Yarrow for internal use beyond brushing teeth is an "as needed" plant ally, not one that we should be taking on a daily basis just because we feel like it.

If I was drinking a Yarrow tea I'd probably not use her for more than 5-7 days in a row. In fact, if I am using yarrow tea and the issue is not severe I'll do an every other day cycle for 14 days. That's still only 7 days in use, but it's just an extra kindness I can do for my body to not push it too hard.

Externally I'd probably not rub myself head to toe in yarrow daily for no good reason. This brings me back to the 'use her as you need her' aspect.

·4·

Comfrey Heals the Bones, But Not the Cynicism.

Another time. Another place. One more ride to Eugene. To say I bounced around a lot is an understatement, often returning to my home town area just long enough to find another way out as if someone had twisted my arm to return. No matter where I have gone the consensus of small town folks is always that their town is cursed and no matter what they always get dragged back. I don't know that it's a curse so much that as humans we just gravitate towards the familiar, even if it's soul crushing.

In my teenage years, the internet was, well, not what it is these days. No smartphones. No instant messaging, not the way it is now. Shit, this even predates Myspace by a good long while. What street kids with Rainbow family ties did have were good ol' message boards where we could find out the 'what's what' of an area and post ride needed ads, amongst other things.

Down at that park he rolled up in his fancy RV, more than happy to pick up a young girl and her dog. Even though I could instantly feel he wanted more than to give me a ride, I just felt the risk of staying in town and spiraling out of control into a full blown meth addiction, which was really the only past time for most of us, was more of a risk than catching a ride with this guy.

We drove all day as he talked non-stop about how amazing he is, and how much of a cunt his ex-wife was. How she never fully understood his needs, his unique tastes, his desires. I remember the whole time watching the miles to go signs thanking God Eugene was really only a six hour drive, but figuring in that slow ass RV it would be 8 hours max. Maybe that would have been the case if he didn't pull in to every damn rest stop, for no other reason than to show me things - like literal things he had in random drawers, like crystals and a big bag of some shitty beaned out weed.

He kept giving me things, each time saying he could tell how grateful I was. I wasn't dumb. I knew what he was doing and how unstable he was, but I also knew then like I know now that it was more dangerous not to act like he was a gift from God and accept every item like it was the best thing I had ever been given. I had seen a sign that said Eugene was only a hundred miles away and made plans to disappear at the next rest stop. Until that is, it began to rain so hard we had to stop from sheer lack of visibility. Again I decided this man was not as much of a threat as hypothermia. He decided it would be best to park there at that rest stop until morning since it was already getting dark. I agreed but had zero intention of actually sleeping.

I laid there on the floor with my dog Spliffard, a barely six month old dalmatian/pitbull cross, listening to him fake snore. It went on for what seemed like an eternity until he must have believed I was fully asleep. Then he slowly got up and walked to the only door in the RV. I heard the sound of a padlock latching, and in that moment my heart sank. I had planned to sneak out as soon as the rain died down and the reality of just how dangerous this man was had sunk in. I quickly recalled the fact that all of the side windows were screwed shut, his explanation being they came open on the highway. I connected the dots of all the creepy things, lying there praying his once again fake snore would turn real.

I fought hard against slipping in and out of sleep until I lost the battle. I woke barely after dawn to the sound of air brakes blaring on the highway. In an instant, I began to look for any way out. I thought of taking this huge piece of petrified wood and smashing out the windshield. I thought of bashing him with it and finding the keys. Then I recalled seeing a skylight in the bathroom propped open a bit when he picked me up, which meant it was not screwed shut. I slowly got up, put my pack on my back, picked up the dog, and walked quietly as I could to the bathroom.

The very first turn of the handle that raised the skylight gave out such a high pitched, metal grinding squeal that I knew it would wake him up if I continued. Frantically digging through the tiny bathroom looking for anything to lubricate the handle I discovered the only things he kept in the singular cupboard were gloves, duct tape, a bottle of ammonia and, of all things, vitamin E gel caps. Like this guy was gana torture the hell out of me, but while he was at he was going to be sure my fucking vitamin E levels were goddamned adequate.

I tried biting the top off of one to get at the oil inside but it just wasn't enough, so I put a whole damn handful in my mouth and chewed. I almost fucking choked to death from the oil blocking my throat, but after spitting it up in my hand it was enough. Pointless, but enough. Spliffard began to bark at the door just as I hit the max level the window could open, which was not enough to get out of. There was a broom in the corner and I began bashing the skylight with it until the prop on the window broke and it swung open. He was banging on the door frantically, and I couldn't fit my pack through the small window.

The thing is a street kid's pack is their life. You may hear me say this often. All I had to my name was in that pack. Not pointless shit either, very needed stuff. I frantically emptied it, tossing each thing out the window onto the roof of the RV. I pulled myself up through the window quickly, shoved the breakable things back into my pack, and tossed the whole thing over the side while kicking the rest over the edge. As I lowered myself halfway through the window to grab my dog by his collar my oily hands lost their grip and I fell face first into the sink.

I remember a ringing sound, the taste of blood and the sound of the door now fully being kicked. I don't really recall how but somehow when sound came rushing back in from reality I was on top of the RV with my dog. I ran to the ladder on the back of the RV and my oil covered hands fucked me yet again with the aluminum ladder and a freaked out dog. The fall wasn't far, but my foot didn't care. The sound of the snap was distinct, but I ran on it anyways. I didn't even feel it at the time. I also didn't grab my pack. I ran so hard, never once looking back to see if he was giving chase. There were trees in the distance and my mind said that the only way to survive this was to get there. The grass was so wet from all of the rain I must have fallen another dozen times as I ran.

Finally, I hit the oaks and in an instant found an old hollowed out stump from a tree that must have been hundreds of years old. I jumped in and Spliffard faithfully followed. We laid there all day not really making a sound. Every human I heard, every car door, every snap of a twig made my whole body react. Day soon turned to night and we both shivered. Somehow I fell asleep, or maybe I passed out. Either way, when I woke up in the morning all of that adrenaline had worn off because I was woken by the extreme amount of pain I was in. I remember not understanding where I was or why I was in such pain.

I ran my hand gently over my closed eye, swollen from slamming into the sink. The sudden sensation of pain made it all rush back and fully woke me to the situation. I could feel my foot was swollen to the point my boot was acting as a compress. I could also feel it would be easier to die than to face this. I think I may have been content with that choice if the damn dog would have felt the same, but he had other plans. The chatter of some chipmunk pissed off at our presence made him shoot out of that stump with a burst of puppy energy, refusing to listen to my stern, but very whispered, commands to return!

He began to bark like fucking crazy and I was terrified it would alert the man to where we were, not realizing in my trauma that he probably drove off right after the whole ordeal. So I slowly limped through the woods trying to get Spliffard to come to me. His chase led me to an old abandoned homesite with nothing more than a foundation and overgrown, fallen over sheds. I finally caught him and decided I would limp my way back to the edge of the woods to see if I could see the RV, and maybe find help.

There was a small stream, swollen to its banks from the rain that had been dumping from the sky all night. I stopped to wash the blood, caked-on mud, and God knows what else off of my hands, then realized my swollen face must be covered too. That swift water ran red as I rinsed my face. I ended up just laying there with my eye in the cold current for a while, it helped so much with the pain.

Sitting at the edge of the woods I couldn't see the RV but I could see one of those free coffee stands that pop up now and then at rest stops in an effort to keep people awake on the highways. I realized I was starving, freezing and injured, so they might be willing to help me. Getting closer, I realized the table next to the booth had all of my stuff on it - my clothing, food, sleeping bag, cookware, books, everything. I walked up and began to put my stuff back in the pack as a woman walked up with coffee and a donut. She sat in on the table and hastily said, "this is all of the help you're getting don't ask for more!"

I didn't speak one word to her just slung the pack over my shoulder and felt defeated in looking for any further help.

Making my way back through the woods I decided to go check out the old homesite - to hide there a while. It became apparent that this was at one time an old ranch sight that the state must have bought to make a rest stop. There was an old bit of canvas tarp sticking out of the long, fallen over shed that I used to make a lean to shelter of sorts against the crumbling stone foundation. I just laid there living off of cat food quality canned tuna and drinking the water out of a can of corn. It rained hard all night long again. I shivered just as hard.

Come morning I woke to the slight warmth of the sun. It was so bright like it was somehow summer again instead of late fall. My eye was bad and my foot was losing feeling, so I decided I better soak them both in the cold water of that creek I had passed. That's when I realized I heard the water in a different direction, too. It wrapped around the backside of the homesite, which I was crazy grateful for, being so much closer. Walking towards the sound I realized this whole area was overgrown with familiar plants and foods. There were still some Blackberries on the vines, the Oaks had begun to drop their acorns, there was a patch of Rhubarb that had long gone to seed, with its now stringy stalks that I chewed on anyways.

But what really caught my attention was the hybrid Comfrey. It was abundant, almost choking out all other plant life in areas. I sat there with her recalling all of the times I had seen those close to me heal wounds with her, and the story my Grandmother Audrey told me about why she was called Knitbone. I slowly gathered up an armful of her scratchy leaves and made my way to the creek bed. I knew once I took my boot off there was a real possibility I would not get it back on, but I needed to see what was going on. There was not much to see aside from a horrendous amount of yellow bruising and that it was dangerously swollen. I was honestly worried that the skin would split.

I sat there with my foot in the cold water as I took two rocks and mashed the Comfrey into a fresh poultice the best I could. I used my knife to cut my sock into two strips of material because it clearly wasn't going back on my foot anytime soon, and used my boot laces to hold it all in place. I remember as soon as that boot came off I could feel my heartbeat in my grossly swollen foot, each throb shooting with pain, but that cold Comfrey was such a comfort.

Digging through the old metal piles scattered here and there I came across a not-so-old metal coffee can. It wasn't even rusted. This would be such a game changer. One of the things I had in my pack was a little propane tank with a single burner attachment. Not only did this mean I could eat cooked oatmeal, but I could also make real poultices and broths. My eye responded the quickest to them, and in a matter of two days, the swelling had basically vanished, although I had no mirror to see the true extent of the bruising or the blood vessels broken in my eye.

As I limped around gathering dried acorns to leach, hoping to make a mush that maybe the dog would be more enthusiastic about eating if I mixed in the tiny bit of dog food crumbs I still had left, I came across a large patch of Miners Lettuce. Instantly I thought of all of the times hunting with my dad, stopping at the bottom of the same canyon every year where the Apple trees were wild. Spring fed and surrounded by these greens we always gathered and ate a little bit, "not too much though or you'll use up all the toilet paper," he always liked to tell me. It was like finding a piece of myself, my homelands when I needed it most. The dog was even willing to eat it once cooked, and I added some horrible ramen noodle "chicken" flavoring packet to it.

The swelling in my foot finally went down with days and days worth of compresses and drinking Comfrey broth, just as my propane ran out. I never wanted to leave. I felt safe here. I knew what was around me. I knew what it could do for me. These plants, this place, were clearly more willing to help me than humans were, but with no propane, there was no way to boil water for drinking, and I had already learned that horrible lesson a long while back. The fear of starting a fire and being discovered was soon outweighed by necessity, but it wasn't wrong. With that very first fire I was discovered, luckily I suppose, by some fellow street kids who had a van. We camped there another week before getting kicked out by state patrol.

My foot was doing a lot better, but still was causing me a lot of pain. When we made it to Eugene I asked for a ride to the emergency room so I could get it checked out. I left my dog in the van. The guy who owned it said they would wait for me, seeing as they had nowhere to go anyhow. It took four hours before my foot was finally x-rayed. There was indeed a break in one of the top bones. The nurse said the doctor would be right in to talk with me about it. He showed up with security to escort me out screaming around that I was a 'piece of shit homeless drug seeker wasting his time!', that it was clear the break was 'months' old, and that I had simply hit my foot with something to cause fresh bruising.

When I got to the lobby the lady that pushes the button to let you through the doors said my friend had left a note for me and handed me a piece of paper that had been folded into one of those triangles that kids did to notes they pass in school. After a ridiculous amount of effort to open this stupid thing, I shit you not, the only words written inside were, "God told me your dog is actually mine."

The van was long gone and so was my dog.

That Comfrey may have healed my swollen face and a broken foot, but it sadly didn't heal my cynicism towards humans and traumas gained.

·5·
Comfrey
Symphytum uplandica x.

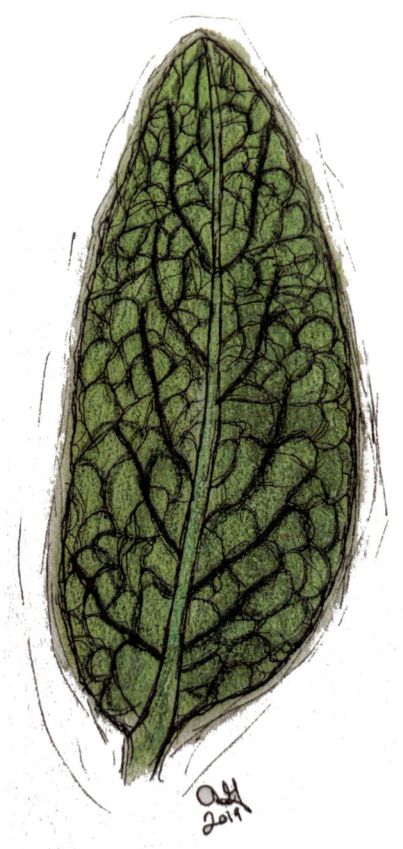

There is so much I could say about you, dear. How you knit my bones back together after countless humans tried their damndest to break them apart. I think in this you do indeed comfort me. I mean, what could be more comforting than knowing not if, but when I brake there is someone there just waiting to graciously put the pieces back together? I also deeply relate to your struggles of being witnessed as dangerous to use, too risky to rely on, too wild to trust should she take root, and vastly misunderstood out of sheer ignorance kept alive by unfounded fears. Yes, there is so much of that I can relate to.

But I also think I found you in such a long abandoned place for a reason, even if it would take me years to see it. After all, it is in these places, rather they be internal or external, where we will find our most potent healing once faced!

But this all my history, my story, my experiences, and that's enough of that. Let's dive into her story, her history, and hopefully this will be the beginning of many other people's experiences with her!

The History of Comfrey:

There are so many stories of Comfrey across mankind's history of broken bones, wounds and illnesses healed over the ages that we will never know, yet the many humans who came before us knew. They called her knitbone, boneset, bruisewort, and healing herb, just to name a few. You just don't earn names like that without truly delivering, and she has been doing so since as far as about 400 BC, we find her first written account by a Greek historian named Herodotus.

By that point the odds are good that wise women had already been using her for a very long time, and around the 400BC mark these heroic healers in Greece picked up this knowledge. From there, her written accounts exploded and her ability to help heal broken bones and beyond was cemented into history when she was written about in the Greek physician Pedanius Dioscorides' famous book 'De Materia Medica' (On Medical Materials), a five volume Greek encyclopedia about herbs and medicinal substances. This pharmacopeia was used for 1,500 years. It is considered by some to be the most influential and important herbal encyclopedia ever written.

She would go on to aid the Romans in their relentless desire to conquer all. Right alongside our dear friend Yarrow, Comfrey would dance through the renaissance ages with grace, as more and more was written. She held strong through the age of "enlightenment" in the 18th century before fear of her use would begin to take root as the side effects of wild comfrey use *(Cynoglossum virginianum)* internally began to be noted.

After this, while she was still praised highly she seemingly fell back to the wise woman and healers that did not follow these books. We'll fast forward a bit here because her history will fill all the pages if we allow, but eventually something beautiful occurred. A man named Henry Doubleday crossed two varieties in a quest to make Comfrey not only safe for livestock consumption, but humans too! His cross between Common Comfrey *(Symphytum officinale)* and Prickly Comfrey *(Symphytum asperum)* created our lovely lady who is often called Russian Comfrey *(Symphytum x uplandicum)*. This cross is sterile, meaning her seeds are not viable and she must be planted by root. She is, for the most part, the Comfrey that is now grown in every garden and on every farm world wide, which I find rather damn impressive!

What's the big deal, you ask? Well, in his life long quest he created a variety of Comfrey that had much lower (pretty much non-existent) problematic alkaloid (pyrrolizidine) levels in their leaves, which is what made her unsafe to consume internally. That is not to say that the utter fear of her does not hold up strong in the heroic healer world. In fact, the great Comfrey conflict is a legit dividing line drawn in the mud between many herbalists. Can you guess which side I stand on? That's right, the side that has drank about four quarts of Hybrid Comfrey infusion a month for the past decade and is tremendously healthier for it! I mean folks, not to blow my own horn but have you seen my skin, my nails, my hair that reaches the ground with ease? Comfrey is a huge reason I'm doing pretty good in those departments after a rough damn life!

The Many Uses of Comfrey:

She would love to help you deal with so many of life's pains and irritations!

Maybe you have been suffering for years with stubborn psoriasis or eczema. No problem! An infused oil will have you covered and finding relief in no time!

What if your gut is absolutely unhappy and nothing you do seems to give any hope? IBS? GERD? Any other abbreviation that means you are suffering at times? An infusion drank regularly will likely change your life in ways unimagined!

What if life has caught up with you and your bones are brittle to the point of osteoporosis? You and comfrey should probably become friends!

How about that nasty sprained ankle from an unfortunate step taken? Maybe you broke a bone instead? Pulled a tendon? Tore a muscle? Fuck that all sounds horrendous, but comfrey want's to ease your pain and cut the healing time in half!

How brittle is your hair? Have a hard time getting your nails to grow? Teeth crumbling? Well, these are all a type of bone so give her a try!

Are you suffering from shitty cartilage in your joints? Arthritis? Any other membrane just making you suffer from lack of it? Comfrey! Comfrey! Comfrey!

Stubborn boils? Cysts? Built up scar tissue from an injury? You guessed it, Comfrey!

But why?

How Can Comfrey Do So Much for Us?

Let's dive right in to the two main compounds found in comfrey that make her such an awesome healer of the ages! She is full of mucilage & allantoin!

So let's talk about mucilage! What in the hell does that mean? Think of something slimy and slippery that coats anything it touches. This is what any herb that has high levels of polysaccharides does. So when dry comfrey leaf has boiling water dumped overtop what's going on is these polysaccharides swell up when exposed to the water and that is what makes it seem kinda slimy!

Sound gross? Well yeah okay, so maybe drinking a cup of something kinda slippery doesn't sound good to you right now. But what if I told you it's that very sliminess that makes her a powerful anti-inflammatory for basically EVERY mucous membrane in our bodies?

Just for fun let's name all of the mucous membranes we have as humans and see how comfrey can help each one!

So the two big ones you are probably aware of are the stomach and every inch of your digestive tract - the areas that most humans have issues with at some time or another! Comfrey is such a powerful healer of these particular mucous membranes because of her ability to coat and soothes alllllll of our inflamed and angry tissue in these areas! One thing that is hard to do is heal the gut/intestines when the issue IS inflammation, because how do we allow it to rest?

When I had a peptic ulcer sure Yarrow stopped the bleeding and even helped a bit with the pain, but it was a thick double brewed Comfrey infusion drank that got that nasty stress induced ulcer healed up in no time. In a way you could think of mucilage as like a "bandaid" for your internal systems, because what that Comfrey infusion did was coat the wound (ulcer) and protect it from my own stomach acid so it had a chance to heal. It took about a week of infusion and a low acid diet, but damned if I didn't treat a peptic ulcer all on my own!

The funny thing is that while you were drinking that infusion to help your stomach you were unknowingly helping a pretty unthought of as mucous membrane known for being your entire breathing, drinking, swallowing and talking mechanisms. You know, your lungs, windpipe, and the mouth that leads to that whole ordeal? This makes her great for anyone who is looking to heal from constant irritation caused by GERD or anything similar, and the same principle as above applies. We are using her sliminess as a bandaid so our body can focus on healing versus defense.

I live in a very diverse area of high mountain desert and within our unique mountain range there are many microclimates. In just a few hours I can be standing on extremely lush soil that is nutrient dense, solid clay that won't let go of water, or on barren alkaline soil that only the tough as nails sagebrush and some berry farms can thrive in.

Not too long ago, a childhood friend was paid to clear strip about 50 acres of sagebrush so a farmer could put in another crop. He had done this too many times to count. He had even done the opposite, where he helped reclaim land that had been put into a CRP (conservation reserve program). Because of this he felt a little too comfortable and cocky I suppose and decided he didn't need to wear his respiratory protection when dealing with that powdery alkaline soil.

It was about 11pm when his girlfriend called me in a panic, saying he was refusing to go to the hospital. You see, as he was out there ripping up sagebrush the soil became even looser and, let's just say we have a ton of wind turbines here for a reason. That gust of wind hit the sage barrens just right and in an instant, he was stuck in an alkaline dust storm and his mask was in the truck he could no longer see his way to. Alkaline burns are serious, especially for membranes because unlike acidic things the alkaline substance is absorbed readily by the body and, in his case, it was his lungs.

Wana guess what had him talking in about three weeks like nothing had ever happened? Comfrey infusion! Should he have gone to the ER? Absolutely! Was comfrey the next best thing for a stubborn person unwilling to go? Sure seems like it!

So let's rattle off the remaining bits of mucous membranes we haven't touched on yet and see how Comfrey can be a great ally for them!

The womb, vaginal walls, urethra (the thing you piss out of), eyelids, oh, and let's not forget every single bit of connective tissue in your body. So, ya know, just the stuff that literally holds your body together. That's all, ha!

Maybe you'd like to strengthen your womb. Comfrey is the gal for you! Does down below seem like it's not as happy as it could be? Comfrey just keeps waiting for you to call her name! Does it always burn when you piss even if you don't have a UTI? Maybe you find yourself just dribbling a little bit, even when you haven't sneezed.

Of course, when using her for womb health we're gana have to drink her, but we can also do castor oil packs, even though her mucous bits we're after won't really cross through. For cheering up that upset vagina I really like using sitz baths from warm Comfrey infusions and even a finger bath (likely exactly what you imagined), especially if the upset is from irritation or tissue that's degrading, such as vulvar dystrophy.

No matter what has you drinking comfrey infusion she will end up coating your bladder with that slime I am trying to convince you to love! Doing this, she again is singing that same ol band-aid song, just giving these hot and angry surfaces a bit of a rest!

So what exactly is connective tissue and how can we visualize something Comfrey can help with in that area?

Okay, humor me for just a second.

I want you to touch your nose. Now your knees. Now the muscles in the back of your calf. Now your ears. Now your spine. Now the muscle in your biceps. Now the tendon just above your heel. Now grab a love handle, or any place that jiggles a bit. Now, last but 100% not least, I want you to knock on your head like your at someone's door.

What the hell was that odd game of Head, Shoulders, Knees, and Toes about?

You just touched all of your "connective tissue" that comfrey can help with!

Bone is the strongest of connective tissue of course, but there are also your muscles, tendons, ligaments, cartilage, and adipose, which is just a fancy word for fat!

Take all of that in for just a moment. I mean, really think about the fact that every time you drink a comfrey infusion you are literally supporting every single aspect of your body that you just touched!

I know many are wary of using her internally, but she can also bring so much healing externally as an infused oil or a compress! This brings me to her allantoin content and all of her amazing uses!

Did you know comfrey should never be used on a fresh open wound? Not because of the comfrey madness scare, but because she is so damn effective at healing wounds rapidly she can cause bacteria to become trapped inside of the wound!

How does comfrey do this? Well, the allantoin has some neat tricks up its sleeve!

One of her "main" functions is to generate new skin cells, which encourages new tissue development. Did you catch that? Comfrey grows new cells... However what I am about to type out will make your jaw drop a little further.

Comfrey, and the allantoin she contains, can clear away necrotic tissue (read hear rotting dead flesh), making way for new cell development.

So when you apply her as a balm, salve, oil, or compress, she is no joke making new skin cells to replace the damaged ones and getting rid of dead and rotting cells! What good does that do if we can't use her on wounds? I didn't say that at all! I said we can't use her on fresh wounds! That means as soon as you have a well developed scab it's fair game to begin using Comfrey to heal a wound!

This has a lot to do with how our bodies heal themselves, really. You see, a scab is like a natural band aid that protects the wound while your immune system gets busy battling off bacteria and generating granulation tissue from the bottom up. The issue with using Comfrey on an un-scabbed wound is that she has a tendency to heal from the top down, which is not hard to imagine because that is where you are applying her! When that happens, IF there were bacteria present the two healing methods have now trapped it in the middle. Trapped bacteria is deadly bacteria. Usually bacteria will go to the surface of a wound since they like air, but when that is not an option it spreads inward, and God help you if it hits your lymph nodes, the superhighway of your entire body.

So now that I am done making you a germaphobe, let's touch on one of her common names - Knit Bone! While you may have thought I was full of shit about her healing my broken foot so rapidly, I promise I was not exaggerating in the least. That is to say, her allantoin content will happily absorb through the skin to a broken bone and encourage rapid healing, so much so that it was actually a stupid idea for me to use her without the broken bone being set correctly first! While my foot does act up from time to time I am usually able to calm the aching from a not so evenly healed bone with a relaxing foot soak in warm Comfrey infusion!

While she was working hard to knit my bone back together, her powerful anti-inflammatory abilities were busy pulling down the swelling I was sure would make my skin split if it got any worse! This ability plays into her role as healer, considering inflammation of any kind is not only hard on our bodies, but it really delays healing on a serious level.

That might be a bit confusing for those who know that inflammation is caused by our own immune systems response, but it will probably make perfect sense to the person who is battling chronic illness due to chronic inflammation. The cure our body creates can actually turn into the thing that causes the disease. Pulling the swelling down in my foot was crucial, not only in healing but allowing my immune system to focus on other areas in need of attention!

Beyond these already amazing things this particular part of Comfrey also acts to soothe our skin, in fact, she can kinda toughen up sensitive skin making it much more resilient to the things that irritate!

Then she swoops in and protects our skin from UV damage and calms down hot angry skin, although I would not use her as a sunblock, but instead as a way to combat the sun's effects! We can't forget her amazing ability to fight free radicals by grabbings water from the air to hydrate our skin! It is really no surprise that synthesized allantoin is found in many high end cosmetics, and even topical medications!

But I 100% would bet my last worn out dollar that a deeply infused oil with her root and leaf will do far more for our bodies and beauty than any synthetic counterfeit!

Truthfully I was lucky to come across her in such a time of need, and over the years my relationship with her has become vast. No matter where I find myself living in the years to come, if I can stick a root of her in the ground I most certainly will feel better prepared for whatever may come, just from knowing she is near!

Where Does Comfrey Grow?

One of the points of Russian Comfrey beyond it having lower alkaloid levels is that she was made sterile. This means that her seeds can not germinate, so coming across her in the wild is unlikely.

It is so unlikely that I have only ever stumbled across her ONCE where there had clearly not been a home sight. Not long ago I was walking along the raging river banks of the Walla Walla River in spring and I came across the biggest Grandmother plant I have ever seen, growing unattended a few feet from the water's edge! My best guess is that at some point a local farmer was growing comfrey as a livestock feed along the river and some root must have been washed downstream. She does prefer a bit of rock and a lot of water, so I was not surprised at how abundantly she had taken hold!

Now that does not mean that you won't come across common Comfrey (*Symphytum officinale*). She was introduced to Europe in the 1800s from Eurasia and continued her journey to North America,exploding on the scene as a very hard to eradicate invasive plant. Why? Well, not only does common Comfrey have extremely fertile seeds that last a long time (until conditions are perfect to germinate), but she also aggressively spreads from disturbed roots.

Meaning if you attempt to dig up her root, so help you, if you miss even the tiniest bit of it she will come back with a vengeance! This meant every time an unknowing farmer plowed a field each broken Comfrey root became a new plant. That is why common Comfrey can be found growing in almost every US state and ALL of Canada according to the US plant database that tracks invasive plants!

While we can't use Common comfrey internally we sure can use her externally, and the best places to look are indeed along river banks, moist soil, ditches, and old farmland. For the sake of finding hybrid Russian comfrey it is best to buy some root crown and plant her in a place you will always want her to be. Then you will know for certain that you have the correct plant ally for internal use, and as long as you don't dig her roots she will never spread beyond where you put her!

When Should We Harvest Comfrey?

I am mindful to only harvest her after she has done a fair amount of blooming, keeping in mind that if I cut her back more will grow and likely bloom, and I must wait for that round to finish up as well. This ensures that her pyrrolizidine alkaloids levels are as low as possible. I also will not harvest her for internal use after any sort of frost has touched her, because there's some belief that the pyrrolizidine alkaloids from the root travel back up into the leaf. Honestly I don't harvest any summer medicines after a frost because my grandmother taught me this is when they want to be left alone.

What Cautions Should We Take?

Fuck it, let's have a fight! That's the first thing that comes to mind when I even think on discussing Comfrey with a good majority of other herbalists. That line drawn in the mud about The Great Comfrey Debate is a very real one. I know that while I will probably get a lot of hate for this book in general, this section will have angry letters flowing (My existence earns me a lot of angry letters. I am either an asshole or I'm doing something right enough to piss people off. Probably a fair bit of both.), because in our current society (2019/20 for the way in the future reader's sake) it is basically a crime punishable by death to have a differing opinion than someone else, but here I go anyhow!

Are you a rat? No, I don't mean did you snitch on someone, I mean like a literal rodent? Seem like a silly question? Maybe, but it is a very relevant one in the grand scheme of things! How so?

You see, all of the studies, including the big bad main study that told us the dangers of Comfrey ingestion, were done on rats and their livers. I know many are appalled at animal testing and many count it as a blessing. We are not here to debate that, but rather how these tests are conducted and how sometimes the results are completely absurd to compare to a human.

Case in point - did you know that a vast majority of testing in regards to the safety of using Comfrey internally was done on rats, and the testing was done in rapid and short successions of highly concentrated root powder that was essentially turned into rat food?

Why is this an issue? A few things.

First, let's accept the fact that rats do not have that long of a lifespan, and the main reason testing is done on rats is because we can see the long term effects on a living organism in a pretty short amount of time. Doing a rapid study on rats indicates that in a matter of a few months they presumed to have enough data to draw a conclusion.

Only the issue is they didn't. Not really.

What they did discover is if you feed a rat Comfrey root - which should never be ingested at extremely high rates, even if it was "only 2% of their diet" - they will get sick as hell! To put 2% into perspective, these rats were ingesting the equivalent of 20 years worth of comfrey root in a matter of weeks. I can tell you right now if you eat ANY herb or commonly bought vegetables in that volume some bad shit is gana happen to your body!

That is not the only study on Comfrey using rats. Another common one used as ammo in the Do Not Ingest Debate is where rats were fed pyrrolizidine alkaloids derived from Russian Comfrey ROOT to study the effects of the herb on the liver.

So while I am NOT here suggesting that pyrrolizidine alkaloids don't pose a real health issue, what I am trying to get across is the point that almost all studies done on the safety or lack thereof of Comfrey have been done with isolated compounds, NOT whole plant matter, and on the portion of the plant that every herbalist agrees is not safe for internal use, in levels that are never realistically going to be ingested by a human.

There is also a pesky fact that in the 1960's - when many of these trials began - the government refused to evaluate the willing humans with no raised liver enzyme levels, even though they had been steadily consuming comfrey for over 20 years.

In one fail swoop because a handful of rats showed liver distress after being exposed to massive amounts of pyrrolizidine alkaloids this ancient ally that has been helping humans for thousands of years was deemed so dangerous that in certain areas of the world she is illegal to work with in any way, shape, or form. In their minds the tiny, if at all present, levels of pyrrolizidine alkaloids in a simple infused oil would somehow (through transdermal absorption) murder your liver.

In 2001 the FDA declared that Comfrey must be pulled out of the dietary supplement market (things you ingest), and is now working hard to heavily restrict her use in topical herbal products.

Does all of the above rambled out opinion mean there are no cautions we should take?

Absolutely not! In general, only Russian Comfrey leaf (Symphytum uplandica x.) is considered moderately safe for spaced out ingestion in nourishing herbal infusions or tea blends, and it is best to harvest after the flowering period. I also strip the leaf away from the stem. Then I use the stems alongside the root for infused oils and other topical creations so there is no waste.

Also, if you are living with impaired liver function or are pregnant I would probably find another option. I always encourage folks to do their own research beyond this book, that blog post, someone's strongly worded opinion, and truly dive into how these conclusions were made. See how your own thought process lands on the matter!

How Much is Too Much?

Well, this is almost a moot section after the last one! I suppose we can touch on the fact that how every human body responds to Comfrey will be as unique as each human! If you should decide to join the side of us who feel like Comfrey has been demonized in a sort of How Dare You Heal Yourself Witch Hunt, I'd say to start slow. Maybe a few cups a week to see how your body reacts.

If I am not using her for a specific ailment I simply add her to my weekly rotation of nourishing herbal infusions, which has me ingesting about a quart weekly (four cups). Because I feel comfortable in my decision and relationship with her, if I had something that really needed more internal help I would probably drink up to two quarts a week max, and be sure the second one was a rebrew of the first plant matter so I can extract even more of her awesome sliminess!

.6.

Dandelion Helps Us Digest Food, but Not Cruelty.

If I end up in hell I'm positive my version will be a long, never ending hill, with nothing to drink and the lingering taste of an expired chocolate soy based protein bar than makes me gag over and over as it relentlessly coats every inch of my mouth, no liquid to swallow with.

I have walked down, hitched down, and ridden down thousands of miles of highways, interstates, backroads, gravel and dirt roads alike. In all honesty, most blend together. In all sadness, I only vividly recall the roads that lead to painful situations. I can recall every curve, every sound, every blindspot, every gust of wind that slammed me in the face from a rig whipping by, stealing my breath with their hot exhaust.

Over the years of dealing with thousands of street kids, Eugene became hostile towards the homeless. The strip was ripped out and turned into a road. The courthouse yard was fenced in. Spare changing and flying signs were made illegal anywhere worth doing it. Soup kitchens shut down. Sleeping outside was now a more complicated affair, as it was essentially illegal to be homeless and sleep.

Many moved on and I was happy to join, as staying still for too long caused my heart to beat erratic with anxiety, which is why by this time in my life I had been to the east coast and back about four times by simply hopping in rigs that were heading one way or the other. I could cling to the notion that travelling is factually in my blood, my very genetic makeup, but if I am being honest I was running from trauma and from facing myself and things that had been done to me as a child.

A mile down the highway we bravely threw up our signs, as on many stretches of road in the United States it is illegal to hitchhike. You can walk down the road all you want, but so help you God should you stick out your thumb or hold up a sign, more often than not staters are happy to haul your ass in and throw your pack in a dumpster, just because they can. We walked south for two days before anyone stopped. It was not a surprise really. There were far too many of us. Five people, mainly guys, who don't often get rides. To be fair, a few folks did stop and offer to give just me a ride, but I never had a chance to say no as the guys screamed to fuck off at the creeps.

Finally, something big enough drove by that could carry us all - a no joke, straight from Mexico prison bus. Two well to do college kids whose diet consisted mainly of adderall and e-bombs had just had it delivered to them all the way in Eugene after winning it in an online auction in Mexico. They were now setting out to make it a rave tour bus. I have accepted many rides over the years that I should have known were dangerous, but didn't until it was too late. This one, however, sent chills down my spine from the moment it pulled up to the moment the gate slammed behind me, clearly locking us all in the back.

They were on their way to San Fran and would happily give us a ride all the way down the 101 to where we were heading. About two hours in, after having stared at every apparent bloodstain and figuring out what the many words scratched in the walls said, they decided it was boring to drive so they would both eat an entire fucking bag of mushrooms. To be fair, I am positive they weren't sober to begin with. I saw the first guy down a bag and I just said, "fuck we don't have seatbelts back here".

It seemingly gave them instant permission to feel superior to us, these dirty, gross, poverty stricken homeless kids they had locked in a prison bus. Really, I think they were just no longer able to hide their true nature. They began ranting about how much money they were worth, about their fathers, about how we were the root of all of their suffering, talked on genocide of all poor people, but not the women of course. They could be of use. That led them into the spiral of asking the guys what they were willing to do for money. More to the point, what were they willing to do to me for money.

This older kid who went by "Just Jeremy" from Montana was very protective of me, the way a big brother is of a little sister. I think I reminded him of somebody he may have lost. When he heard this suggestion he snapped and began kicking the front gate. He was not a small person, easily 6 '3 with the weight to match. The rich kid not driving pulled out a gun, and we spent the next two hours barrelling down the highways with self entitled privileged college kids tripping fucking balls on mushrooms, telling us how they can do anything to us and if they did get caught it didn't matter because their dads could get them out of trouble.

During that entire time, we didn't say a single word back to anything they had to say until the one with the gun opened the gate and stepped through with his fancy looking fucking book bag. The driver decided to pull over onto a wide shoulder to watch. I hid behind Jeremy watching as this guy put a gun to each person's head as he made them eat huge amounts of mushrooms, which I knew would easily kill me since at the time I maybe weighed a whole 87lbs on a well fed day, and it was never a well fed day. Jeremy fought so hard that they broke his tooth shoving the gun in his mouth. I wasn't crying, but I was pleading. Pleading for them not to make me eat as much. I was terrified, tears just didn't flow. I was locked up, not that I think it would have made a difference. The smell of chewed mushrooms and vomit filled that space as I watched all of these humans so much bigger than me vomit, like one often does after eating mushrooms of this variety, but on such a different level.

I just kept saying with my face shoved into the ground "I've already eaten an eighth! I've already eaten an eighth! An eighth is enough!", knowing that was the max amount I'd likely not overdose from, he yanked my head up by my dreads and I pleaded one last time that I had eaten enough. He stuck that gun right in my face, touching my nose. I don't know if it was the mushrooms kicking in or just pure shock, likely a bit of both, but I began to laugh hysterically. I could see the words stamped into the barrel perfectly. It was a fucking bb gun. They had removed the bright orange plastic tip from it that lets you know it's not a real gun.

As soon as Jeremy could understand the words I was trying to get out between my uncontrollable laughter and vomiting, that the gun was fake, he rushed the guy with the bb gun and everything just happened in a blur. The other kids began kicking the shit out of the guy. The other one stood in a corner and legit pissed all over himself. It didn't feel like reality. Shit, it still doesn't. Time was slipping. Suddenly we were off that bus and it was driving away. Suddenly we were setting up a makeshift camp off the highway in some Alder trees. The only thing I felt sure I knew was that there were Alder trees and they would keep me safe.

I remember being terrified to fall asleep. I didn't want to wake up in that place I did so long ago. I remember cop lights and hearing someone say "HIDE, APRIL!" I remember a little cave-like structure the alder trees had made with their bent over branches. I remember watching Jeremy and two others getting hauled away. I remember falling asleep, much to my terror.

I woke up the next morning to a horrendously sharp pain in my left kidney and instantly vomited what little liquid I had in my stomach. There were only two left after the cops got done. A kid named Seth who just fucking despised my existence for I don't know, being a woman is what it felt like, and a kid named Jones that would happily watch my back if I spread my legs for him. I asked if the stater hauled the other kids off because of what happened thinking those college kids had called the cops or some shit but it was just dumb luck of the cop seeing our camp and the others having warrants out for their arrest. I knew I'd never see Jeremy again. It absolutely broke my heart that he was gone, which was surprising to me. That was honestly just how it was back then, living this kind of life. You only have your friends in the moment. Once they are gone, they are gone. There's no number you can call, no house you can visit, no social media you can look them up on.

We just began to walk, and we walked for hours. Seth had a small jug of water that he refused to share with me. He said he didn't want my disgusting lips to touch it, refusing to even dump some from a distance into my mouth. Yet again the only food I had was cat food grade tuna fish. The food box places handed that shit out by the metric ton no matter where you were. I knew I needed to eat, it was just so fucking salty and was canned in oil.

It wasn't long before I was shitting myself violently down in a ditch. At this point, both of my kidneys were fucking screaming and I'm sure my liver was hating on me plenty, too.

After a few hours of walking, I flat out begged Seth for his water. He stopped walking, unhooked his jug from his pack, looked me in the eye and said, "sure", as he dumped it all out onto the ground. He hated me so much he was willing to suffer too just to hurt me. I went quiet and walked, stopping every fifteen or twenty minutes to puke nothing or shit pure bile, having to run to catch up since they wouldn't wait. It might be easy for you to think, "Fuck that. I'd just let them leave me behind." or something along those lines. The reality is that when humans lead a life like this we revert back to the pack mentality I have mentioned in so many ways. We know that no matter what, more so as a woman, it is more dangerous to be alone on the highway or streets especially if we have not been posted up in an area long. Even if the group treats us like shit we keep the fuck up, because the devil you kinda know is better than the devil you don't know who may pick you up all by yourself.

Finally, a conversion van pulled over and offered us a ride. We piled in. The guy was nice enough but had no water, and was clearly OCD about germs. Bless his heart for suffering our very dirty existence as long as he did. I just wished he would have suffered us for five more miles. I could finally smell the ocean, lying there using every muscle in my body to resist the urge to shit in this mans very clean van, when he pulled off the shoulder at the base of a hill, saying, "I'm sorry, I don't think my motor can handle carrying such a heavy load over this hill."

"It has a one ton motor. It could pull a fucking trailer full of cattle over that hill, let alone three half starved kids." I thought to myself as I jumped out of the van.

I just stood there looking up at that hill. It was the kind of hill that you can't really see the top of. It just keeps fucking going with too many winds and bends. There was no real shoulder to walk on, which is dangerous as hell because some folks like to pretend they are gana hit you. Sometimes they do. At the base of the hill was a fancy cedar fence, eight feet tall at least, with many hidden half million dollar cottages built behind it. I just leaned against it and cried. I had not eaten anything but hallucinogenic mushrooms and salty canned tuna in days. I had not drank water in over 20 hours, maybe more. I'm honestly not sure. It was not long before some security guy came to chase us off. I asked him if he could fill our jugs with water. He said we weren't worth losing his job for, and that there was a spring at the top of the hill, about five miles.

A five fucking mile long hill? There's no way I could make that treck, I thought to myself. Maybe that guy was just pulling a number out of his ass. I mean, could a hill really last that long? I just wanted to sleep. Across the road was a small field with some trees. I tried my damndest to convince them we should camp out over there, but it was barely noon and they weren't stopping for me, that was for sure. So I kept walking. My pack was always too heavy for my body weight, riding on my kidneys. It wasn't safe to walk up the hill in a zigzag pattern to make it easier with too many cars and motorcycles barreled down it. Out of all of the places to pick up a hitchhiker, a huge damn hill should be one of them. An hour in and my vision became a bit tunneled and I tried to ignore it. I thought it was from low blood sugar and begged Jones for one of the protein bars I knew he had stolen from a store many towns back. He tossed me a chocolate flavored one and said if I can choke it down he knows I'm equipped to choke down a dick, too. Asshole.

Luckily, I didn't pass that test. I could not swallow this thick, triple soy chocolate thing sent straight from hell. I gagged and almost suffocated from the film it left in my mouth as I chewed it and then puked it back up. I couldn't even wipe the bit I got on my hands off, so I'm sure my face, I, looked brutal. I wouldn't pick me up either. I just kept walking. I was too dehydrated to produce tears, or even cry out from the pain that now shot all throughout my body. I am pretty sure my kidneys were shutting down. I began abandoning things from my pack just to gain any kind of release, like some pathetic trauma filled bread crumb trail. I did feel pathetic. I remember that distinctly.

Yes, these guys were cocksuckers, but I felt so weak like I was some burden being suffered instead of a human who had just like them gone through a horrible trauma. I was supposed to be stronger than this, I thought to myself. Maybe this is why they hate me. In the end, all I had left was my sleeping bag, a few books about herbs, my empty water jug, a small tarp and my tiny propane cooker set up. I had never been so happy about a sideways coastal downpour in my life. It was getting dark and from the signs, we knew we had one more mile to go to "The Hilltop General Store". The whole time I walked with my mouth open, finally getting the chocolate flavored soy coating out some, but I couldn't really get enough to take a full drink. By the time we reached the top, it was pitch dark and we found some bushes to hide out in. I just laid there, trying in my exhaustion to use the tarp as a funnel to guide water into a gallon jug as I slept instead of using it to stay dry.

I slept really deeply, I'm sure from sheer exhaustion. I seldom don't wake before the sun rises, but on this day I woke up with it high above my head. I knew it was at the very least noon. In a matter of moments, I realized I was alone. Those assholes stole my tarp and, I thought, my water jug until I looked over and saw the jug filled with what I thought was rainwater. I read what was written on it:

"I wouldn't have taken your tarp if you would have sucked my dick, but Seth said we should at least leave you with some water from the spring so we don't get blamed for your death."

I was so thirsty that I didn't taste it until I had chugged the top half of the jug. This wasn't fresh crisp, drinkable spring water. It was sulfured out spring water. I had now just drank a fucking quart of sulfur heavy water after being critically dehydrated. Kidneys and sulfur do not play nice together on the best of days and this was not a best fucking day.

My body instantly purged. I laid there thinking on what horrible things must have occurred to those guys to make them despise women so much, or what I had done, again thinking of how pathetic I was for not being as physically able as them. But I also wondered how in the fuck do you treat another human like this after going through what we went through together on that bus. Maybe they were upset that they didn't die. I have always thought that people like that are angry about having to be alive. I thought a lot of things while laying there waiting for I don't know what. I didn't want to die, I just didn't want to move. Finally, I did, my head that is. I stopped staring at the sky and looked to the left as though I expected to see a long lost family friend.

In some ways I did. It was an entire field of Dandelions. Most had gone to seed. I realized I was laying in them too. I knew they were edible and I instantly hopped on my hands and knees, shoving bitter but moisture filled leaves into my mouth. I must have looked like a crazy ass grazing animal to anyone who would have seen me feasting, puking a little bit and eating more. I remember sucking on a mouthful of chewed up leaves and swallowing the "water". It was like some bitter healing nectar sent from the Gods. I hid in those same bushes that night and read by dying headlamp all about Dandelions and their roots' amazing ability to help restore proper function to the kidneys and liver. I had for sure drank a lot of tea from her roots growing up, and I suddenly remembered why as I drifted off to sleep with a gut full of this plant ally.

I woke, terrified as someone shook my foot saying, "APRIL!! APRIL!! ARE YOU DEAD??"

Out of all people, it was Jeremey. The jail was too full and he got matrixed out. Catching a ride halfway up the hill, he said, as soon as he jumped out of the rig he saw something in the ditch that didn't look right. It was a waterlogged book I had recommended he read, so he picked it up and kept walking. Following my discarded possessions, he was positive Seth had fucking choked me to death when he saw me in the bushes. I had never been so happy to see someone in my life and instantly asked him for water he said, "I just filled my jug up at the spring!" I freaked, warning him of the sulfur, and he looked baffled. There was no sulfur in that spring, but we discovered there was indeed a sulfur hot springs another 7 miles down the road. That guy fucking hated me enough to go fourteen miles out of his way to make sure I drank poison water. I would not be surprised if that man if he's still alive today, has killed a woman or two.

We found a place a little further back off the road that allowed tent camping for $4 a day. We didn't have any money, but those slips are easy enough to alter to make it look like you paid far enough back for multiple days and they assume the money had already been collected. We spent the next few days living off of Oatmeal and Dandelion roots. We made broth with them and we roasted them in some old foil. In about a weeks' time of daily digging the field looked like a gopher had declared war, but my piss was clear and the pain was gone. I have no doubt that my kidney functions were critically low from dehydration, starvation, a massive dose of psilocybin and a far too heavy pack riding on them.

During our time together I learned that Jeremy did actually begin traveling to find his little sister that ran away after a Rainbow Gathering came through his home town area. He said a body was found a few years later but he did not believe it was his sister, even though the dental records matched. Eventually, we ended up parting ways. Our roads of looking for something or someone led us in different directions.

My dearest friend Jeremy, if you are alive and reading this I hope you found your sister or the courage to face her loss. I hope you know how grateful I am to have had your friendship for the short amount of time we spent together. I hope you know that you, out of the thousands of humans I have met living this life of mine, are one of the few truly kind and generous ones that I will never forget.

You had an impact on me for the good, and that's just not something I can say about many people.

·7·
Dandelion

Taraxacum officinale

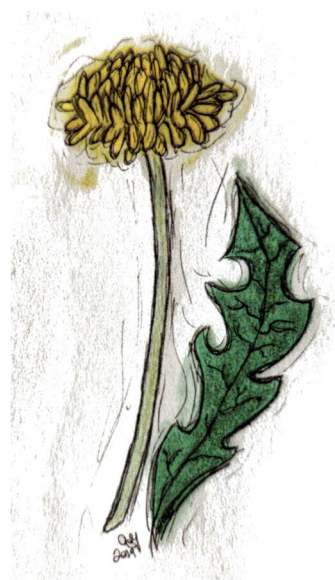

I'd like to think that the roots of this humble yet powerful healer run as deep as that glimmer of meaningful companionship has throughout my life. Yes, I am going to believe her tap roots are endless, because for me that feels right.

I also feel like I would be short sighted if I didn't make the connection to how hated I felt by mankind at the moment - who seemed to be hellbent on my eradication - and the eradication efforts that our beloved ally Dandelion faces every single day the sun is shining.

Sometimes I wish this story had sharper teeth to match the appearance of those leaves chewed, and that I could say I was so much more courageous than I truly was. Maybe that is the lesson she would like us to remember though, eh? What lesson is that? The one where we assume ourselves to be fierce, but are actually rather gentle in nature. This does not make us weaker or lesser. It makes others who would seek to destroy us weak and lesser from their own hatred directed at something they can not seem to grasp. All of that could be bullshit though, so let's talk about why to this day me and Dandelion have a deep relationship.

The History of Dandelion:

This ally has not hopped to so many different countries by sheer happenstance. No, quite the opposite is the case. You see, this now reviled weed that takes over the wasteland of pointless waves of green grass now consuming first world nations was once a vital food crop for many cultures ancestors - especially if your ancestors came from one of the many differing cultures of Europe or Asia, as these places are where the common dandelion originated from.

Because of this, and the fact that my mind might be a little quirky, I see the deep irony in how hard most humans who are usually in one way or another from these areas now work to kill off these gentle and giving allies. To me, I link the dandelions with ancestors trying to be remembered and current day humans trying their hardest to rip out, poison, and eradicate all notions of where Self came from.

Dandelion (and how much she has given to humans of all walks) predates most written languages, and has been traced back to about 30,000 million years! We can get started in the 10th century though, as that is when Arabian physicians referred to her as a type of "endive" that was good for just about everything under the sun! Later she would be talked about by the Romans who, while they had a deep penance for brutal genocide, also had deep understandings of how a plant might heal us. She even reached as far as Egypt, became revered there as well! Greece would write of her many healing ways, and I'd dare to say Rome likely picked up a fair bit of what they knew about her from there, but one of the longest continually recorded histories of detailed use comes from the Chinese, with the better part of a 1000 year relationship!

Of course, this ally does not care who you are or where you come from, it is just important to understand how long of a relationship she has had with humans.

Her name Dandelion is derived from the French word "dent de lion" which means "lion's tooth", which is not hard to imagine when looking at her very tooth like shaped leaf! In fact, I would say this is one of the main ways to properly identify her! There is also some debate that her name comes from the Greek word 'Leontodon' which also means "lion's tooth" in English. Of course just like every other plant she has many other names, such as priest's crown, Irish daisy, monk's head, and blowball, to name a few.

Mama had a baby and it's head popped off! If you don't know what I'm talking on you likely a.) Think I am crazy as fuck and b.) are substantially younger/from a different generation.

Random thing to think about if you do know what I am talking on. No one really knows where that came from or what event in history created a chant such as that, but to this day it is always done across the world with many variations, always using Dandelions!

A few think it *may* be linked to the french revolution but can't be sure. I bet the Dandelion knows as she has been around longer than us!

I will give you one last thing to think on that elaborates our utter disconnect from this ally:

She was once so revered in Europe that poems were written on her behalf. She was considered one of the most beautiful flowers. She was planted in landscapes and fields alike for her nourishment, medicine, and beauty. In Japanese culture entire horticulture societies were formed just to appreciate and study her existence - no other plant, just our beloved Dandelion!

Now companies make millions of dollars creating chemicals to kill her. They always fail, as she knows how to persist.

The Many Uses of Dandelion:

This lion toothed lover has so many uses it is a little shocking to see her viewed as an enemy, especially when she does no ecological damage to the lands she is not from, unlike any other invasive species. Meaning she does not choke out other native plants. She does not hurt wildlife. She does not poison wildlife or livestock. In fact, she improves soil, strips contaminants from it, and is a main food source for both native and honey bees in the spring!

She would love to ease your aching muscles and breasts alike!

Need a hand improving digestion? How about encouraging your kidneys, liver, pancreas, and gallbladder to function optimally?

Got a sour stomach? Sluggish colon? Want to digest more nutrients from all the other foods you eat?

Maybe you really need to kick up your vitamin levels or lower your blood pressure?

Facing cancer and want to slow the cellular growth? Need an antioxidant boost?

Inflammation? Diabetes? High cholesterol? How's your immune system?

How about eczema? Psoriasis? All around angry skin?

Any of these things a factor in your life?

After reading all of that Is it really any surprise that her Latin name Taraxacum means "disease remedy"?

How Can Dandelion Do So Much for Us?

She has so many compounds that her leaves, blooms, stems, and root all have similar and different ones at once! Remember how I said I want to keep this simple for ya? Well, for the sake of that we are only gana name drop a few of her main compounds and talk on what they are great for!

Taraxacin, eudesmanolides, Taraxacerin, Inulin, sesquiterpene lactones, phenylpropanoids.

That's a bit of a mouthful, huh? Well, that's okay because so is a sip of her as a nice bitter tea! Speaking of her bitterness, that mainly comes from her Taraxacin properties, but this is the GOOD bitter that helps really get digestive juices flowing. Anything that is a friend to healthy digestion is also a key component to getting your liver, gallbladder, and pancreas running to the best of their ability!

This is why she is so often mistakenly labeled as a plant that can "detox" our bodies. I want to be frank with you - your body is not dirty. your liver is not a car filter that holds onto toxins and more people get injured from following dangerous detox trends than you likely realize!

You see, she does not detox your body and neither does your liver. Well, not in the way that so many would lead you to believe. Allow me to get sidetracked here and break down exactly what your liver does for the sake of clarity!

The liver is probably one of the most misunderstood organs in the herbalism world anyhow, with so many thinking it acts as a run of the mill "filter" as mentioned above When we think of it as a car filter we are assuming like a car filter that it can somehow be dirty and needs a change every few thousand miles.

The truth is what your liver mainly does is convert the nutrition we get from our food into a form our body can actually use. It stores said nutrients until our body requires them. This is also why liver is such a nutritious food. So, to recap, your liver takes vitamins and minerals from your food and stores them. Then as your blood passes through the nutrition is released as needed. That bit right there is where the misconception comes that our livers can "store" toxins. HOWEVER, if the proverbial they would have taken a few more moments to read, they would have known that the liver has another really neat function.

That function is making sure any substance our body does not know how to process or does not need is turned into a harmless substance or - and here is the important bit - secreted into our digestive tract so we can (you guessed it) leave it behind in the toilet! Are there substances our liver can't handle? Absolutely! Is our liver ever dirty? No, not in the way that you imagine it to be, and honestly considering the cellular turnover rate our liver has you will do more damage attempting to clean it versus supporting its function for 150-500 days. Sure that number is wide, but it depends on the health of your liver to begin with. If you are a long term alcoholic and are not past the point of return according to your Dr, I'd say the 500+ days would be expected for full or best possible recovery from damage, but if you have no real liver issues that are known to you and you have just fallen for a detox fad, I'd day your liver is just fine and would be even better in the next 150 days if you drink Dandelion root tea daily!

While that may have seen like an odd ramble that did not have much to do with Dandelion, it actually gets me to how Dandelion is able to help you digest more nutrients from your food. Actually, she doesn't do that. I lied. What she does is support optimal liver function, and when your liver is really happy it does its job better, which is primarily to extract nutrients from food eaten and deliver it to your bloodstream. This is also why she is considered a blood builder and, by proxy, I suppose she is!

What exactly about her helped out my kidneys though? It's all about those sesquiterpenes lactones that really get us pissing. This is the main compound that all of the science-based folks believe acts as a natural diuretic. Beyond making our kidneys function optimally - which is what makes us really get to pissing - there is also a compound that is believed to act as a powerful anti-inflammatory, which takes us down the rabbit hole of how she acts as a pain reliever of sorts, both internally for sore muscles or breasts or internally from sore joints and non autoimmune arthritis!

Why didn't I mention rheumatoid arthritis there? Well, when we have an overactive immune system that is causing issues in our bodies, the last thing we want to do is give our immune system a boost, and that is exactly what our lovely lady dandelion does! How? Because she is an amazing source of vitamins and minerals, such as vitamin A (1,400 units per 100g), as well as lutein, beta-carotene, and a ton of potassium. She is also a source of fiber, iron, calcium, magnesium, phosphorus, thiamine and riboflavin. Oh and let's not forget sodium, vitamin C, vitamin D, and a shit ton of phytonutrients!

Vitamin A has a pretty big role in our immune system's function, as well as just about every other aspect of our body. It hunts damaging free radicals and kills them, fights inflammation off on a serious level, plays a critical role in brain function, skin, heart, kidneys, lungs, vision, and of course the health of our immune system.

Something I think is beautiful about most safe simple plant medicines that are also in the food realms is while yes, they do have specific compounds that do specific things in our body, so very much of it comes down to the deep nutrition that they offer us!

That list of vitamins and such in their natural state really marks so many things off of our "How does she do that?" list from above, and this combined with her somewhat unique to her and sometimes not compounds truly make her a little sunny miracle! I just felt like showing some deep appreciation to this savior of mine!

So beyond being bitter how is she helping our digestive tract? Inulin! What is that? Well to give a visual to at least a handful of ya have you made a tincture yet and got kinda worried when, for some reason, there is like a white residue at the bottom of the jar? I know more than a few of you have. This is probably one of the most common kinda panicked messages I get from folks, asking, "Did I do something wrong?" Inulin is basically a type of fiber found in MANY plants that our digestive enzymes can't digest.

Now that might sound like a bad thing, but it is actually a very good thing! In fact, our digestive health relies on inulin surviving our digestive enzymes! Why? So when this particular type of fiber reaches our lower digestive tract it acts as food for the good bacteria, and when they feast we thrive! This is why inulin is considered a prebiotic! Just to put a touch of importance on this, if you're taking probiotics but are not actively ingesting prebiotics you are basically wasting your hard earned money on those pills or effort on that homemade sauerkraut, because without good levels of inulin in your diet those little bugs you are eating are essentially starving to death!

Beyond that, the fact that she is an indigestible fiber means our digestive tract has an easier time eliminating waste and keeping things moving as they should, which is key for not only firming up loose stools, but for dealing with chronic constipation also! Of course inulin should not be the only source of fiber in your diet, but she is one that needs to be present for optimal health!

This type of fiber does something else though that's also pretty neat. If you are living with high blood sugar, insoluble fibers are a powerful tool against these issues! You see, indigestible fibers slow the uptake of sugars from your digestive tract, and in doing so result in more stable glucose levels. Then - because inulin is just this awesome - if you have high cholesterol it's going to lower your bad levels (low-density lipoprotein). Just because this tough little fiber keeps giving, it will also help reduce blood pressure and inflammation!

One real large problem any human who does not have regular access to food knows all too well once they do gain access is loss of appetite. You find yourself in a vicious cycle of being so hungry that your body gives up on sending hunger signals. You adapt to low blood sugar levels and then when you do eat you feel like shit, which only serves to make you at worst avoid food and at best eat the bare minimum to survive. This is something that is deadly for anyone, but as a tiny woman I suffer from this behavior rapidly. This is why Dandelion with her eudesmanolide levels are invaluable to me. This compound is proven to increase not only appetite but the signals that tell us we are hungry!

All of these things jabbered on above already make her a pretty powerful ally in the prevention and the battle against cancer so I don't feel like I need to dive crazy deep into that aspect, but her phenylpropanoids levels and the compound's ability to not only halt, but reverse the growth rate of tumors and cancerous masses is pretty astounding! This particular action seems to be most helpful for breast and prostate related cancers.

How crazy that this is all just the internal stuff she can do, huh? The same actions apply topically in most cases, making her ideal for dealing with skin conditions. Of course, I believe using her internally alongside of externally for angry skin is the best route to take because after all, our skin is usually a huge indicator that something within our body is not overly happy.

Maybe now you see why I think it is a symptom of mass disconnect to wage war on this ally that presents herself to us so freely, especially considering how many are suffering from these issues on a regular basis while they do all they can to kill the very plant that would offer them sincere relief!

Where Does Dandelion Grow?

I think it will be easier to talk about where she does not grow than where she does grow!

I'll do that, but first let me toss out a few places you can start the hunt, just in case! Your front yard, back yard, side yard, parents' yard, friend's yards, abandoned yards, parks, cemeteries, meadows, growing out of the tiniest cracks in the middle of a highway.

Almost anywhere her seed touches soil she will grow and multiply with her wish granting puffballs!

Actually, we need to create a new challenge called find a place in the world that Dandelion doesn't grow. So far there are records of her growing in the Antarctic, which is - just to put this into perspective - a solid landmass of ice. Oh, think maybe you won't find her in the other Arctic (North Pole)? You'd lose that bet because she's taken hold there, too!

She prefers rich moist soil, so maybe she would not be found in someplace like oh, I don't know, the Sahara desert? We just lost our last dollar because she is also found there, and in many deserts around the world (albeit different varieties)! Of course, this does not mean she will exactly thrive in these places, but what it does tell you is that if you happen to live in a more commonly survivable climate you, with a little bit of effort (or actually not much at all), will more than likely find some Dandelions growing near you.

When Should We Harvest Dandelion?

She is an all seasons lady really, especially if you live somewhere where deep freeze doesn't happen, but let's take a second to talk about which bits of her are best when.

Clearly springtime is bloom time, but it is also the best time to harvest leaves for eating, especially if you don't plan on cooking them! After this, she becomes very bitter and somewhat tougher. Now, I know come spring we are really eager to get to harvesting roots, but the truth is most roots that are dug in spring are empty of nutrients and most medicinal properties.

Why? Think about it this way: A root is a plant's "root cellar." This is the place she works hard most of the growing season, especially after seed has set to store up sugars, starches, minerals, and all of the healing compounds we are after so she can survive the winter. This is how roots survive cold temps and no sun! So when we dig a root in spring when the plant is just barely hanging on waiting for those first rays of sun we are digging something depleted up!

Also, with Dandelion specifically,the inulin levels skyrocket in fall, with a whopping 25% more than spring dug roots! I prefer to wait until the first gentle frost before I dig. This sends a signal to the plant to finish up and pull in anything she has been building up before a deep sleep. If you don't get frost just give it a week of cooler temps before you begin to dig.

There will be many folks who don't agree with me on this, and there are certain roots that I only dig in the spring as I want them to not be so potent, but for the most part I firmly believe that most root medicine is fall medicine, and should only be dug then to make the most of killing a plant by digging her roots.

What Cautions Should We Take With Dandelion?

While she is considered a safe food type plant ally, this does not mean she is safe for everyone! If you have a latex allergy it's pretty important to avoid her if you are not able to tolerate natural latexes, since the highest amounts will be found in the roots.

If you have an obstruction of the bile ducts, gallbladder empyema, ileus, or gallstones she may not be the ally for you.

Because she is a bit of a natural diuretic - this means you may piss out medication faster than your doctor intends - be sure to see if you can safely take diuretics alongside of any medications you may be taking.

There are also a few studies that show she does not play well with Lithium and tends to make the side effects somewhat worse.

How Much is Too Much?

It happens to the best of us. We drink that first cup of deliciously nutty and bitter roasted root tea with our creamer and we can't help but have another cup, and maybe just one more after that, and suddenly you feel a bit of a twinge and you need to get to the bathroom!

Yeah, this is because she does have the ability to make us go with her natural latex content. Also, if you are severely lacking bitter foods and/or inulin in your diet (found in a lot of plants), the results can be explosive if you drink too much too quickly.

I always recommend with the root to start off with a light brew and a small cup. As time goes on you can brew it thicker and drink more. After that, she usually won't do much more than stimulate your natural need to go, but that is a good thing.

.8.

Plantain Soothes the Burning, but Not the Fear.

I can't really explain the feeling of contentment that a fire on the beach, or anywhere for that matter, brought me when it was surrounded with like minded folks, other 'kids' that for uncountable reasons simply had to be free, even if that cost of freedom was daily suffering, damp feet, and the bramble bush hack we all got from breathing in that smoke.

It didn't matter because I was happy. I was also a very young traveller. Not many were out on the road at my age save for the lot kids with mom and dad's money to enrich their experience of being 'houseless', as so many liked to call it. My young age and even younger appearance was a blessing when I flew a sign for money that said 'I could be your daughter', but it was a curse when I was seen as a target for abuse in so many forms that, if I felt inclined, I could make this book thicker than the Bible and twice as heavy.

I was just sitting there laughing around with a group of kids that had invited me to their early morning fire for a breakfast of sand covered questionable hot dogs they had found left on a picnic table when, out of the blue, a man named Blue from Nebraska I had run into and was 'with' once more began to yell at me to get back to the tent. The whole group of kids just went quiet until one spoke up asking if I understood that I didn't have to go with him? In that second I remembered I indeed could just hop groups/people/paths whenever I goddamn wanted, and this guy who I had been dating for a few months now could go fuck himself.

In that same split second of realization, my arm was yanked out of my socket back towards the camp, as he ranted and raved that I was free to go, but he'd be taking my pack and all of the crystals in it to the Tucson mineral show with or without me. That pack and those stupid fucking rocks were my life, in a very literal sense. Without these few small things, my already hard life would be even harder. Barter was a large part of my existence, but that aside, crystals and the wire wrapped jewelry I turned them into made it possible for me to get a hotel room now and then. They made it possible to eat when flying signs was not possible or as profitable as needed, especially in this area where, like Eugene, the homeless population had worn out its welcome, and flying sings or even spare changing was no longer permitted within city limits.

So you better believe I got in the car. I remember seeing those giant trees finally slip away from sight as we headed towards Arizona, and for the first time in a long time being on the move did not make me feel safe, but saddened. He had it in his head that I could somehow sell my crystal collection at this vendor's show and buy double what I had, and that we would just keep flipping these crystals for profit along the rock and mineral show circuit like it was a fucking dead show and the rocks were grilled cheese or some shit.

It was all a blur of highways and shitty little towns where I flew signs for hours in the now increasing temperatures. It was realizing that anything in Southern California marked "National Forest" on the atlas was now million dollar homes behind million dollar gates. It was realizing anywhere we parked to sleep it was not long lived before we were chased off again and again. It was watching the green life of plant allies I was familiar with give way to the ever expanding death and dryness that is desert. Deserts never stop growing, I thought often. It was cold nights sleeping in a car while I laid wide awake in anxiety attacks, wishing I could go home. Wishing that I could escape this man. Pleas for help written on the windshield all steamed up from my rapid breaths for any stranger that may pass were wiped away as quickly as I wrote them. By this point, I knew that whoever may have 'saved' me could likely be who ends up killing me.

When you measure your travels by how much gas you have in your tank a simple two day drive can take weeks. We would get just enough gas money to go just enough miles, like some fucked up game of Spare Change Leapfrog. I suppose the upside of this is that I got to truly see any given state I was travelling through. All of the little towns and all of their people, for good or bad. I saw it all. Usually, there are entire groups of kids flying signs, although you may only see one when passing. We are either posted up at different key areas or taking turns, especially if the weather is harsh. This was not the case for me. This man's pride could only afford to have my face seen - my quickly burning, covered in sweat and likely desperation face, standing at corners holding up a piece of cardboard for hours with no luck, somewhere past L.A. I told him it was pointless in areas like this. Big cities and the people that reside in them have become numb to sights like me. This girl and her sign may as well be invisible.

There are of course exceptions to this invisibility. The ones who want to throw glass bottles always see you and the ones who feel like having a lot of money means they can pay to fuck you always see you. I saw them too. Seldom did the bottle hit me and I always saw the beamer coming, slowing its pace, $100 dollar bill hanging out the window from what seemed like a block away. He pulled up with a story locked and loaded in broken English. He was in the country for a business trip and his wife was very sick and he was very lonely. Somehow, in all of my glory, I reminded him of his daughter. She also had a wild and free spirit so he wanted to give me this money. You learn over the years to take the money but not engage. They almost never have the balls to outright say what they want when you are not clearly a prostitute. They want you to connect the dots on your own. To be so grateful or fucking awestruck by their wealth that you will get into their car as if money equals safety.

So when you take the money and quickly say thank you and disengage from their attempts, they can become one of two things - embarrassed and drive away, or enraged and entitled to your body. I had slipped away quickly into the store's parking lot, heading towards the car that contained the devil I knew. It must have taken this man a while to build up his rage, or maybe it just took him time to navigate traffic to get into the parking lot. Either way, he was livid when he almost hit me with his car. I'll never forget the smell of burning rubber from his hard braked tires on that hot, freshly laid, choke you asphalt. In a flash, my face was slammed into it. This man jumped out of his car and had me by the back of my hair, screaming "I PAID YOU GET IN THE CAR! I HAVE MORE MONEY!" with a fist full of cash waving in the other hand.

His shoes were so goddamn shiny the sun was blinding me with the reflection. It was such an odd thing to notice. His tie kept waving in front of the glaring light. As I grabbed the side of his leg I thought his suit was so soft it must have been silk, and probably cost more money than I had ever had in my entire life. I heard someone in the background say, "Ohhhh shit!!" and laugh. I thought a million and one things in those few moments until his tie brushed my face one last time and my hand, on its own damned accord, grabbed it and yanked. His face hit the car and he made a choking sound. The money he was waving hit the ground just as fast as I had moments earlier.

Suddenly I was in the car, a handful of money and Blue looking at me all wide eyed saying, "I was wondering how that was gana play out!" We now had a little over five hundred bucks and a straight road ahead. We drove all night, only stopping for gas and to indulge in fast food. By morning we rolled into Tucson and he was excited about the gem show. I was still in a state of dissociation from the shock I had endured, and nothing looked real to me.

So it was just fucking great when we rolled up to the address and there was no sight of anyone or anything. The show was in February. In that moment I collapsed internally. I could have stayed on that beach. He could have just taken this stupid bag full of rocks himself. I didn't have to have road rash all down the side of my face. I didn't get to feel sorry for myself for long, because it very loudly became my fault the show was not during the dates he expected. I remembered when we heard about it. We were sitting around outside a soup kitchen and some kid talked to us about it, just for a split second, and I had said something about how it would be cool to see all of those crystals in one place. I guess from that encounter I was supposed to be an expert on all things Rock and Gem Show.

It became pretty apparent that this was not a good place to be homeless. It was easily over a hundred and ten degrees Fahrenheit during the day, so I pulled out the atlas and began plotting a route. Anywhere greener, anywhere cooler. I just read the word 'Mountain' and my heart assumed it was like my mountains from home, that there would be pine trees and medicines. As we drove towards the national forest I imagined Mount Lemmon and what it was named after. There were indeed pine trees, but they were so few and far between at the base. It may have been considered a mountain in this place, but to me, it looked more like what we call foothills back home. I secretly hoped it would be as familiar as home so I could just walk off into the hills, leaving this man far behind.

But that would not be the case. Instead, I plunged headlong into the isolated desert lands that may as well have been another planet compared to my homeland. I remember being grateful as I looked at the map - at the very least there was a river. It was pitch dark as we arrived, and we hastily set up camp under some low hanging trees. I hoped they would shade us in the little draw I had chosen. The next morning I woke to the tent being shaken by a forest ranger, saying we could not camp there. I was utterly confused. It was a national forest and a free campsite. Half asleep, I was extremely defensive, spouting off all of the national forest rules. When I was done eating my foot he simply said, "That's great you know all of the rules, but you still can't camp in the river bed." The draw I had chosen was indeed a nice shady spot. It also happened to be the bone dry river bed. These stones may not have seen water in a millennium from the looks of them.

Dragging the tent out I heard the first rattle. You see, we also have that sound on our Mountain. I knew it better than the sound of my own voice. Rattlesnakes. I noted the ranger was wearing snake boots. I was in a pair of cut off filthy Dickies and sandals that had long fallen apart. I put our tent as far away from the rocks as possible, way out in the open so I could hopefully see any, should they come my way. A picnic table, a few extra lengths of tent poles, and a ratty tarp were the only makeshift shade we had. By the end of the day, Blue had begun to panic about needing money. Somehow we only had enough for one more tank of gas, and that wouldn't even get us out of the desert, he proclaimed. We had planned to head towards Colorado, to a regional Rainbow Gathering that was most certainly going on, and where I felt things would be okay. I was wrong.

I woke up the next morning just as the Sun was just creeping over the Mountain. The second I unzipped the tent to find Blue every muscle in my body tensed up. The car was gone. His stuff was gone. The water jugs where gone. I figured in a matter of days I would be gone from the heat, too. He left a note that said "Went looking for work. Will come back when I have money. Took the water and food because you know about plants." I could already feel the sun burning my skin and my mouth drying out as two things wandered through my head - my grandmother always told me if I left our mountains I would die, and how the fuck does me knowing about plant justify taking all the food and water? Like in his mind could I just transform the few plants around into water like some goddamn magical act of alchemy?

I sat there all day in that bright blue shade cast by the tarp, hopeful that the ranger would be coming back through. Hopeful that anyone would drive into the camping spot, but not a soul. Soon I was thirsty beyond ignoring and decided to search the campgrounds for a water spigot of any kind. The thought slowly crept in that it would not be the heat that claimed me but the damn snakes. Walking to the primitive restrooms off in the distance to check for water was like walking through the Valley of the Shadow of Death with an encore of rattles to welcome you to your end. As soon as you made it past one snake's warning you heard another. I have never walked the center of a path so perfectly in hopes of staying far enough away that they would not reach me with a strike, like a tight wire act that reeked of fear and adrenaline. I can't completely explain the terror these snakes put in me, and I believed it was the first time I felt bloodline trauma stir on a cellular level. You see, my Great Grandmother was bitten by a Rattlesnake. It reached her heart and killed her. My Grandfather was just a child and witnessed this happen to his mother all alone. Terror passes on.

There was no water at the glorified outhouse. There was no water at any of the campsites. There where only snakes. When I got back to my tent I saw, clear as day, the tracks of a snake that had crawled into my tent through a rip in the bug screen. The red dust covering everything that had made Blue freak out had saved my life, or at the very least prolonged it. I hit the tent with a stick I had been carrying and a fucking snake instantly struck the side of the tent, which means he was just chilling in there already coiled up. He could keep the tent. All I really wanted was my sleeping bag. The heat was not the only threat. At night the temps dropped very low, and when Blue took off with the car he took my pack. The only clothing I had was what I was wearing and it was not enough to keep me warm. With my long stick, I ripped a hole in the bottom screen as wide as it would go, hoping the snake would take the hint and exit, then laid on the picnic table whacking and shaking the tent with the stick, hoping the snake would runoff.

He didn't budge and the Sun had slipped below the Mountain. Curling up in the old ratty tarp that was once my shade, thinking if I die from a snake bite while wrapped up like a trash burrito at least the disposal of my body would be easy enough - already wrapped in a tarp and all. I woke up to the sound of Coyotes howling in the dead of the night and for a second I thought I was home, but it didn't take long for me to realize they didn't sound quite right and the air smelled different. Shivering, I looked up at the Mountain peak that blocked the expansive view of stars and decided if I was going to live through this someone would have to find me.

Someone did find me. It was barely dawn when, from what seemed like a mile away, I heard tires hit gravel. I instantly woke up thinking it must be Blue, but before long a huge luxury line RV pulled up. I'm talking about the kind that you see bands tour in. Jet black windows, sleek design, fancy gold scrolling - the only thing missing was a random band name painted on the side. I laid there for a few more hours as the morning sun brought heat and I played out a million possibilities in my head of what, who, and where these people were heading, and if I could make it onto that bus.

Like a magic trick, an automated awning came out of the bus, providing highly in demand shade. The door opened just as smoothly and out stepped a man who I looked exactly like fucking Santa Clause. I don't just mean fat with white hair and a beard. I mean this guy could have been the same damn actor that played on all of the old Coke commercials! I waited for more people to come out but he seemed to be alone.

He walked around placing caution cones on all four corners as if someone would miss this massive thing and run into it if the cones were not placed just so. He took out a big roll of green astroturf, a few lawn chairs, cooler, and a little barbeque then went back into his portable mansion. Hours passed.

That stupid fucking snake was still in my tent, and the slightest wind would blow my tarp shade over. I began a conversation with the snake. I asked him what his name was, if even though he needed the heat to digest food if it was ever too hot for him, if he had always been a carrier of bad medicine or if someone made him that way. What was his side of the story? Did he think when the guy came back out and started to cook he would give us some?

Eventually, I did not have the energy to keep putting the tarp back up and, although I knew it was dangerous, I hid under the picnic table in the shade. I kept hitting the tent with my stick sporadically now, making sure that the snake was still there versus coming to kill me. Just then I heard the door on the RV open. I did not move until I heard his footsteps getting closer. I popped out from under the table and saw the neon glow of a liter of mountain dew, dripping with condensation. My jaw ached with saliva just looking at it.

He said, in the most hilariously high pitched voice I ever heard for such a large man, "You look like you're a little thirsty. Had you dropped your pride and knocked on my door you could have had all of the food and drink you could imagine, but now to learn a lesson in humility you only get as much as you can drink by the time I count to five". I feel like I have to say this pretty often - it would be easy to imagine what you would or would not do in these situations, but the truth is the better off will always test the limits of what someone under them is willing to do for any amount of something they need.

He started to count as soon as the hiss rang out from the bottle being opened, and I opened my throat and squeezes the bottle. "...four...five..." knocked the bottle out of my hand, screamed "You cheated!", then stormed off with the bottle. It was fucking obvious now that I was stuck in the desert with the worse devil I didn't know. I could feel his anger like a pulse in that hot air, coming from the RV. I laid there again praying to the land, to my Creator, to the snake, to anyone that would listen to bring Blue or the ranger back to me.

I was once again wrapped up in my tarp, defenseless to anything but the sleeping snakes when the smell of smoke and lighter fluid woke me up. He had come out once more and was getting the barbeque going, spraying the lighter fluid bottle, making flame light up the whole area in an obvious attempt to get my attention. From what must have been a Mary Poppins cooler he pulled out endless amounts of sausages, burgers, steaks and I watched as he burnt them beyond edible until he had a whole serving platter full and approached me.

Yet again he blamed my pride for not knocking on his door and asking for food, but this time he said, "If you don't learn to ask me properly things will get much worse for you." It was a dominance thing, so I decided that the only way to win was to refuse to speak. He dumped the plate of burnt food behind his RV and took a few moments to kick dirt over it, thinking that because it was burnt and dirty I would never touch it.

I waited about two hours before dawn, then I went and dug up that pile of burnt meat. I was now not just suffering from extreme dehydration, but a hunger that even my well shrunk stomach could no longer ignore. He did not burn these things as bad as he had hoped, and I sat there until the sun came up eating the center out of anything that I could. When I heard the RV door open I ran up the hill and hid behind a rock. I heard him screaming with anger as soon as he discovered I had eaten the meat, and then a gun fired. At that moment I heard something more terrifying - a rattle that was too close to escape from. This huge rock had a large crack in it that made a perfect den for the snake, now coiled and at face level.

I have never at any other point in my life been able to meditate. My mind is simply not wired to not think. This does not always mean that my constant thinking, especially then, was well founded, but in that moment out of pure survival, my mind and body went quiet. The high pitched screaming from the man that I had "broken the deal" and the constant unloading of his clip all faded away. The only sound I heard was that rattle and my heart. With every slow and shallow breath I took she would sound off. Eventually, it became the rhythm of my heart - my breath and her warnings.

Moments of rhythm turning into hours. My skin searing under the sun, feeling cracks form in my lips as they rose with blisters. I heard her age in her deep and full rattle.

I opened my eyes.

The sun had slipped behind the mountain and at some point, the snake had either gone on her way or retreated further into her den. At that moment I felt the depth of my sunburn wrack my body with shock, and the man was now singing, "Come home little chicken." That was the song. Over and over, just those four lines, again and fucking again. Eventually, the heat gave way to freezing temps and I, in my delusional state, decided if I ran to the highway he would find me. I would have to run up a well marked hiking trail that spoke of what sounded like a lodge where humans might be.

As quietly as I possibly could I made my way to my tent, only to remember a snake had made it it's home. I grabbed my tarp and an empty water bottle and limped towards the trailhead when I heard him scream, "You're gana die up there and no one will care!" I didn't necessarily disagree with him but figured I'd rather have these strange lands finish me off than let him have the pleasure of making me beg to die, which was clearly the direction we were heading in.

I don't know how long I walked for or how many times I tripped and slammed into the rocky ground, but eventually, I had to stop or the next fall would be where I laid to die. The trial was following the dried out river bed, and fuck the ranger. I was gana sleep in the river bed and pray for a flash flood to claim me. It didn't.

To my surprise, I woke up. For the first time since this whole ordeal began, I was able to really look around. I wouldn't say that the desert is not brimming with life, just that I did not know this life - those trees, that weird looking lizard, or how these Poplar looking trees endured this lack of water. I do come from a desert, but high mountain desert is such a different world. It gets this hot and I can burn this bad, but it stays warmer in the evening and there is moisture filled life all around, even in the 120*F heat.

It didn't take long before my movement began to set off rattles all around me, and I wondered how in the world humans were able to come here. How were people not dropping dead every tourist season from a fucking snake bite? Suddenly I had an idea. I would cut some bark off of a tree to guard my legs. Then I remembered my knife was in my backpack.

So with the flattest, sharpest rock, I could find, I cut off sheets of bark. They naturally wanted to curve around my leg and went all the way up to my knees. I cut a part of my tarp into strips and used the strips to tie the bark in place.

I had made myself a pair of 'snake boots' out of a random - what I assume was poplar - tree's bark. I had even attached some over my sandals so my feet were not as exposed. It felt like a small victory, even if I looked like some backwoods version of the tin man.

I don't know how many miles I had walked up that trail since there were no markers like some trails have. I did know I had clearly climbed in elevation. I could smell the difference in the thinner air, and my lips were already so cracked that they began to bleed. The snakes did not seem to be as bad on this trail as there were below, that being the only solace I had.

I just wanted to sit down. I was dizzy and no longer sweating. The bark had dried out, making it hard to walk in and cutting my legs all up. The trail was rolling, meaning I went up a hill then down a hill, over and over. I remember thinking whoever cut this trail in was a real fucking asshole, and that they just wanted to extend the job they were paid to do. I suppose it was better to think about those things than the reality I was certainly walking to my death.

Soon I could not walk with the left leg bark on, so I tied it to my belt loop. Walking, walking, walking, flat out stepping on a coiled up baby rattlesnake. It gave no warning as it had no real rattle yet, stepping on it with the unshielded leg, it instantly bit into the bark on my still shielded leg. It stuck there, biting over and over again. I took that sharp rock I had used to cut the bark and cut off its head, then put the other leg shield back on and his still squirming body, that would now be food, into my pocket. That thing twitched for another solid fifteen minutes.

At the bottom of a dip in the trail, my senses exploded to the sight of fresh green growth and the smell of moisture. There was a spring just below the surface that was bubbling up into a little pool. I drank until I vomited and then I drank some more. There were so many plants I didn't know, but as I laid there in that cool oasis I honestly questioned was real I saw a shade of green in the distance that felt familiar. I crawled through those thick Willows to find a huge patch of Plantain Major thriving in the shade of this almost marshy land. I began to pick and eat the newest growth and it made my jaw hurt so bad from salivating that I screamed out. Quickly I realized tiny mosquitoes inhabited this place, and they were as excited about me as I was about finding water. I made my way back to the water and curled my severely burnt body that needed very real medical attention in that cool pool of water and just cried.

After about an hour I pulled myself up and began making mud to smear on my skin, in the hopes it would fend off the mosquitoes so I could truly get at that plantain. I cut a big piece out of the ragged tarp to carry the leaves I would harvest. The mud gave some semblance of protection from the millions of mosquitoes swarming my body as I frantically ripped and pulled at those leaves, shoving them in my mouth and filling the tarp. Back at the spring I sat there choking down stringy plantain and smashing it up with a bit of water, trying to cover my shoulders - they were the worst off all - hoping for any relief, and to maybe ward off infection since I had decided to put desert mud that does not decay into the burns. As the sun went down I started a small fire with the lighter I had in my pocket and cooked that snake on a stick. There's no good way to eat a snake, and I personally believe it should only be done for the sake of survival. I still have his little vertebrae as a reminder.

That entire night I dreamt of horrible, dark things that lived in those hills and that the snakes worked to push you down certain paths so they could swallow you up in their caves.

In my dream, I was caught watching these things and was chased up the mountain to my death, where I saw them eat the marrow of my bones. I woke up with a gasp and a pounding heart. I have never been one to discount the importance of dream messages, and firmly believe eating that baby snake all wild with venom, on top of not eating or drinking for days, allowed me to glimpse something I was not supposed to know about.

I sat there all that day, thinking on the man that abandoned me, the man that chased me up a mountain, the snake that stole my tent, the one that allowed my mind to go quiet, and the baby that died to give me the dream that still shakes me.

As hydration set in and food of a sort hit my digestive tract I realized there was no survival in front of me, and the only way out was to hope that someone may see me on the highway. I could only pray that that someone would not be a bat shit fucking crazy Santa Clause. I took some willow branches and fashioned the tarp into a sort of umbrella, filled an empty pop bottle found on the trail, tied up the plantain in the other bit of tarp, put on the peeled bark I had soaked in water to soften up again, and headed back down to the campsite.

Slowly making my way back towards that uncertainty I could smell smoke. Although my fire had been long dead, I second guessed myself and was worried I had set the fucking Mountian on fire. Worried, with all of my lifelong luck, of being chased by flames, I walked a little faster. A snake raced out in front of me and I took a step backwards. The whole way down the trail I had just walked the day before was covered in snakes.

Soon enough I made it back to the campground. The RV was long gone, but sure as fuck there was Blue, posted up with, I shit you not, a whole encampment of teenage boy scouts working on getting their Eagle badges. He's just sitting there, clearly spun out of his damn mind on dope pretending to eat pancakes, like it was no big deal he just left me in the fucking desert with no food or water, or that the tent was here but I was nowhere to be seen.

Here I am covered in mud, burnt to death, decorated in bits of tree bark and blue tarp, and he, with no concern whatsoever, said, "I've been waiting here for almost half a goddamn hour. You're lucky I didn't leave you!" The boy scouts, who were all years older than me, had concerns and were out there to learn about desert survival. Their scout leader took me into their RV allowed me to shower and found clothing that would fit me. He offered to take me to the emergency room, but my fear of not having a way out of the state consumed me. He did, for "educational sake", talk me into allowing him to set up an IV he had. It probably saved me more than I realized.

Food was eaten, and plantain was mashed with the aloe gel they had gifted me. Here is the part where you're hoping for the inspirational bit of the story - that moment when I realized he too was a snake or the monster from my dreams that was draining my marrow.

That I had learned some amazing survival skills or that I didn't get back in the car with him. But those of us who have lived in abusive situations know how easy it is to rationalize away our own need for safety and to justify just about anything done to us. We also know distressed teenagers don't make the best choices in any situation.

It took me another year, a horrendous miscarriage, almost freezing to death in Nebraska and a very long, cheap, kicked-down, cocaine fueled train ride to escape this man. I hold no shame about it.

.9.

Plantain
Plantago major

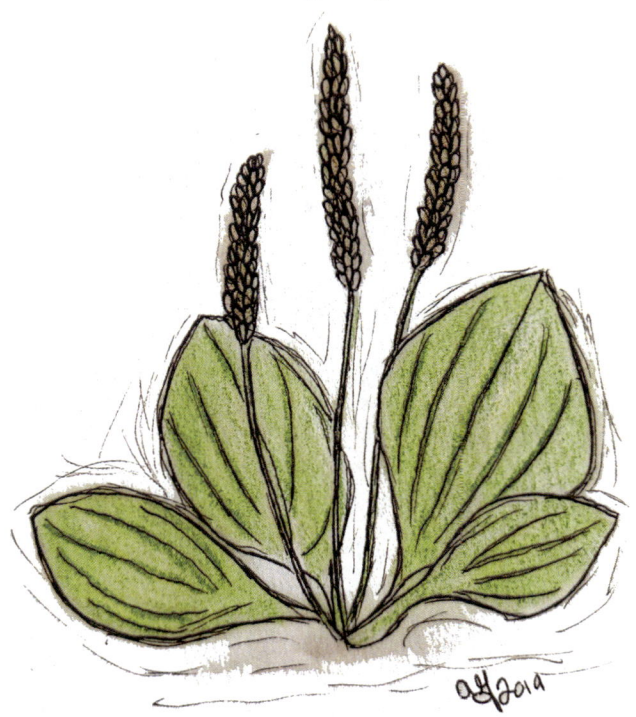

That story could have continued with a few more weeks of healing from such severe burns, and how utterly amazing that Plantain was at healing my burns. How for the next few weeks I hunted down more and more patches once we hit the Colorado state line. How it not only healed my burns, but left little to no scarring.

I mean, I should have sought medical attention. My severely deep blisters should have become brutally infected, especially when you consider I was lucky to shower once a week if even that. I should have called the cops about the murderous Santa Claus. I should have abandoned Blue at the gathering.

We 'can', 'could have', and 'should have' ourselves all we want and it won't change a damn thing.

Plantain became yet another savior for my Searching-For-Pain teenage self, and she remains a steadfast friend to this day. This is why I think you should look up to this plant that you so very often walk upon!

The History of Plantain:

Before we jump in any further let me clarify in case you skipped ahead to read this chapter. I am talking about a plant that grows low to the ground commonly referred to as Plantain, not a certain variety of banana that is also called Plantain! While rubbing a banana peel all over your skin probably won't kill you that is not what I'm suggesting you do, ha ha!

We can start there though, huh? With her name, or I should say her many names, like Ripple Grass, Waybread, Slan-lus, Waybroad, Snakeweed, Cuckoo's Bread, Englishman's Foot, and White Man's Foot, just to name a few.

The last two names on the list truly speak to her ability to spread far and wide. She was seen as a symbol of English colonization, and she LOVES to grow alongside people, no matter what land she ends up in. I am at the same time always amazed and yet not surprised when I am deep back in the cuts far away from roads or trails and I find a healthy little patch of narrow leaf plantain growing happily!

She has been used by mankind for thousands of years, not just for her medicinal values but as a pot herb too! That is to say, she is the type of plant that was commonly tossed into soups and she was often used as a natural thickener.

Her native ranges cover just about every western European continent, and many regions in Asia. She was once regarded as a sacred medicine by most of these cultures because of her sincere ability to feed and heal at the same time.

She was considered such a blessing to travelers in Russia that her seeds were often sewn along trials as prayers for safety. There are even accounts of her in the *Lacgunga,* a 10th century Anglo-Saxon herbal anthology, so it's not too shocking that when colonization of North America took place she was brought along for the journey.

I would dare to say that in those times she was more deeply understood as the powerful soother that she is, because when you have that close of a food based relationship with a plant ally... well, I suppose it's much like the difference between a lover and a friend.

These deep relationships even made their way into the theater, as love for her endured and she was seen worthy of a place in not only one but two Shakespeare pieces, Love's Labour's Lost and in Romeo and Juliet. Of course, her roles in those and many other pieces had quite less pain behind them compared to the story I have told here!

I have no doubt that this enduring ally that can take more walking upon than most will continue to weave her way through human history and beyond!

The Many Uses of Plantain:

So while I am sure some reading this know that Plantain is a great ally for bug bites, stings, rashes, and calming down pissed off skin issues such as eczema and psoriasis,having a deeper relationship will grant you so much more healing from this giving lady!

Do you have a nasty cough? Sore throat? Need to hack some crap out of your lungs?

Maybe you have chronic diarrhea? No? How about chronic constipation?

Hows that tummy doing? Heartburn? Sour stomach? Low stomach acid? Ulcers?

Got water retention and really need to get to pissing? Kidney's acting up?

How's that liver doing? Bleeding more than you should?

What about sincere inflammation or even cancer?

It's pretty clear that this walked upon lady has so much more to offer than folks assume!

How Can Plantain Do So Much For Us?

It really comes down to a few little compounds that, when combined as a whole, make her so capable.

Catalpol, iridoid glycosides, aucubin, apigenin, baicalein, asperuloside, flavonoids, mucilage , tannins , phenolic acids, saponins and flavonoids.

That's quite a list, and while we won't cover all of it for the sake of redundancy, the main actions of said list are anti-inflammatory, antioxidant, antineoplastic, hepatoprotective, hemostatic, antispasmodic, antiviral, vulnerary, expectorant, diuretic, demulcent, astringent, antiseptic, and alternative.

Her anti-inflammatory abilities are without a single doubt what calmed down my serious sunburn. Beyond that this action is what makes her so ideal for an array of inflamed issues, and while we could just leave it at that her ability to calm down inflammation on a deep level is worth having a chat about!

Okay, so when you think about inflammation what comes to mind? An infected wound? Swollen ankle? Maybe arthritis? What if I told you (I think I may already have, I don't know, it's a long book.) that a majority of studies conclude that most disease is caused by, or at the very least deeply fueled by...you guessed it, inflammation. Sure, this makes her amazing for healing up most skin conditions that are really problematic such as eczema and psoriasis, but I think folks are really overlooking her ability to combat some serious diseases when used internally, especially those related to our digestive tract.

What I should mention - but won't go crazy deep into - is that Plantain, just like Comfrey, has a lot of mucilage to her. Remember, that means she's a good kind of slimy that not only coats our stomach and intestines, but acts as a band-aid of sorts, protecting our inflamed linings from whatever may be doing the inflaming. The only reason I'm not going into this aspect, even though it's an important factor, is I deeply covered the amazing ability of these slimy plant aspects when we learned about Comfrey.

Anyhow her slimy nature combined with her anti-inflammatory nature is what makes Plantain ideal for coping with sore throats, burning stomachs, ulcers and, to an extent, constipation. The part that many folks may not put together is her ability to move beyond our digestive tract and into the battle against inflammation. The Catalpol in her is a type of iridoid, which is a sciencey word for a compound found in plants that is giving pharmaceutical anti-inflammatory meds - such as Ibuprofen and other similar classed drugs - a real hard run for their money in the battle against inflammation that doesn't end up giving us all sorts of side effects from long term use.

Well actually, there are some side effects from using Plantain as an anti-inflammatory, but I don't think you'll mind one bit! A really big one is that she inhibits oxidative stress on a cellular structure. What the hell is oxidative stress?

In a super tiny nutshell, oxidative stress is when your system is all out of whack from an imbalance between free radicals and antioxidants in your body. Free radicals are not always the enemies folks would have you believe them to be. In fact, free radicals are a good thing to an extent as they help fight off pathogens (infections) and such. However, when they run a damn muck in our body and outnumber our antioxidant levels, some serious things begin to happen, such as...wana take a wild guess? Inflammation.

I really love how all of these things that do one thing link us into another thing. How if you stand back and look at a plant, a situation, how a body functions, and finally how they react when joined, you get this big beautiful picture of a whole symbiotic relationship. This random segway is gana throw us into talking about what else oxidative stress does, and I'm pretty sure it won't take you long to see where I am going with this.

So let's talk about the fact that oxidative stress can cause cellular damage at a genetic level, and what do damaged and or mutated cells have the ability to turn into?

Cancer.

So this tosses us down the path of how Plantain also acts as an antineoplastic, which in regular human words means to inhibit, prevent, and or halt the growth of tumors, cancerous or otherwise. Let's just take a moment to absorb that singular sentence and how massive that it. There's this plant that's basically so safe it's a food, and it is taking over lawns, gardens, abandoned lots, dirt roads and beyond, and it has the literal ability to stop the growth of cancer.

Now there is a fair amount of debate as to which part of her has the most potency in this matter, and I always kinda laugh as folks declare it's her seeds, or her leaves, or her roots. Why are we looking at her as something to be separated when all of her parts are capable? It's a symptom of breaking things down for drug-like reactions versus seeing a plant (human) as a whole and valid just as they are. Not to say that there aren't specific parts of Plantain or any other plant ally that don't have the capability to do different things. It can just be a damaging mindset to hold when attempting to work with safe simple healing, as it edges us into that "herbaceutical" mindset.

Okay, so we've kinda talked on some serious things there, right? Seems like there's not much left to jabber about beyond the fact that some folks shit too much and others not enough. But these are pretty serious things too when you consider our digestive tract is the front line in nourishing our bodies, and when it's not doing so great we're usually suffering a good bit aren't we?

Here's a random fact for your enjoyment. Did you know that the main ingredient in most dietary fiber supplements is psyllium, which is derived from the seeds of *Plantago ovato*? That's because her seeds, and the seeds of any Plantain, are an excellent source of fiber, and fiber is key to a healthy digestive system. Fiber can slow down loose stools and loosen up hard ones. Add this to the fact that Plantain has those slimy aspects and the ability to soothe sincere inflammation and she is an ally anyone suffering from IBS, Chrones, ulcerative colitis or chronic constipation should truly consider as a nourishing herbal infusion or even added to your soups and such. Of course, you won't get any fiber from drinking an infusion of her, but the healing aspects will be extremely available.

Beyond fiber, she has another ability that really does go hand in hand for digestive issues. That's her natural ability to act as an antispasmodic. Ya know when you suddenly get a cramp in your lower "stomach"? This is actually your intestines. The stomach is just below your ribs. Most of the time that sudden pain is from literal spasming or twitching. This can lead to real issues, such as chronic diarrhea and severe pain. Basically with things like IBS, if you're not addressing the spasming you're missing out on a whole area that needs to be tended to. I mean, that all sounds great, but what is actually going on the dries up loose stools? Sure, fiber is good for acting as a binding agent and no more spasms can really help, but it's her tannins that pull it all together. Tannins basically dry up excess moisture and tighten up loose situations.

So we know she's capable of some pretty serious relief, but how did she prevent my severe burns from becoming infected while I was homeless level dirty? Well, aucubin is yet another type of iridoid (yeah, there are different kinds) and this one in particular does a neat little trick once she makes her way into or bodies or onto an open wound. Once metabolized she becomes a powerful antibacterial compound called aucubigenin. How potent? I'm talking potent enough to outright slaughter some heavy hitting bacteria such as Salmonella typhi, Salmonella paratyphi, Shigella dysenteriae, and Staphylococcus aureus. Recognize that last one a bit? Yep, that says Staph. If I was gana catch a life ending infection in that desert it would likely be Staph because the dry hot conditions actually prevent animal fecal matter from decaying and turning into soil. It just turns to dust, but is still actively shit! That's why way back in the day folks who became even moderately injured in the desert didn't really have great survival rates!

So talking about the desert made me think about those poor humans who end up having to drink their piss out of desperation. That took a hard left turn, didn't it? Ehhh, it got my mind to the next bit I'd like to jabber about - how, as a diuretic, Plantain likes to support kidney function and really get us pissing. Of course, just like those folks in the desert who are dangerously dehydrated, if you're not taking in fluid to replace the fluid you putting out you won't be doing your kidneys any favors! This makes her a great ally though for anyone who suffers from hot UTIs, because with her slimy bits, antibacterial bits, and ability to make you piss, you can really push out the bacteria and soothe the inflammation.

This brings me to another organ that you really want to be functioning optimally, and that is the liver. You've probably already heard me talk on how the liver is not a car filter, your body is not dirty, and detoxing is dangerous, so I won't go into it beyond that, but those good ol catapol levels and their natural hepatoprotective actions would love to protect your liver. You see that's pretty much what hepatoprotective means - a substance the literally protects your liver from damage, but this also means that she supports optimum function which in turn makes her a blood building ally.

While we are on the topic of blood, let's break down her hemostatic abilities. Now for whatever trauma laced reason, I'd like to let you know that human blood freaks me out. It's not the sight of it, it's thinking about it. I'm fully aware of how quirky that is. I bring that up because I am glossing over this section a tad because of it. Deep breath, and here we go! Basically hemostatic means that she has the ability to prevent hemorrhaging, so while honestly she's not the first ally I reach for to stop bleeding if she was nearby, I'd not put my nose up by any means. While she has this ability externally, she also acts as a hemostatic internally, but that's more to due with her really great vitamin K levels. This also has a big role in her being a blood builder. I mean, keeping it 'thick' and in your body is a good qualifier as a blood builder, I'd say!

Yep, that did it. My skin is fully crawling, but it is such an important aspect to know about this incredibly soothing and underestimated plant ally. The next time you're chewing some up to spit onto that bee sting or mosquito bite, take a moment to really be amazed by what this truly enduring little plant ally is fully capable of!

Where Does Plantain Grow?

While she is a native inhabitant of a vast majority of European and Asian countries, she has become naturalized to just about every other temperate landmass in the world. In fact, if you live anywhere in the Americas, whether far north into Canada or way down south into Mexico, you will find one variety or another growing. Speaking of different varieties, there are over 200 different ones, and while a large number of them are considered medicinal, the most common varieties used over time are broadleaf plantain *(Plantago major)* and narrow leaf plantain *(Plantago lanceolata)*.

One of the reasons she was called White Man's Foot, beyond the obvious colonization/invasive plant connection, is that she LOVES to grow along well worn paths. I often wonder if this is due to the connection of her being sewn for protection by many cultural beliefs, and she simply continues that tradition. Maybe she was so heavily planted and humans tend to walk the same paths for time immemorial until pavement is put down, so she is just there. Actually, she doesn't care about your pavement because she can still exist in the cracks!

There I go, lying again. I know exactly how she spreads along paths but sometimes it's nice to think of things like that. Truthfully, her seeds are so tiny the wind easily blows them, and since foot paths are often blessedly free from obstacles the seeds and the wind take the paths of least resistance. Beyond that, when she gets wet her slimy nature turns into a sticky nature and clings to any passing animal feet, including our own. Some birds eat her too, but if I had to guess that's probably not the top way her seeds are spread compared to wind and feet.

Alright, back to where you will find her. The first place you can look is any and all grass that may be growing near you. Of course, you will find her on footpaths, but I'd not gather from there if you can venture off of those paths and see if a nice patch has established a safe distance away.

She really will grow in just about any soil type there is, excluding severely alkaline soil, but then again ya never know! I've seen her in the scorching desert of Arizona all the way to an

8,0000-foot elevation mountaintop where there are maybe two months of warmth on a good summer!

Really though, finding Plantain is just about as easy as finding your own feet. Just keep looking down in that direction and soon enough she will be underfoot!

When Should We Harvest Plantain?

This is one of those situations where it truly depends on not only what you're wanting to do with her, but what climate you live in. She doesn't really go dormant unless you get a good amount of snowfall, and even then I have gone out after a warm Chinook wind in February and harvested her from patches of melted ground. For the sake of adding her to your food spring is best. If you're feeling fancy and intend to use her roots (this will kill her fully), fall would be my choice to dig.

As far as gathering her leaves for the sake of making nourishing herbal infusions, before she sets all of her energy into making seeds would be ideal, but after that she's still perfectly fine for making an infused oil or the like. To gather her seeds you will want to wait until they are fully mature. This is pretty easy to figure on, just run your hand up her seed stock and if a bazillion seeds fall into your hands she's ready!

What Cautions Should We Take?

While she is safe and considered a food, like with any herb are precautions to consider. For instance, if you are on medication to keep your blood thin using an herbal ally that thickens your blood is not a great idea, assuming you want your medication to do its job. The same goes if you have a disorder that causes you to clot too much.

Remember how she's great at lining the stomach with her slimy nature? I mean, she is REALLY good at doing this, which means at times she can even prevent the absorption of certain medications, such as lithium and some heart medications.

Also, because she is a natural diuretic (makes you piss), if you're on a prescription diuretic that might lead to far too much pissing, and you could end up potassium deficient.

Last but not least, she's great for stimulating digestion, which means if you suffer from over productive stomach acid she may or may not make it worse. I have seen it go both ways.

How Much is Too Much?

All things in moderation until your body is used to her and she is used to you. That really needs to be the rule for any plant ally, honestly.

Most plant allies that have high levels of mucilage tend to have the same effect if you go a bit too quickly. What is it, you wonder? Well, you're gana spend some time in the bathroom as she empties out your colon! Although this usually takes a good amount and a system that is not used to much roughage before it happens. All bodies are different.

It usually doesn't happen more than once, maybe twice before your body adjusts, and while I don't think your body is dirty (because it isn't), I'd rather have you shit too much from Plantain than do a coffee enema any day of the week!

.10.

Elderberry Keeps the Flu at Bay, but Not the Human who Carries the Virus.

I have been hit by plenty of men, plenty of women too. I have been spat on, both physically and verbally. I have scars, weaker bones, and cynical eyes to go along with many stories of what-in-the-actual-fuck situations. But not a one of them, not a single moment of all of the moments, has ever been as long term damaging to me as gaslighting has been. Being told what I know deep in my bones is not true, being told what I see with my own eyes did not happen, being told what I heard with my own ears was not heard. Eventually, you cannot trust the very words that come out of your mouth. Did I say that? Didn't I? Am I actually hungry? Am I actually sick? Do I actually know anything?

I had been uniquely groomed for years to accept abuse from humans. I questioned if they were actually abusing me. Can I really trust what I think I know is happening? I don't even know how to start this part of the story, as it spans so many years and encounters. I could begin when I was ten and I first heard the music playing from the upstairs apartment next door. I could begin when I was twelve, heading upriver in your shitty boat of a car for the hundredth time. Just trying to decide brings me back to the chronic indecisions a deeply gaslit person has to live with.

It was such a long and lonely pregnancy I was forced to endure, not knowing I didn't need my mother's permission to have an abortion. At least I had my best friend "K" by my side throughout those long, hot months. We were inseparable, so much so that on the rez the long standing joke was that "K" was the one who knocked me up. I must have read those Ina May books a hundred times preparing for this birth, but nothing prepares a teenage girl for a shitty OBGYN deserving of a lawsuit and a 10 pound baby. But this is not a story about the birth of my first child, nor my best friend.

Once the baby is born it's not that fun to hang out anymore - when I am laying there for two months recovering from the over two hundred stitches caused by my vaginal birth because that bitch used suction against my will on a full head of hair, or when I am laying there unshowered for days with sincere postpartum depression. I don't blame him for not wanting to witness that at seventeen. I sure as fuck didn't want to witness it. I was alone in that basement. My baby hated me, bonding to my mother as she fed him my breast milk and I rotted away of no further use. I could talk about all of the times I tried to hit the highway and never made it more than a few hundred miles before I came running back to that 24/7 screaming kid, or I could talk about the sheer torture that is unchecked anxiety, afraid to stay and afraid to go - in some perpetual Hell.

I would walk all over town, going no place, in particular, I walked past houses where friends once lived, where parties once happened, where people once knew my name, just hoping to catch a glimpse of my old life, even if it was all haunted by traumas. Crossing those tracks I immediately recognized the way you walked, and it made my heart beat out of my chest. At the time I believed you to have been my first love. For years (as a literal child) you were the only human I thought about (you kissed me), dreamed about (you touched me), did everything in my waking power to be with, in any way possible (you kept me close by). So much so, that when you left me without even saying goodbye my conditioned brain could not handle it and it made up a story that you had died so I could cope. This fed your ego - utter worship on a level I'm sure to this day you still don't fully understand - having a "woman" live for your very existence, let alone one that seemed so much older and could keep up with the drinking and smoking, but young enough to bend to your will so easily when no one was looking.

So I suppose when you saw me, grown, with breasts larger from having been full of milk and a lonely look in my eyes, there was no doubt in your mind that I was finally good enough, truly malleable enough to be yours publicly. I can't even remember the entire conversation, beyond that you were back from Arizona, now a 'certified shamanic healer and herbalist', and you forgave me. What I do recall vividly is the awkward sex that night, as your crooked dick, pierced and uncircumcised, hurt like hell, and when I told you so you said, "No, you are not in pain. You just need to relax and fully accept the experience." At that moment I slipped right back into being the ten year old girl who was so well groomed versus the outspoken, go fuck yourself teenager who had lived through and seen bigger monsters than you coming from a mile away. I was yours to manipulate at will, and you damn well knew it.

Weeks, maybe months went by. I was paying $100 a month cash and all of my food stamp card, meant to support my child, for us to sleep on the floor of your friend's cockroach infested apartment. You had fully separated me from my son at this point while making sure I still felt the guilt of not being able to be a good parent - like you would be whenever you actually found someone worthy to have a child with. I swallowed it hook, line, and sinker, all the way to the very bottom of my soul. I had been working at an elderly home - one of the longest taxable jobs I had ever held down. The pay was less than $7.00 an hour and the kitchen was so dam crowded that I perpetually slammed my hip bone into the fucking stainless steel counters that matched my hip height perfectly. Who would have thought such a small thing would give you the final tool you needed?

It must have been three in the morning when I woke up screaming. Terrified, I instantly recalled when I was younger and had OD'd, but that was not happening. It was my hip, likely a combination of it still closing back together after birth six months back and slamming it over and over into the fucking countertops. Suddenly the roommates were standing there, very angry I had woken them, and he was pulling out his bag of herbs to rub some arnica gel on my hip. The woman had offered me a vicodin, which was way more realistic than store bought arnica for this level of pain, and he loudly said, "NO! She needs to feel this pain so she can accept the responsibility!", never making it clear exactly what fucking responsibility I was supposed to be finding in the pain that now had me vomiting.

By early morning the pain had finally subsided to a dull ache. He gently stroked my hair, proclaiming me healed by his hands that mere hours back rubbed a small amount of arnica gel on me, and that to show my gratitude I should have uncomfortable sex for the last hour before work instead of sleeping. I should be grateful for that too, as orgasms release pain relieving endorphins, even if it's just the man who cums. That's what his scientific data being rattled off anyhow. While I was pregnant with my son I hustled my ass off to buy this big ol' one ton chevy conversion van, even though, having spent my whole life hitchhiking, I didn't really know how to drive. In my mind, it would be a home for me and the baby as soon as I learned how. Like it was any other morning, he dropped me off at work. I had not slept, I had not eaten, and I was never wet when he was fucking me, so I was sore.

I was mixing up a two gallon batch of ranch dressing and trying not to vomit from the sheer volume of mayonnaise involved when I looked up and saw a stray bottle of Cayenne powder. I set out to make a simple paste to put on my hip with olive oil and the powder, as I had seen my grandmother use hot peppers this way in the past. I held it in place with saran wrap wrapped around my waste. It burned slightly, but it was not long before my hip didn't hurt at all. I was so damn ecstatic I thought on it all day, and could not wait to tell him when he picked me up in the evening. You see, the one thing I delusionally believed we had in common, something that bonded us, was our love for plants and helping others heal. That big bag of herbs he carried around called me in like a moth to a flame, but those moths always get burnt up, don't they?

I hopped in that van so full of energy, pulling that hundred pound door shut with ease and telling him all about the paste I had made - how I bet if we got some beeswax it would make a good salve and I could have it on hand if my hip acts up again, and that my grandma used to make a salve that was bright red and it was the best stuff in the world and I wondered if I could one day get her recipe book. My mind was going a million miles an hour with pure wonderment until I realized he was as quiet as the dead. I stopped talking, knowing I was not giving him time to answer back with what surely would be shared excitement. His reply was so calmly spoken that it had to be the truth. He had to be right, I thought. I could have hurt myself. I don't know what I am doing. My grandmother probably did hurt a lot of people by pretending to know what she was doing. Maybe I do need to go to an herbalist school like he did because I really could have hurt myself, right?

Months went by and it became apparent that all I knew was just a delusion. He made it apparent that I, in fact, knew nothing. My anxiety was to a level that I can't explain. For months now he was demanding sex two to three times a day, and there was something wrong with me for not enjoying it. Somehow marriage had come up, and I sewed a wedding dress by hand out of patchwork, lace & brain tanned buckskin while we set off, in my van, to the 2003 National Rainbow Gathering in California. I was so excited to be going to what was home to me. These people! I knew every kitchen's name that would be set up. I knew where we should avoid. I even knew where to hang out if we wanted to eat meat while we were there!

It was so hot out for the end of June as we drove through the desert wastelands of Southeastern Oregon. The van began overheating so we blasted the heater on high. I became dizzy, clearly on the verge of heatstroke. "No, you're just having an anxiety attack." Oh, I guess I am having an anxiety attack. We slept in the desert and I woke in the morning to horrendous pain, and what looked like blood in my piss. I knew it was a kidney infection like I thought I knew the back of my hand. "No, you're still just having an anxiety attack, so your body is tense." Miles went by with the heat blasting, drinking warm, green, off-brand gatorade so thick it felt like cough syrup, each drink him insisting I take. I don't really recall how it happened since I was going in and out of consciousness, but suddenly I was in a little hospital. He was telling them I was having an anxiety attack, and I saw them put something in my IV, which I now know was lorazepam.

The nurses didn't even question this man with a tiny girl carried in unconscious. They just drugged me at his request.

I was floating down that highway now, thinking about iced Dandelion tea and how good it would taste right then, especially if it had sweet cream in it. I honestly believed it was my subconscious, screaming for the medicine it knew my kidneys needed. But I was just having an anxiety attack, what did I know? Suddenly the radiator blew its cap, and he decided we better drive home before the van broke down for good. I was so overjoyed at this decision, but sad too. I truly wanted to go home, but not to the home we were heading to. Not the home where I knew nothing, where I was a failure, a horrible mother, and so broken that I didn't enjoy having sex three times a day like every other woman did, I was assured.

So when we realized a different van full of mutual friends were heading down we jumped at the chance. Before leaving he had presented me with his verbal findings - that gluten was likely the cause of my anxiety attacks. In 2003 Eastern Oregon, which is deep wheat country, gluten free was not heard of, or even really a thing. I was hungry again like in my early teen years, but this time it was different since there was plenty of food in the van, but none of it was gluten free. The whole ride down I was lost in the laughter of life long friends, one being my sister's boyfriend at the time and who has always been a brother to me. We rolled up to the gathering, driving past the federal agents and forest service right into A camp as usual. I had followed these events across the country and back, but I could tell right away this would not be home as I remembered it.

Nonetheless, being around these people sparked me to remember, created a ripple under my skin, and I began to question. Not only was this man I was with full of shit, he full-on embarrassed me at every turn of the trail. We had a Rainbow Gathering wedding as friends and strangers danced around us, trapping us in a never ending fucking drum circle in the horrendous heat. At that point, I, without a doubt, was having an internal anxiety attack. Sometime after it was all said and done I went for a walk on my lonesome, looking for friends from a different life, familiar faces from some highway, some soup kitchen, something. I saw my son's biological father, who I had not seen since he got me pregnant. I didn't have the courage to approach him and give him the photo of his curly haired son, who was now crawling like a pro.

Trade Circle was spread out along a long trail instead of a circle. The monks were not in attendance to serve food at noon out of those huge cauldrons. The kitchens were at literal war, poisoning each other's food with dog shit. The land was being trashed beyond repair. There where more Weekend Warriors, high as balls on God knows what, than I had ever seen at a National. There had been four rapes in the two days we had been there. A child molester got his head beat in with a rock a few hundred yards from me. And now, out of the blue, the man I had just Rainbow married decided to take a shit, freestyle right next to a kitchen in front of everyone. As they all screamed at him, "DON'T SHIT THERE, MAN!!" I walked off into the trees towards the sound of running water.

I thought about my son, and about the Catnip plant, I saw that someone else had shit on top of. I thought about my anxiety attacks. I thought about how fake it all is, these people are, how I can't believe I was having to learn this lesson again, what I had gotten myself into again, about the sex I didn't want to have that night, or any other night really. An old woman came across me sitting there. She was easily in her late seventies, with long beautiful silver hair, and she asked me sternly, with a very familiar backwoods drawl, what was eating at me. I told her I didn't think any of this was right, but I just didn't know. She laughed and said, "Oh, you damn well know girl, it's just time you remembered." as she handed me a joint and went on her way. I don't think she could have fathomed how much of an impact her words would have on me later in life, once I finally woke up.

The time had come to head home, and I did not want to leave. I knew the real gathering began after the 4th of July was over and all of the college kids leave. Then the real die-hard family shows up for weeks of clean up. Maybe I could head to a Regional after this and come back home in a few months. He quickly crushed any self confidence or remembering I had done. I would, as usual, be a piece of shit for abandoning my son, lose my job, and besides, I would absolutely have an anxiety attack on the highway and have no one to help me. So I got in the van.

Not too long after getting back, he got a job at a local farm and we moved into a small two bedroom apartment. I was excited that for the first time I would have a place for my son to be besides my parents' home, but he said it would have to be the music room too, and my son would have to sleep through that - "A good mom would get her son to sleep through that." I wasn't a good mom. He had taught me that well, so when I realized I was pregnant the lessons became sterner. My body was dirty and needed to be cleaned if I was to carry his blessed child. My anxiety was my fault for not being close enough to God, or the 'Great Spirit' - it shifted as often as the wind - but an OHM tattoo on my chest would solve that, no matter if I wanted it or not.

You would have to be a better mother, a better woman. More sex was important. These herbs will clean you. Your body is too dirty to carry the baby, bleeding out is your punishment. We still have to go to my work picnic. Please don't embarrass me by bleeding through a pad, that's disgusting. I didn't want to have children with someone so weak anyway, so the Great Spirit answered my prayers - to kill the baby if you were not strong enough to support such a powerful life.

As summer turned to fall he started taking his wedding ring off. He would drive to his friend's house in a neighboring college town for the night and he didn't want to "lose it". Any concern I might have was met with being assured all of the women in the house where lesbians - but I could not come because my "homophobic ways radiated off me and my straight white privilege would make them uncomfortable". It was very close minded of me to only be attracted to the opposite sex, and the ring served as a blatant smack in the face of these women who could not yet legally marry.

We entered a cycle that I can't really put into justifiable words. He would get home from work, filthy, criticizing that I had eaten an unfair amount of food - even though it was my food card used to buy it. Then he would fuck me, unshowered because in his dirtiest state he was still cleaner than me. I cried the entire time, every time. Most nights he would wake me up suddenly from a dead sleep, just to tell me he didn't want to be with me anymore because I was such a horrible, clearly unintelligent person, then go right back to sleep. He'd get home from work the next day, make me beg to take him back and explain how I would be better, do better. I would admit I was a horrible mom, a shockingly stupid person, then he would fuck me, pass out, and the cycle would begin again. During all this, the childhood friends we visited on a regular basis had no idea this was going on - none of it. He was, after all, a great spiritual shamanic healer, so fun to hang out with, to jam with, and he had my van they could all drive around in.

I would get glimpses of ways out now and then. People would come to visit that didn't know my story, and I thought maybe they would see me and think I was worth something. Once it was two young kids, who were, in reality, my age. One had a guitar, and the song he played was so sad, forlorn, and vulgar. He didn't give a fuck how this song made anyone feel, or so that's how it seemed to me, and my soul absolutely related to his music. He sat in the hallway of all places, and this set the man I have yet to name off, so he responded passively aggressively, as usual, by beginning to play a horrendously racist "Gaucho" song he wrote for the Hispanic groundskeeper of the apartment complex, with a voice so bad that it once got him kicked off an open mic stage, so many customers were leaving. He suddenly stopped playing and asked this kid to leave, saying his energy was "upsetting" me, and I was prone to anxiety. Just to put this out there, that young man is now my husband. He did not make me uncomfortable.

One day a woman came over to get help from this "Master Shamanic Herbalist", as that was what he was now calling himself, but he was not home from work yet. She began to talk to me as if I, an uneducated woman, would know anything about why she was cramping in her first trimester or what she could do to ease her horrible morning sickness? I was so shocked that she looked at me and saw someone who could know anything. After all, it was not my name on the dollar store framed certificates on the wall - no, I could never afford such things. But when I am nervous I talk. I scan my brain for anything that will appease the person making requests of me so the interaction will be short and painless.

Suddenly, so much valid real life experience information was pouring out of me. Like the fact that cramping, as long as she is not bleeding heavily, is pretty common in first time pregnancies since your muscles are literally stretching as your womb expands. These pains usually don't last past the second trimester. I recalled reading this in Ina May's books, and I certainly felt those pains when I was pregnant with my son. That adequate protein, especially animal based protein, was vital for helping with morning sickness. Oh, and Chamomile was a bit safer for constant use during pregnancy than Ginger was, and could help reduce that pain a little bit! We were going back and forth and her stress was melting away, and for the first time in a very long time, I felt joy. It was not long lived.

He came through the door, knowing she was there waiting for him and proceeded to consult her. She began quoting things I said and he instantly and aggressively dismissed me, saying I liked to pretend to be an herbalist because now and then I look at his books. The books HE got while HE was becoming a certified herbalist, even though, just to set the record straight, there is no such thing as a 'certified herbalist in the United States. I watched her body tense up and he told me I was making her uncomfortable, so I went to sit in the hallway and listen. He told her a wonderful herb to help strengthen her womb and take away the cramps was Pennyroyal, to drink three to five cups a day, and take warm epsom salt baths. This was so wrong it made my chest burn, but my tongue was trapped under the weight of not believing I knew anything. I saw her about three months later in a grocery store. She had no life growing within her and she avoided eye contact with me.

That fall I had gathered a ton of Blue Elderberries, like I had done since childhood with my Grandmothers, knowing they made good tea to keep flu and colds at bay. When I brought the bag home he took them from me, saying that this was a perfect example of my ignorance to the world of herbs, that they are full of cyanide and I could have killed myself. But I have made tea with these my whole life! But I know these are safe, aren't they, as long as they are cooked and we don't eat the seed? "No, they can damage your kidneys," he proclaimed, as he put Goldenseal down my throat. It was such a long winter, and my kidneys were angry most of the time, drinking foul tasting teas and tinctures that would "clean" my body.

Spring came in like a lamb, so mild and beautiful. All that was on anybody's mind was camping way up there in the hills, all around the mushrooms and tender green shoots. But spring brought the stomach flu to our area, and my son had that flu. My sister decided to play with him, lifting him up and down in the air, and he puked on her face. Now my sister had the flu. She kissed her boyfriend, who shared a pipe with all of us. Now multiple friends had the flu. This flu spread fast like flu often does.

We were way up there on that Mountain with two groups of people. The first group were all the good ol' boys I had grown up with, drinking and shooting at cans, that sort of deal. The second group was his female friends from the college town, and they, every one of them, were hardcore vegan, to the point we were not allowed to share a fire because they did not want meat cooked over their flames. They gloated how they were blessed to have cleaned their bodies enough to no longer bleed monthly. I so badly wanted to be at the other fire. I heard them all laughing, being vulgar, screaming around about how delicious the deer they were eating was with wild mushrooms. Instead, we had brick tofu, sliced then and barely heated, with mushy rice and nutritional yeast flakes.

I felt ill, and then I felt iller. I begged him quietly to take me home, even though we had only been there for about an hour. He pronounced loudly so everyone could hear him that I was just having an anxiety attack, and he would not be taking me home. Suddenly this uppity, self righteous, deserving of the word cunt laid into me that my anxiety was caused by my stomach being a graveyard, that the terror I felt is the terror of all the animals that have been murdered, and that the only way for me to be free of my sins against the world was to fast, deeply detox my filthy body, and learn to have a conscious. This entire time she was up in my face gripping my shoulders, and I was too weak to break away while she unstably ranted at me with sobbing tears and snot running into her mouth. My body reacted, and I projectile vomited all over her chest. I had a hamburger for lunch, with way too much ketchup on it. I also had the stomach flu that was going around.

He still insisted I was simply having an anxiety attack, and as his obvious lover bawled her eyes out, while swallowing a hand full of xanax to deal with what she labeled as "trauma of death energy touching her", I had to tell him I would have sex with him any way he wanted, if he would just take me home. It was a sixty mile drive of constant beratement. He brought me to my sisters. She and I were so ill we were vomiting and shitting all over ourselves. My mother was doing her best to keep us alive while tending to my son, who thankfully was nearly recovered. My sister's boyfriend who had been at the other camp also came home that night vomiting.

To no one's surprise, he came back the next day. I was laying there half dead in a pool of my own vomit and my sister was on her couch puking into an old cooking pot when he decided it was time to collect payment for the ride home.

My sister, with her weakened voice, said as loudly as she could manage to leave me alone, but it was useless and I was in no position to fight it. It took me a long time to come to terms that this was rape. He raped me, while I had the flu. The only saving grace was my sister's boyfriend, who came running out of the bedroom towards the bathroom to shit himself, causing this thing I had gone numb to, to come to an end. He pulled his pants up, threw the blanket back over me, and pulled a thermos out of his bag, pouring himself a cup of steaming tea. I knew that smell anywhere even in such a state, that familiar friend I had been missing so sweet and healing and it made me weep. I rolled over and asked him, "Are you drinking Elderberry tea?"

He looked me in my tear-filled eyes and said, "Of course I am, I'm not trying to catch the flu!"

I began to laugh hysterically, and like the fucking scene from braveheart or some shit, I screamed "HYPOCRITE!" with energy I did not have.

He replied, "I have the proper training to use these berries safely. Do you?" Then he stormed off in my van.

As I laid there slowly recovering from this virus, the damage that had been done from the virus that is an ego driven heroic "healer" came to the surface. I remembered everything. It was almost like in such a weakened state my brain did not have the energy to uphold the conditioning this man had worked so hard over vast portions of my life to instill. This was finally the beginning of the end. I told him that I was leaving him, but like a true virus, he would not be that simple to shake.

He had, to my delight, moved out of the apartment when my son's biological father contacted me, after two years of not a word spoken, and came to meet his child. At this point the unnamed man had decided that no one could have me, coming in drunk at two in the morning, screaming he was going to cut my throat, killing my plants and smashing what little stuff I had, until he heard my son's father - this man who grew up in varying Chicago boys homes - say, "Man, I don't even gotta put my shoes on to kill you. You sure you wana be doing this?" I had never seen him move so fast as he scurried out the door like a reptile.

The next day I got an eviction notice. He had told my very religious landlord that I was a witch, and was giving illegal abortions to emigrants in the apartment. I only knew this because the landlord screamed it at me as I walked up on him throwing my already broken shit out into the driveway. It took months for him to stop showing up to my family's home, to stop coming to holiday dinners he certainly wasn't invited to, to stop telling vicious rumors in our tiny little town about me. As social media became relevant the onslaught continued for years, blocking accounts as he and his hoards of heroic healer female friends he collected like found pennies attacked me relentlessly.

It has been almost fourteen years and I still suffer daily from the damage this man's gaslighting has done to my self confidence, self worth, self belief and beyond, and the only thing I really have to say to him is this:

"God" is not liable for putting that deer in front of my van, asshole. You still owe me $2000 for a new radiator and a busted up grill!

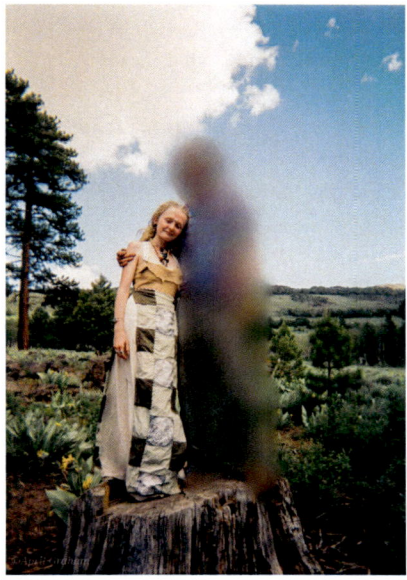

.11.

Elderberry
Sambucus

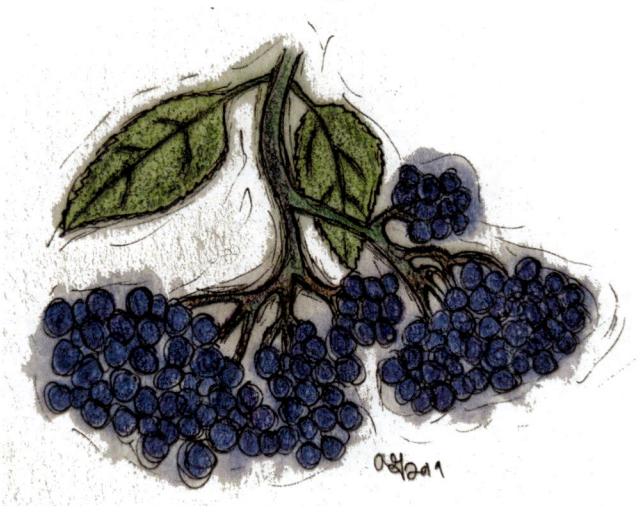

As an odd ritual, each fall I swallow a few uncooked Elderberry seeds as a reminder - a reminder that there is more death to be found in human nature and the cruelty that can seep into our bones than there is in a handful of often misunderstood Elderberry seeds, but also to remind me that I damn well know what I know.

For some time afterward I actually rejoiced in how many folks were uninformed about the toxicity of Elderberries. Those beautiful dusty blue berries hung so thickly on our trees that branches would snap. I could gather abundantly, the critters could eat their fill, and come winter there would still be huge amounts left to hang frozen on the trees.

It was never really about having them all to myself, so much as it was the undisturbed and plentiful relationship I needed to heal from such lack of self allowed.

It would be easy I suppose to think that this story didn't have much to do with Elderberry. I guess in a way you're right, but she is the first ally that showed up as a child and the first as I remembered not only am I valid, but that my knowledge is valid as well. That money is not required to attain it or a qualifier of it.

The History of Elderberry:

She floats through thousands of years of human history like music on the wind. That's what came to mind when I was thinking of how to start this section so that's what we'll go with, because it's not only beautiful but accurate. You see, while there are many different varieties of elderberry they all have one thing in common.

Their genus name: Sambucus

While many land-based cultures had long standing relationships with her prior to the issuing of Latin names and plant genus documentation, when she was named after the Greek Sambuce (a type of flute) they truly tapped into something that all cultures who had a relationship with her knew. She could not only be a source of food and health but music, as her pithy branches make for easy hollowing, giving way to the creation of beautifully melodic flutes sure to entrance the listener.

Yet there is a debate. Did she actually earn her genus name from the Greek word Sambuce, or was she possibly used for yet another instrument with the ability to entrance? In Greece there was also an instrument called a Sambuka, which was a harp. You see, her wood is also very bendy and would give way to beautiful strings plucked. I always find these debates to be somewhat funny. In the same way that she can be food as well as medicine, why couldn't she be a harp as well as a flute and the name or even use simply varied from one area to another? One thing I dislike about Latin names is that they give zero room for fluidity and all of the space to rigid debate and sides taken.

When we, or at least I, think of flutes and harps it brings me to imagined sounds of Celtic ballads and forlorning flute notes bouncing off of grey, ocean-battered rock on some distant shore. Of course that might seem a bit imaginal, but it would be impossible to talk about Elderberry without touching on her deep history in most Celtic and European lands. Folklore references too many to count make note of her healing, as well as magical abilities.

We do know that the oldest (to date, anyhow) evidence of elderberry, not just being used but actually cultivated, comes from a Neolithic (2000 B.C.) pole building in Switzerland, where it was evident they were storing their elderberries like any other crop harvested to sustain them through winter. Take a moment to think here with me about that. Sure, 2000 B.C. was a long time ago, but the Neolithic Era was the very dawn of people switching from hunter gatherers to more settled farm based communities. Here's what I'd like you to think on - What would these very new to farming ancient humans begin to cultivate first? The food they already knew well. So while the only evidence we have of an actual timeline of use puts us at the 2000 B.C. mark, it is absolutely absurd to think she hasn't been in use much longer than that. Especially when you consider it was likely when the Ice Age began to recede around 9000 B.C. that her seeds were drug across as the ice receded to Europe, North America, and Asia.

Fast forward a few thousand years after that ice melted away and she explodes into the world with her deep healing abilities from Greece, to the Americas, to Egypt and so far beyond that there are now hundreds of different types across the entire world. She has been shown great reverence in many ancient medicinal texts, an important one to not being the Historia Plantarum. This book series (10 were made, only 9 recovered) dates as far back as 287 B.C., and is considered by many to be the most important and influential book(s) of natural history written in ancient times. The author Theophrastus had done something entirely new in the history of Botany. He explored each and every plant's structure, how they reproduced, and went into intricate details of their growth. He then applied this to the vast varieties of known plants around the world at the time and linked all of this to their medicinal uses. This series of books would majorly influence the world of healing, and Elderberry had a front row seat in its pages.

From ancient humans to clinical research seeing if she can save us from the next flu pandemic, Elderberry has stood strongly beside mankind. No matter how our beliefs about her ebb and flow she is there, even when we don't think we need her.

The Many Uses of Elderberry:

I'd be willing to bet my last dollar that about 90% of you reading these pages have heard a thing or two about Elderberry's ability to help keep the flu or the common cold at bay but not much else, and I would probably be correct!

So, of course if you're wanting to keep the flu and colds at bay Elderberry is a good choice for most, but she, and other parts of her beyond her berries and blooms, have so much more to offer!

Got a nasty fever?

How about some stubborn seasonal allergies? Sneeze be gone! (That made me laugh)

Maybe you suffer from chronic fatigue?

How's that body of yours feeling? Back pain? Leg pain? Nerve pain?

Any arthritis going on that's not caused by your own immune system functions?

Do you suffer from chronic sinus infections?

Is your blood sugar through the roof? Does your heart need some tending to? High cholesterol? High blood pressure?

Need to piss a little more often? Have some water retention you'd like to shake?

Maybe you need some help being regular in the bathroom?

Family history of cancer?

Struggling with your skin's health?

Do you bruise really easily?

Find yourself struggling with low moods now and then?

How high are your uric acid levels? Got a good bit of gout going on these days?

That's quite a list, isn't it?! How'd I do on that bet? I'm still feeling pretty confident that most folks don't consider her much more than a cold and flu remedy. I'd even go all in and say a lot of herbalists could be in that category too!

How Can Elderberry Do So Much for Us?

So now I've gata back up the Why, right? Yeah, that's the usual pace of things! As with every other plant ally, it comes down to what compounds those berries, blooms, and other bits of our lady Elder contain.

For the blooms we're mainly dealing with triterpenes alpha- and beta-amyrin, ursolic acid, oleanolic acid, betulin, and betulinic acid.

The berries are different creatures all together, with a host of compounds such as quercetin, kaempferol, rutin, phenolic acids, anthocyanidins, and phytonutrients.

Deep breath out, drink of tea. Okay, let's do this.

Maybe that tea I was drinking was of the Elderberry variety, The school year has started and those first cold fall nights tell me that illness is coming, as we cram little and teenage humans alike into confined, poorly vented rooms, their teenage level hygiene letting them pass around germs like notes (sadly, I think smartphones killed the art of note passing, but you get what I mean). The last thing I want is to fall victim to a rogue virus that will make being a mom and the million other hats I wear harder to manage than they already are.

What's really in that tea, besides probably too much sweet cream, that's gana help me ward of the child gifted influenza barrelling my way?

Phytonutrients and anthocyanidins are the Who, What, Where, and Why of keeping the flu and other viral nastiness away, but let's step deeply into the flu aspect for a moment, since that is the common use of her.

Swirling in that cream, phytonutrients that once acted as a protector to berries from sun, insects, and pathogens are now passed onto us as we drink or eat them in some fashion. In fact, phytonutrients from Elderberries are what's being studied worldwide in the battle against the flu, with tremendously exciting success. Imagine a castle. Your cells are the king in a tower and enemies are rushing every gate, window and door. Phytonutrients act as guards to each entry point in your castle (body), preventing an invasion. But as we all know, sometimes a siege is inevitable. It only takes one man (virus) to get past our best defenses and the castle can fall.

But here is where Elder's unique phytonutrients are causing waves in the medical world. She not only continues the attack on the influenza virus, she rallies with an astounding battle cry and tells our immune system to send out every single resource it has, resulting in significantly subduing the virus' ability to replicate. In less fantasized terms, IF the influenza virus manages to enter our body, the phytonutrients literally guarding our every orifice triggers our cells to release cytokines. Cytokines act as messengers, which allows the immune system to communicate between different cell types. When this happens our body is able to coordinate a more efficient attack against an invading pathogen.

This is why people almost never die from the flu. Wait, what? That sounds like an absurd statement, considering that between 291,000 and 646,000 people die from complications of influenza worldwide yearly. Want to know what those complications are? A huge majority of the time it is your immune system being a ruthless and overly efficient attacker of the virus that is invading your body. In a desperate attempt to protect the king of the castle your body makes a fever so hot you die. Your body attacks the virus in your lungs so aggressively that your own lung tissue is too damaged to take in air and you often, as fucking morbid as this is about to sound, drown in your own blood.

Even when one's own immune system is not the cause of a flu related death, the flu virus still is not likely to be why someone dies. Instead, it's a secondary infection alongside your immune system's overzealous response. Your body is now taxed. All white blood cells have been spent and they cannot send reinforcements to the likely bacterial infection that is setting into your lungs, so you succumb. There is also the possibility of organ failure, often caused by your own immune system or whatever infection it is now, yet again, too weak to fight off. Super fun stuff.

That hard to read and likely germaphobe enforcing bit is why Elderberry is best used as a **preventative** for the flu versus alongside the flu, especially if you don't start using her until your immune system is already making you very sick. Remember those cytokines and how they allow you cells/immune system to communicate more efficiently? Yep, that's like giving your already overreacting immune system an unstoppable fully automatic weapon during the dark ages. That sort of attack can become something we are not likely to survive. This is not making you feel very comfortable using Elderberry, right? Wait, didn't I do this exact thing I am saying not to do? I did, and if not for one different thing it could have killed me. You see, the part I left out of the story was how I didn't have the flu. Nope. I had the "stomach flu", which actually isn't even related to influenza, but is called the flu ALL OF THE TIME. It's actually norovirus.

In fact I have never once in my life had influenza, and neither have my children, my mother, or sister. I am fairly confident this is because my great grandmother somehow survived the Spanish flu while pregnant with my grandmother, but that's a theory for a different time, and also an insight as to why I find the flu so interesting.

So let me reign in your fears about dying from the flu and Elderberry being the final blow that kills ya. The thing is, by the time you are so ill that Elderberry would potentially be deadly you're not going to be willing, let alone able to take in liquids, and you'd likely already be much closer to death than you're realizing. I would feel perfectly safe drinking Elderberry regularly during the flu season, or if folks in my house had it and I was hoping to prevent it, even if I had just caught it and wanted to keep it from getting any worse, and I wanted to recover a bit more quickly. I definitely would not use Elderberry if I was already 2-3 days into influenza and my symptoms were horrendous. This is the time when your immune system is already halfway killing you in an attempt to kill the virus, and it really does not need any further ammunition.

I didn't really mean to write a terrifying castle scene that morphed in an article on how Elderberries and the flu can at times be a bad idea, but there you have it, ha! Let me reign myself in and get back to why phytonutrients are actually amazing at preventing the flu, and how when used with a touch of knowhow can stop all of the above madness from happening in the first place. An amazing study conducted by the University of Sydney showed that phytochemicals from Elderberry juice applied to a cell infected with influenza were not only able to stop the influenza virus from infecting most cells in the first place, but they are even more effective at stopping the spread of the virus when the cells had successfully been infected!

That fact is pretty amazing really, because most things stop being effective at the door, so to speak. Finding out that a humble little berry can not only prevent the flu but prevent the viral load from replicating after you have already caught it is how we survive the flu. That means if we can stop the virus from getting out of hand our immune system will regulate it's response accordingly, and that's the difference between a few shitty sick days and drowning in our own blood. This is why it's so important to have Elderberry in your body well before you get sick. If she's already there right off the bat the virus you pick up is not going to be able to replicate on a level that will cause your immune system to lose its shit!

Taking a sharp left turn, now we can talk all about anthocyanidins and how something as simple as color is so crucial to the health of our immune system. Color? Yep. You see, anthocyanidins are what give berries and some veggies their color. How Elderberries are black or blue, or how a strawberry or a tomato is red - that's all anthocyanidins! All of these colors have an astounding effect on our bodies. As an immune supporter she also is able to attack viruses, while having amazingly powerful anti-inflammatory actions. Not only is this how Elder is helping with most of our aches and pains, but this little trick is actually really helpful for the regulation of our immune system - especially once you put two and two together and realize that damn near all inflammation in your body is caused by your immune system attacking something. When we pull this response down we can calm our sometimes murderous immune functions down!

But what are anthocyanidins beyond "color"? Flavonoids, which are a sincere source of antioxidants. That's a recurring theme here in a lot of these plant allies, isn't it? We covered the extremely impressive abilities of antioxidants in the chapter on Plantain, but let's touch base a bit again on how antioxidants fight free radicals, are anti-viral, and play a huge role in the battle against cancer. Let's actually dive deeper, because shallow water can be dangerous when we're jumping in head first, right? Because she's full of anthocyanidins making her rich in flavonoids, and because those flavonoids fight free radicals, she also reduces (you might have guessed From the Plantain chapter) oxidative stress! Did you know that oxidative stress is a huge factor in heart disease? That's how you connect those dots to heart health, folks. We also know that she's capable of lowering blood pressure and cholesterol.

As usual, some guys in white lab coats (I imagine them wearing coats, anyhow) started feeding some Elderberry extract to some very sick mice, which in turn helped reduce cholesterol levels and improved HDL function. You wana guess what the main reason was? The high levels of anthocyanins! From there they decided to give some rats high blood pressure and, wouldn't you know it, when polyphenols extracted from the berries were administered to rats that had been given the gift of hypertension, their blood pressure was substantially reduced. Researchers are now suggesting using polyphenols to lower blood pressure. Isn't that funny? They do a study that shows Elderberry is capable of doing all of these things and their conclusion is to cast aside the whole plant in favor for the few compounds they believe responsible instead of asking how less effective this would be without all of the other beautifully complex properties, so perfectly put into place by our ever giving Elderberry ally?

Sometimes when I am stressed out I give way to the call of copious amounts of sugar, which I will dearly pay for in skyrocketed blood sugar. After years of starving and subsisting off of cheap, often somewhat spoiled food and readily available sugar highs in between severe hunger, I am extremely susceptible to high blood sugar. While you'd think staying away from berries (natural sugar is still sugar) would be wise, I have found when I do finally cave and eat not just one but all of the cookies, an infusion made with elderberries then simmered down a little thicker gets my blood sugar to stabilize rather quickly. Why? Because she has an amazing ability to regulate blood sugar by stimulating glucose metabolism and insulin, helping lower our blood sugar levels.

I'd like to imagine the rats the scientists made diabetic had a good time getting there being allowed to eat all manner of delicious things, but I think that is just wishful thinking. In any case, they gave some rats diabetes and then fed them extract of Elderberry. They discovered that Elderberry lowered insulin resistance in the rats with type 2 diabetes. Honestly, this is a combination of her polyphenols, which are flavonoids, and phenolic acid, which plays a major role in moderating blood sugar.

I'd say the most painful thing out of the What Can She Do list would be gout. I'll be honest here, I have never felt the pain of gout. I have seen my father suffer from it, and heard the wailing of pain he made when a pillow gently rolled onto his foot. This is a man that does not tell you he's in pain and refuses pain medication at all costs. I'm talking three days post-op from removing a cancerous kidney he refused to take any more pain medication. He had that type of pain tolerance, but a pillow on a gout ridden toe made him cry out like a banshee.

Gout happens from the buildup of uric acids that are failing to break down in your bloodstream and that you're not able to piss out fast enough. These crystals often end up settling in our joints, most commonly in the big toe but any joint can be struck and cause arthritic conditions. Wana know something else uric acid does? When our levels are high our blood pressure is also high and our odds of heart disease increase. Elderberries lower the levels of uric acid by increasing antioxidant enzymes in our blood.

So what about the actual health of our veins? Rutin, another factor of color. I'd like to take a moment to note how beautiful it is that the compounds that create stunning colors for us to gaze at are the same things that are here to heal us. There is something about that that truly moves me. Rutin is a bioflavonoid - a pigment found in certain plants and fruits, such as Elderberry. Sounds simple enough?

Not in the least. This little compound is a powerful supporter of healthy circulation while helping to strengthen and promote flexibility in blood vessels, such as your arteries and capillaries. When our blood vessels are strong the same can often be said for our overall health. Why? Because strong blood vessels prevent or ease up issues such as easy bruising, spider veins, and varicose veins. While I'd not solely rely on Elderberry for this, rutin can help a bit with hemorrhoids (which are for the most part just swollen veins) since she shrinks up your veins. This helps reduce some of the pain and burning you may be suffering with.

On the subject of pain, it's her anti-inflammatory abilities that help us cope with nerve related pain, but we also know that rutin is pretty damn effective at helping with arthritis because she also helps reduce oxidative stress, getting us right back to her powerful antioxidant and anti-inflammatory abilities. Sometimes it's an unknown build up of uric acid that is causing discomfort and Elderberry is a fantastic ally to try for joint and knee pain, so long as you don't have an autoimmune issue like rheumatoid arthritis. We don't want to be stimulating your immune system any more than it already is.

Sometimes while writing this I feel like a broken record. I mean, when you consider that many plants with the ability to heal us more often than not share similar compounds, I could write the same paragraph again and again. Now toss in the fact that some compounds act extremely similar to other compounds, or are simply a different branch of a type of compound. Take phytonutrients as an example. There are over 25,000 different phytonutrients found in plants. I bring this up because within our juicy Elderberries we will also find kaempferol and quercetin ,which are phytonutrients.

So kaempferol and quercetin are basically the most important flavonoids on the face of this planet, and these two little compounds that are heavily found in Elder act as antioxidants, which we've talked on a lot already, anti-inflammatory which you know pulls down swelling and irritation, antimicrobial so they can kill bacteria, and anti-cancerous (that one's pretty self explanatory). They're also a cardioprotective, which means they keep your heart happy. We also can't forget about the neuroprotective aspects that support and repair our nervous systems, antidiabetic (which we can all likely guess what that means). Oh yeah, they're also antiosteoporotic (a super fancy term that means it counters osteoporosis), analgesic (all about helping to relieve pain), antiallergic (what's gana help you with seasonal allergies), and last but in no way least anxiolytic.

That last one has a powerful meaning. Powerful in the way that it can help with a current crisis most first world humans (I'm not excluding anyone else. It's just this thing I'm about to touch on statistically affects humans in places like the United States more than it does other areas.) are deeply suffering from and highly medicated for via the benzo epidemic - anxiety. You see, anxiolytic means something that counters anxiety, and that horrendous feeling of panic, disparity, and inability to see what's really going on as our adrenals flood our body with fight, flight, puke, scream, cry, and shit hormones.

There was always a horrible chicken and the egg theory that plagued me before I came to acceptance with my fucking array of traumas. Does anxiety cause my depression or does depression cause my anxiety? I remember setting in a counselor's office meant to help me through crippling anxiety while pregnant with my daughter and this man (who ended up being a stalker, no joke.) talked for the entire appointment about this 'which came first' dilemma, and I'll never forget the look on his creepy rat like face when I just began to laugh. It truly doesn't matter which is causing which because if we are able to alleviate either we are making not only forward movement but room to take in a fucking breath, and in that we find room to heal or at the very damn least find space to learn coping skills.

So we know that elderberry has the ability to promote a calm state, yeah? So what if in this calm state we also find ourselves with the room needed to feel an elevated mood? Seemed to work for some mice that were clinically depressed. I imagine they were just naturally that was from the general lab setting existence, but who really knows. Anyhow, in one study Elderberry extract (high in quercetin) was given to two mice that were so depressed they were in the little to no mobility stage (we've all been there). Within 48 hours of use they were up and about, better than the mice who had been given a random antidepressant specifically for lab mice. Now, do I think Elderberry is the answer for severe depression? Nope. Do I think it'd be helpful for those low stages the precede existential dread? Yep. Even if Elderberry isn't the end-all be-all for depression, odds are good your body won't begrudge you the kindness of a cup of warm tea when you're feeling your lowest.

Now, this is gana sound shallow as hell to some, but we'll jump in it anyhow. Sometimes when we are moderately depressed by making ourselves look nice (as much as a struggle as that can be at times) we end up feeling better about ourselves. Some folks would call this vanity, but I don't think it's as cut and dry as that. I mean whether humans like to admit it or not we are just animals, and ALL animals groom themselves. Growing up on a farm off and on and around many wild animals, there's one thing I can tell you. If an animal stops grooming itself something serious is wrong, and it's not always illness. There was once this mean old Appaloosa horse named Blue who was only nice to me. He'd take anyone else under a tree branch or under a clothesline - anything to knock you off. He'd chase dogs with his ears back and come at cows with severe aggression. Blue was old and had been rescued from a slaughterhouse. Besides the 50 lb child named April his only other friend was another horse named Toby. That year, after hunting season had come and after the roundup was over, school started as usual and I didn't get out much to see Blue. Toby never came down from the fall cattle drive, and after wolves were spotted in the area feasting on a horse it was clear Toby was gone.

Blue refused to eat. Blue was filthy, and that's saying a lot for creatures that like to roll in the dirt. Soon enough it was evident that he would die, according to the farm vet. My dad took me out to see Blue one last time, and as soon as he saw me he began to run around the field with excitement you'd not expect to see from a dying animal. For a solid week, I skipped school to feed Blue, to brush him and to spend time with him. He was dying, but it wasn't from an illness. It was from grief and depression after losing Toby and a little girl going back to school. He lived another happy five years when new horse companions brought in and really all it took was getting him moving, grooming him, and making sure he was eating.

How is depression in a human animal any different? We need to get up, remember to eat, and take time to groom our bodies as a deep act of self care. How the hell does Elderberry play into this beyond maybe some sort of food? Well, her blooms are an entirely different creature and while this is just gana keep getting longer and longer with no chapter break in sight, it's all going to be worth it. Knowing these things is worth the read.

I have always noticed the appearance of a depressed person's skin. You can tell they haven't cared to wash or splash any amount of water on their days-long unwashed faces. Why bother? Because you are worth it. You are also worth the rich and caring feeling of a fatty infused oil to feed your depleted skin.

My Grandmother Audry used to tell me that Elder blooms are what our ancient ancestors (who got the name "faery" from the invading Celtic peoples to our original lands) used to give the appearance of everlasting youth, saying "It's not that we lived forever. We just aged with the grace of Elder." I have always loved that simple little sentence from my Grandmother Audry, and it's something I think about often as I watch age set into my well-lived face.

Each tiny little petal that cascades through my fingertips into a well used mason jar is packed with triterpenes (alpha- and beta-amyrin) who at first glance give our skin the gift of reducing inflammatory conditions, but this compound found in those little blooms should not be underestimated when it comes to genuine healing of our skin. Of course we know that inflammation causes red, hot, puffy conditions on our faces, but it can also open us up to infections which lead to even further inflammation and, if you are human like I am (you are), you may now and then have a hard time keeping your hands off of popping that pimple or not picking the scab. The good news is triterpenes have an impressive ability to reduce the healing time of any and all wounds. The faster that sore heals the less time you have to pick it, and the less likely you are to have a scar. I really want to drive home how effective triterpenes are at healing wounds. From 1910-to date there have been over 2181 studies on varying triterpenes, and everything from simple wounds to complex surgical wounds were healed in half the time!

While we have yet to fully unlock the "why" of triterpenes, we know that a lot of it has to do with the fact that they are able to encourage new tissue development, reduce cellular damage, and encourage collagen deposition, which is a vital part of a wound healing. But that word 'collagen' likely sounds familiar to anyone who's into skin care products, right? Sure, because the beauty industry tells us collagen improves skin elasticity, reduce wrinkles, and boosts skin hydration, but what they often leave out the technical why. Basically, it increases the density of fibroblasts, which is fancy talk for cells in our connective tissue that produce collagen. So to wipe away the complications of understanding that triterpenes encourage collagen, we can simply say collagen is what young beautiful skin is teaming with, and Elder blooms encourage your body to make it!

There's this old wives tale that the first dew of the morning could remove the curse of freckles or dark spots from a woman's face, but I always heard the story different from a culture that is often proud of our freckles! I was not overly close with my grandmother Audry since it hurt her too much to be around me long. I looked exactly like an uncle of mine, a son of hers, that was murdered by the police in cold blood. What time I did get to spend with her was always full of enticing stories about who we are, the place we come from, as well as hard stories of oppression endured. My favorites were always the ones that, no surprise, involved plant superstition such as, "It is important that a Traveller woman be mindful to never gather Elders blooms in the dawn or the dew will wash the freckles from your face and your people won't recognize you as any different from some settled woman!" The funny thing is this Traveller's tale is not all that untrue!

You see, ursolic acid found in her cream colored blooms truly does have the ability to fade dark and age spots. Albeit a bit of morning dew won't likely do the trick, but maybe my ancestors gathered A LOT of elder blooms and were just utterly drowning in the morning dew, ha!? Regardless of how that saying came to be, take a moment to think about that level of connection they had to this plant ally and her blooms? To have worked with her so much that they knew without even knowing the "why" that she was capable of such an act. Indeed the ursolic acid can lighten up these spots, but she is also is yet another collagen producer when used on our skin, which means she is great for fine lines, wrinkles, and giving us the gift of a youthful appearance.

Just like every other compound, ursolic acid has many other faces and actions, such as her stunning anti-inflammatory abilities, sincere antimicrobial, antibacterial and antifungal properties, which help prevent or resolve the growth of bacteria fungus (acne can be bacterial folks) and encourage rapid healing of just about any external issue. She also has the ability to act as a photobarrier, so kind of like a sunblock. She's not going to prevent a sunburn but she does prevent the everyday damage that the sun's rays can do to our skin. This also applies to the free radicals that float about from pollution, no matter where we live.

These things might sound superficial, but what if instead of acne we are dealing with skin cancer? Here's the thing - ursolic acid has shown herself to be pretty damn remarkable at outright halting tumor growth and skin cancers when applied topically to (you guessed it) rodents who had tumors and skin cancer. While we have mainly been talking on Elder blooms for external use, it's important to note that she is safe to use internally as a tea or a tincture. All of the things I have been talking about can, for the most part, be of pretty good use to the insides of us too!

Sometimes, well all of the time, I believe we are made ill from the separation. The separation of a compound of a plant, the making of a vitamin, the chemical extractions that leave behind or casts aside. It's not hard to see that many of these compounds that are ALL found within Elder blooms kinda sorta do the same thing, but this does NOT mean that any one thing on its own will be anywhere near as effective when used in it's naturally occurring state within our plant allies.

So sure ursolic acid is amazing, but I'm not touching her on her own because I/they/you don't know better than the plant does.

On that note, oleanolic acid is next up on the to talk about list. Wana guess what her abilities are? She's of course packed with great antioxidant levels, is yet another antimicrobial powerhouse, for sure an anti-inflammatory, and with her ability to fight off free radicals is a legit anti-aging friend to all. She also shines at firming skin from even more collagen production. She does really pull the heat out of skin more than others though, and is why I think anything Elder bloom is ideal for those prone to heat flushed skin.

Wana know something I'm thinking about? It's hard to just write about how her blooms are helpful to our skin. I'm having to stop myself from drifting all about these pages as my mind drifts through archived bits of info I've read here and there. I could easily talk about how betulin and betulinic acids are so effective at halting the growth of cancer and tumors, that there are entire studies being funded to use these compounds as a chemotherapeutic option. Now that that's out of my mind we can talk about how on a skincare level they're going to act as a serious barrier to free radicals (on a 'radiation from the sun' based level), going to help you battle eczema, gana murder the bad bacteria on your skin that's causing acne or even staph, all while being an anti-inflammatory and vastly improving skin elasticity because (of course) she also helps to create collagen in our skin. Didn't see that coming at all, did we?

This ally is deeply ingrained into my genetic makeup, and while my life circumstances may not afford me to age with the grace of many others, I can at the very least hope to age with the grace given to me by the Elders.

Where Does Elderberry Grow?

At one or three points in time, actually probably thousands of times, Elders will try to lure you to an untimely death. You see the ripest, most beautiful bunch of berries you have ever set you eye upon hanging just over that cliff's edge, growing just so out of the side of that steep hill, way down in the bottom of some dangerous sharp rock ravine. These berries are for the birds and all other manner of flying creatures, not you.

You will want to look in open fields that stay green for about half of the summer. She LOVES moisture, so you won't find her in bone-dry lands. This also means it'd be a pretty good idea to look along river banks, lakes, ponds, and springs. Sometimes marshes too, but she will be at the edges not within the boggy waterlogged areas.

I also, at least in my area, see her chronically growing alongside railroad tracks. There are a few theories to this. Perhaps it is because the deer that feast on her low hanging berries use tracks like highwaysm so that means they're shitting out berries all along the track as they go. Makes sense. My grandmother Ruby, however, would have said it's because during the great depression when poor families migrated anywhere there were crops to be worked they were always made to set up camps by railroad tracks, out of sight of the better off folks, and of course they often relied on any source of food possible, wild foods being no exception. So they'd be casting aside seeds and stray unused berries, even taking shits with seeds in them. For me, I land on it being both things - the suffering generations of the great depression brought the seeds to the tracks, the trees grew, and now the wildlife spreads them.

Of course, don't gather near tracks that have been in use in the last decade, as that ground is heavy with oils and at times herbicides, since the railroad can't have aggressive plants taking over the tracks. But sometimes finding her just so you know what she looks like is a good step to take in finding ones you can safely harvest from!

So as far as where she came from, in the grand scheme of things she is primarily native to all of Western Europe. I mean, pick a country (Dear American, Europe is an area in the world with MANY different countries/cultures. Just to put that out there.) in that area of the world and you won't find one she's not native to and where the local folks don't/didn't have a relationship with her. She is also native to the North American continents and a vast majority of the different tribes, stretching from the high reaches of Canada down into nearly South America.

She has become naturalized in every other area of the temperate world, so while you will have to get out and do some real looking for her, I am feeling pretty certain you will eventually find some variety of her.

When Should We Harvest Elderberry?

Come spring when her blooms first unfurl is the time to be extremely watchful. With her blooms there is a dance to be had. You don't want them when they are not fully bloomed, and you don't want them when they are still in bloom, but going to berry stage. There is this perfect in between moment of about 3 days that is ideal to harvest. This is when fostering a real relationship comes into play. You will have to watch her, to check back in daily. If you skip a few days of saying hello you may have missed your window for this batch of blooms.

She is forgiving though, and usually offers late season blooms that will never have time to turn into berries. These are ideal because you can harvest freely without having to be mindful - in the way that in spring what you take off of the tree will be what berries DO NOT show up for the wildlife or for you. With this in mind, it's very unethical to take blooms AND berries from a wild tree in the same year.

If you took blooms. Hands off berries.

If you didn't take blooms. Gather berries.

Didn't take blooms. Gathered berries. Lucked out on some late season blooms.

That is what ethical harvesting looks like folks.

So it's late summer and you see those berries starting to turn dark. Before you fill your basket it's important to make sure that the berries are actually ripe. Locally I have Blue Elderberries, and come July they are a beautiful blue ashy color and look prime for the picking - they aren't! If you get close you'll notice that some of the berries still have a green hue to them and that the bloom tips are still hanging on good at the base of the berry. They might still be firm, like a grape.

The best time to harvest Elderberries for making jelly or other foodstuffs is when there are NO visible green berries left on the tree. Note that I said tree, NOT the individual bunch of berries. Of course, this excludes those late season blooms that have tiny tiny super tiny green berries on them. I'm talking about all of the clusters that are hanging heavy with fruit. At this point, they are nice and sweet and perfect for cooking.

But if you're in this for her medicinal values let's talk about those squishy, boozy, frost kissed berries, because those are where it's at! I'm talking when the cold starts to set in and the mother tree (wanting to give her seeds the best chance at germination) sends one last push of sugars, starches, and all of those compounds we talked on into her berries. Then there's this neat thing that both the cold and slight alcohol does to these late season berries that takes the Elderberry cake! They break down the cellular structure of the berry. This is a great thing, as her nutritional and medicinal values are locked up in these cells and when we do things like make tinctures or teas our goal is to break those cell walls. When this is already done for us we're coming out the gate winners and our tinctures and teas will be that much more potent!

What Cautions Should We Take?

The first caution that needs to be taken is figuring out which Elderberry you're working with as there are many different varieties! While really only the red Elderberry (Sambucus racemosa) is considered poisonous (she's still usable), knowing who you're working with is important.

Okay, let's jump into the terror that many have over ingesting a seed, seeing a bit of stem floating in their tincture jar, or a bit of a leaf that boiled with their jelly.

It is both founded and unfounded fear. It lives in that place of fact, but the fear comes from not really understanding the fact. The big bad word is: cyanogenic glycosides.

Just to add some more fear of Elderberries after I talked about drowning in our own blood (haha), this compound means it can turn into cyanide in our body. "Oh, Jezuz!" is what most folks' reactions are after hearing that, but that gets morphed into "Elderberry seeds contain cyanide!" No. No, they don't. They contain a particular type of glycoside (a lot of plants have these. Some are good. Some are bad. It just depends.) that if digested often can build up in our bodies and be converted into cyanide. That did not make you feel any better after reading itv, right? Okay well, how about the fact that they don't actually build up in our body. They easily pass through, so for you to get high enough levels in your body to do real damage you're going to be needing to consume raw Elderberries on a regular basis. I'm talking big amounts daily. Did you catch how I used the word raw, though?

That's an important catch. Why? Because these scary body killing bits are rendered inactive when we cook them. Fun fact: Tincturing in alcohol is cooking. Dehydrating is cooking. Simmering for tea is cooking. Making jelly is cooking. Infusing in vinegar is cooking. Fermenting is cooking.

Just like that this thing that people hold a lot of fear about is hopefully gone.

Does this mean we should eat the seeds after cooking or fry up a bunch of elderberry leaves? No, don't do that!

Does this mean if we have a bit of stem on a berry here and there in our cup of tea or tincture jar that we are gana up and die or make someone sick? Nope.

Still not convinced? How are you enjoying that Apple juice? Does your kid really like it? Maybe it's all of those inactive cyanogenic glycosides that give it such a satisfying taste! Yep apple seeds, stems, and leaves are teaming with cyanogenic glycosides, and just about every juice company in the world presses the whole apple (seeds and all) into a fine puree to get every single drop of juice. Then they pasteurize it, making the cyanogenic glycosides inactive.

Beyond those things the main cautions are if we are already severely ill from the flu. I'm talking if we are 2-3 days in and considering going to the hospital we don't want to reach for Elderberry because all of those scary self drowning in blood reasons I talked on earlier.

Also, if we have any sort of autoimmune system situation going on that makes our immune system attack us we REALLY do not want to be touching Elderberry with a 10-foot pole! This includes rheumatoid arthritis folks, so before you offer her to your parents or an elderly person be sure this is not a factor.

How Much is Too Much?

While Elderberries are so safe cooked they are considered a food, some folks can experience nausea and even a bit of the shits if they go too hard too fast. So if you have never used Elderberry start with one cup of tea that's not too strong, or maybe only a half dose of the tincture, and even though that syrup is really good, let's just try no more than a teaspoon worth, huh?

Stay at these low doses/weak brews for the first week or so, and pay attention to how your individual body responds. From there you can increase how much your using, or if you do feel a bit off you'll know to back off a bit.

I take elderberry every day that I am able to, and prefer the tincture since it is so shelf-stable and I can easily make enough to last me from one harvest season to the next. Don't let that stop you from trying her tea with some sweet cream!

.12.

California Poppy Calms the Mind, but Doesn't Grant Sanity.

At the time I had no concept of bloodline trauma or even my own. Just an overwhelming feeling that if I stopped moving, stopped running, stopped travelling I would die, be found, caught, captured and contained. So I hopped from one car/train/bus/rig/truck/van right after another. There was even a stretch of time where I could only sleep when barreling down the highway. I swear, as soon as I felt the speed drop below fifty-five my body instantly tensed up, pulling me out of the dream ether with utter fear of what would be waiting once I stepped back out onto the pavement. This is how by eighteen I had been to every state within the lower 48, at least twice. But the west coast was always my home base.

I hopped out the back of that truck the second it pulled up to the plaza, not even giving the kids I was travelling with a moment to say goodbye. I was in my mind, the final leg of a thousand mile journey spent having barely survived the Dakotas and the rampant sex trafficking in the area. I was not really processing what had occurred over the last few weeks, and completely ignoring that I had been feeling much worse than usual. Maybe I did notice and just wrote it off to my infected gums from the lip piercing that was slowly eroding them away over the past six years.

More likely I was in denial.

The rain had begun to fall, and I had not even been there long enough to finish rolling a smoke when the van pulled up, instantly catching my attention. When he stepped out I recognized him from what seemed like a lifetime ago. He walked right up to me and said, "Hey chick, you still know about plants and shit?" They were on a mission, one that would easily be a four hundred mile round trip, and they were leaving right now. Every single bone in my body knew what we were about to do was so very wrong, and that what I was about to be a part of, what my agreement to help, would truly mean.

What I didn't expect is how severely and swiftly I would be shown the errors of my ways. The reality is when you live this type of life morals simply have to take a back seat to the prospect of earning real money. Money that equals food not eaten from dumpsters, a warm dry room to sleep that guarantees you won't be raped in the night, a shower, new socks because the old ones aren't washable. Money that can get you the fuck out of a situation, should the need arise. By no means do I justify my actions for the sake of making a dollar. It's just important to understand as humans we tend to only have values and morals when all of our basic needs are met. It's easy to say "I would never do that" when you're safe, warm, and full.

The rain was pouring so hard now that drowning while standing felt like a real fucking possibility, so I hopped in that van and we hit the highway. It had not even been an hour since I jumped out of the back of the last truck, and I was on my way to Southern California to rob a cactus farm.

When most people think of Mescaline they think of Peyote, when in fact there is another very ornamental cactus that is prized for its looks and contains far more Mescaline than Peyote if one knows how to extract it, and from a lifetime of fucked up experiences involving hallucinogens and plant medicines I was very capable of doing so.

The entire drive down I was battling car sickness which, was a new thing for me. I was restless and I was crampy, and when they decided to stop in LA at some hole in the wall Vietnamese restaurant, the smell in that place turned me green and, for the first time in my life, I said no thank you to a free meal. I waited outside by the van, puking up foamy bile that burned the back of my throat and lips so badly. You learn to hide your sickness from fellow travelers because they will leave you behind quickly, and LA was not somewhere I wanted to be stranded! I had told them that I had a bad experience once with Vietnamese food so I was just going to hang out outside while they ate. A woman who saw me attempting to puke out all of my organs must have felt bad for me and, to my surprise, she gave me an entire bag full of what looked to be homemade tortillas without saying a word.

It would be two more days of slow travel. The van kept overheating, as they often do. It would be two days of hot as hell sun, plastic tasting gas station bathroom water, violently shitting myself, vomiting, pus filled gums, and the only thing that I could slightly stomach was the tortillas, which I had hidden away and secretly ate. I did not want to share the one resource I had. All the while not a single person in the van knew I was going through this. We talked on what supplies we would need, how to despine the cacti, how to get them refined enough to put into gel tab form. We would need to sell it all at once because, unlike weed, people only want hallucinogenics once in awhile. It was vital to sell it in bulk. We went over every factor like we were in some fucking bank heist movie.

The farm was a good two hours past LA in some remote little town on a dusty back road, so driving by it to look was problematic, I explained to the others, who did not grow up in small towns. We would instantly be noticed driving by in a van they had never seen. It was a magazine article that had caught the 'leader' of these kids' attention. It had mentioned that these particular cacti where once used in rituals, and that got him reading more at a local library's free internet, so all we had was a printed map in hand and a magazine with a few photos of the front of the farm.

What we didn't have in the pitch dark of a tiny town with no street lights and packs of stray dogs, was the knowledge that these particular cacti where grown behind tall adobe-type fences with legit razor wire atop of them. We knew they were there because those plants towered over the six foot walls. I ignored the feeling of my heart sinking, realizing these allies were well over a hundred years old. Their first idea was for me to go over, as I could, according to them, 'maneuver' over or through the razor wire somehow. I instantly said I was too short to make it back over the wall and, even if I could, these would be very heavy bags once full. I'd not be able to lift them while trying to climb!

Ripping the carpet out of the bottom of the van, we threw it over the razor wire and over they went with ease. It was not long before I heard the cracking and breaking of limbs that took more years to grow than I had been alive. The first bag came over, then the second bag came over. Then the third and fourth. I said that we had enough, but the slaughter did not end until the eighth bag came over and in an instant we were driving way too fast down those old roads, racing towards the interstate. The entire trip back I talked with her, this plant ally. Begging her forgiveness for how we collected her, for not leaving any offerings, for what we intended to do with her. I begged her to understand that I needed this money, that I needed her help. "Can't you help me?"

In a matter of days, we were at an old farmhouse in a remote little town of Humboldt county slowly and carefully pulling off the spines, removing the skin, breaking down, adding chemical solvents, simmering down, straining, straining, straining. At this point, there was no real food anywhere in that house. I was eating condiment packages and some chickweed I found outside and had a wad of Yarrow leaf in my lip on my massively infected gums like it was chewing tobacco. I believe it was this pure hunger that made the others impatient and me cave once again. It was not ready to be laid out into small doses. It still needed days of reducing, but the only thing standing between us and the money it would take to truly eat were those days. The group decided they would just use the gelatin meant to make the tabs to make jello and we would hand it out at a fucking rave that was planned for that night in a remote industrial zone of Eureka.

I need you to know that I hate rave music. Techno, dubstep, electronic, soulless, computer based shit fucks with the neuro pathways in your brain on a very deep level. In no way shape or form did I want to attend this rave, but we all got a tray of the "jigglers" and each of us had to earn our own damn money, so the hustle was on. I could hear the thumping as soon as we pulled up, and I could see the subtle flashes of light escaping from the windows that had been boarded up. As we walked up those steep, dank, dungeon like cement steps with old rusted pipes for handrails the sickening smell of fake coconut washed over us, and a fog machine flooded the confined space with its poison.

Thump, thump, thump, thump. So loud it shook my teeth. The strobe lights were giving me an instant headache. I just wanted to get the fuck out of there and I saw about four miles back was a best western or some shit, so I fantasized about a room and I hustled my ass off. This rave, in particular, seemed to be mainly women, so when they had a choice between eating the jigglers off of a tiny, nonthreatening dreadlocked girl's tray versus a big, for-sure aggressive looking guy's tray, well, you can guess who they decided to buy from. That and I am a born hustler. Shit is in my DNA. I was selling it for half the cost because quick money earned now was better than dreams of tons of money that never comes.

Thump, thump, thump, thump. It was so fucking hot and my stomach was cramping from hunger and anxiety. I was dizzy and so desperate to hand out these very tiny squares of jello that I had made a forever life changing mistake. I didn't put gloves on before handing out this potent drug all night. As I was sweating with my pores wide open from the heat, I massively dosed myself with mescaline transdermally. There was a whole table of oranges there, all sliced up and I was starving. The thing about mescaline, unlike other hallucinogens, is that you don't know you are high, or at the very least you just don't realize how high you are unless someone tells you. Since I did not knowingly ingest the drug, I was completely oblivious to myself gorging on the orange slices. I was just so hungry, and they were so flavorful - juicy and cold from the ice they were resting in that seemed to never melt. I didn't think I was eating an unreasonable amount until a concerned college student stopped me.

Thump, thump, thump, thump. Suddenly I could not see the people I had come with and there was panic as my pack was back at that house. Racing around in the flashing light trying to find familiar faces was impossible, and the light quickly became claustrophobic. It was so loud and the bodies were so tightly packed that when I animalistically screamed at the top of my lungs not a single human noticed me drowning. The incessant beat stopped for a split second and then the speakers blared "Don't worry, about a thing, cause every little thing, gonna be alright" the intro to the Bob Marley song 'Three Little Birdies' and I remember thinking, "Oh thank God, they are going to play some Bob Mar........", but before I could finish the thought it became a horrible techno remix that just ripped the song apart. That was the end for me.

I sat the almost empty tray down and pushed my way to the door, flew down those stairs, and as soon as the cold outside air hit me I collapsed into a fetal position. Rain began to pour from the sky. Before I knew it was by the van, vomiting up entire Orange slices, rinds and all, almost choking as they came up. I saw I had not even chewed a majority of them. I looked up at the sky, I guess to see where the rain had come from. Every single drop was a different color against that dark sky, some colors that do not exist, and suddenly every drop that landed on me felt like it was as heavy as the whole world. Each drop brought me pain like I was being burned with cigarettes again and again.

Somebody threw me in the van. I am pretty sure I was begging to be taken back to the house while I vomited because my pack was there. Reality was flashing in and out of existence, or maybe I was blacking out. Maybe I was slipping in and out of dimensions, who knows? The only thing I clearly remember from that point is crawling into my sleeping bag in the middle of the living room floor, while an ecstasy, meth, and mescaline party raged around me. I hid in that dark space until it slowly began to glow green. It reminded me of the glow I had seen during my overdose a lifetime ago.

In reality, it was the early morning light landing on my green sleeping bag. In an instant, my stomach cramped up, and I ran to the bathroom, tripping over various people that were sleeping on the ground. I shit and puked for what seemed like an hour, and was grateful the bathroom was set up to where the toilet was directly next to the tub, so I could do both at the same time. In the end I realized, as usual, there was no toilet paper to wipe with. To whom it may concern, I am sorry I ruined the socks you left on the bathroom floor.

Stumbling out of the bathroom, still not sure what was going on but not being able to pinpoint what was different, I rolled up my sleeping bag, threw my pack over my shoulder, and headed down the road. By that afternoon I was back on the plaza, trying to recover from a night I barely remembered. As I blocked it from memory like I so often did with traumas, Food Not Bombs - an organization that feeds homeless kids - was making their way towards me. They always banged pots and pans loudly to announce themselves, and it sent me into the worst anxiety attack I have ever experienced in my life. Instead of eating I ran and took shelter in a little gazebo. Over the next five days my life was a living Hell of discovering everything I loved about this hard life, the little things that gave me joy, now threw me into anxiety. Yet I still had a burning drive within myself to try and do them.

Food was sparse since I ran from human interaction more and more often. My energy levels where so weak I don't know how to fully describe it, beyond it felt like my life force was being drained out of my very bones. As I sat on a bench on some random trail way up past Redwood Park eating a bag of uneaten, thrown away, kinda wet sunflower seeds, just spitting out shells, an older man walked by without saying a word or making eye contact. Then he turned around and sat next to me, asking if I was okay. I said I probably wasn't qualified to answer that question, but I had been feeling very odd the past few days, or was it weeks? I was not sure how long it had been. I could not figure it out so I had stopped trying. The quick and short sentence uttered from his mouth as he pulled something out of his day pack made my world collapse. It kinda felt like a vortex closed or I went back into my body. "Honey, I think you may have taken some drugs. Would you like half of my sandwich?"

I sat there and ate a soggy tuna sandwich, more pickle than tuna, with him in silence until he just stood up and walked off, wishing me well. When that vortex closed I saw it all. I remembered the oranges and horrible music. I reached into my hidden inner hoodie pocket and found a stack of money and the fucking gloves I forgot to put on. Jezus Christ, I had been tripping balls this entire time and would continue to do so to some degree for another two weeks straight, but at least now I knew why. While I'll not say I was ever 'in control' of this situation, I now didn't try and fight the waves of terror when they flooded over me, and I finally understood why things looked different.

The fear I had of encountering situations that I loved remained real and made me flee often, stuck in perpetual flight mode. Much like when I was a very young child I began only feeling safe around the plant people, and I began to make camp further and further back from town, from people, and from the well known trails. I had found a knockoff red flyer wagon at a park and it enabled me to go further, carrying the weight of my pack, food boxes, and supplies to a dead hollowed out redwood stump I had made my home. The vomiting continued like clockwork, as did the pain in my abdomen. Walking seemed to be the only thing that helped the sharp and sudden pains, even if I had no spare energy or calories to burn.

One morning I just kept walking after leaving the primitive trail. I thought I heard a person coming and my adrenaline carried me for quite some distance. I came across a clear cut opening. It had a huge rock outcrop that I found particularly odd, considering the area I was in, and it was covered in an orange looking plant that I could not make out in the distance. I felt a pulling in my chest - almost a burning to go towards her. It was a huge patch of California poppies, growing out of the cracks and such in the rock. As soon as I laid hands upon her it was as if electricity ran through her to me, enough that I remember feeling my heart skip a beat. I instantly had the thought, "She can help me with my pain!" I am sure at some point in my life before then I had read about her in passing or heard one of my grandmothers speak of her since she too grows natively in Oregon and is all over my home town area but at that moment it was as if she talked directly to me. Who knows, maybe she did.

I fully trusted the thought I had that she could help me. I left the last of my stale top tobacco and filled up an old grocery bag as much as I could fit. Even this large amount didn't put a dent in the patches' size. Heading back to my camp something changed. More than ever before I noticed each and every individual plant and could, to the best of my ability to describe, feel their unique energy, like a personality. Some didn't want me to touch them, some screamed to be noticed. Some had fear and some had joy. All had that same glow I had seen so many years back. After brewing what was essentially broth - since the plant was still wet - on my little single burner camp stove, I took that very first drink of pungent California Poppy brew. It felt like the hug I had never truly gotten as a child.

It had no expectations of me, no deep seeded resentment. The healing it offered was not out of obligation. I was not taking up its time. I was not a bad girl for getting hurt, for what happened to me, for getting sick, feeling overwhelmed with a situation or making stupid choices. It was okay to be going through what I was going through when I was going through it - no guilt. It also slowed me down, calming my mind that was racing 24/7. It eased my pain both physically and emotionally, allowed me to sleep, to feel my nerves settle, to come the fuck down from a damn near month long unintended mescaline trip and, for the first and only time in my entire life to date, I woke up feeling better.

Not just feeling better from an illness - it was more than that. It was a real pain off of my chest. The same pain those first raindrops made me feel. I packed up my camp with confidence and headed to town with the expectations and utter childlike belief that everything would be okay now I could continue along my fucked up path like nothing had ever happened. As I'm sure you guessed that was not the case, and as soon as I returned to society all of the terror came flooding back in from the things that I wanted to be doing, but something else was there this time. Rather, it was that something was missing.

That was it! What was missing was my ability to block out the bullshit I had been subsisting in, to ignore how fucking fake this all was - listening to one more motherfucker tell me I can solve all of my problems by buying a crystal or pretending to be happy all of the time. Smoke some more herb. Listen to one more horrendously long Phish song. Screaming 'Fuck the system!' as we begged others within the system to give us their money. The things I thought I enjoyed were actually killing me or at least allowing me to block out the traumas I had gone through.

Just then some chick with 'instadreads', store-bought patchwork, brand new shoes, all clean and well funded on her 'houseless experience' with her parents money before beginning college next summer, as was the case for most people in Humboldt county who were 'homeless', forced an unwanted hug on me - an utter stranger - and said, "Good morning sister bear! Boy, it can be rough being houseless sometimes, huh? Last night the hotel wouldn't give me a room because they wouldn't accept my debit card unless I left my ID at the front desk!" I replied, "I'm not your fucking sister," and walked away.

As mean and judgemental as that sounds, a majority of the street kids I would come across in towns like Eugene, Arcata, Berkley, and beyond were nothing more than privileged children that always had some backup plan. They never once ate out of a dumpster, got beat on, poisoned, drugged or raped, and then wake up the next morning and move forward like nothing happened. No, they would have gone home - one singular wild cautionary story from their youth that somehow as an adult qualifies them as an expert in surviving trauma. And then they'll happily sell you the sacred crystal or oil you need to heal yourself for a nominal sum.

I never had the privilege of not having to fight to survive daily or of having just one trauma to survive, and this was the case well before stupid teenage years. I sure the fuck have nothing to sell you that is going to replace the work of facing up to the shit that has happened to you, that eats away at you. So I suppose I got what I asked for when I pleaded with that cacti ally to help me. I just didn't realize the help I needed was to wake the fuck up, or that it would be such a long and hard journey from that point forward.

My actions abusing that ally rippled through the area with sincere devastation. The bags full of cacti could not be processed without my help and the guys I had robbed the farm with began simply selling it raw to the above mentioned 'houseless' kids. I could not keep my mouth fucking shut, and I screamed around about how disrespectfully we had harvested her and then adulterated her, and how this is not something to just get high with. I honestly felt it could rip your soul away - never mind the fact that the skins have problematic alkaloids that can damage organs - and these people were just eating it like it's a fucking cucumber.

A dog that was fed it died a violent death, puking and shitting blood. A few kids got looped out of their minds and ended up being hauled away to the mental ward for evaluation. A handful more got violently ill. An almost cult like following sprung up of kids who became obsessed with the high, and they sure as fuck didn't like the words coming out of my mouth. I held myself responsible for it all, so against my better judgment, I snuck into the camp where it was being sold from and stole the last remaining bag full of rotting cactus, catching a ride to the beach and dumping it into the ocean. Later that evening they found me there on Moonstone Beach and beat the fuck out of me, kicking me in the stomach, ribs, and face, demanding to know where it was.

They didn't seem human, or at least their cravings for it were inhuman. I was expecting to be violently raped and killed by the time they were done, but a feeling came over me that I had never experienced before. The urge to defend something, but what I had no idea. I hunched over on my hands and knees waiting for the next blow, pretty much blind from all of the sand in my eyes, felt a big round rock and blindly swung it. It hit one of them square in the face and I heard a sound like someone spitting out a drink from laughter. Then he just began to scream, "MY TEETH!! MY TEETH!! MY TEETH!!!", all gurgly sounding. Instantly they were all running to the van.

I laid there all night, freezing and listening to the tide. The day before I had bought myself four bottles of California Poppy tincture from a local herb shop since it was the only thing that kept my mind steady. When the sun came up I made my way back to my tent hidden in the brambles, dug out one of the bottles, and drank it down like a shot of liquor before sleeping the entire day away. The next morning I was very slowly and very painfully, with clearly broken ribs, packing up camp when I noticed my entire tampon pouch was full. It all just clicked, right down to the unknown wave of feeling defensive of something other than myself while I was being kicked in the gut the night before. I was pregnant this entire time, and this poor child had endured more in the first three months of his life within me than the average human will ever experience in their entire life span.

I sat there and just bawled my eyes out. At a young age - after a very violent miscarriage that nearly claimed my life - I was told I could not have children, and that I would always miscarry the same way around three months. That was something I could not survive by chewing up a fucking plant and spitting it on it, so I took the money I had left and bought a bag of trim. I picked out the popcorn nugs and began to hustle, selling it cheap and fast so I could get the fuck out of there. So I could get back to the place I had run from my whole life to the place I was never really welcome. The place that first taught me hunger, fear, sexual abuse, and all of the traumas that made me run. I was headed home to lose the child growing inside of me.

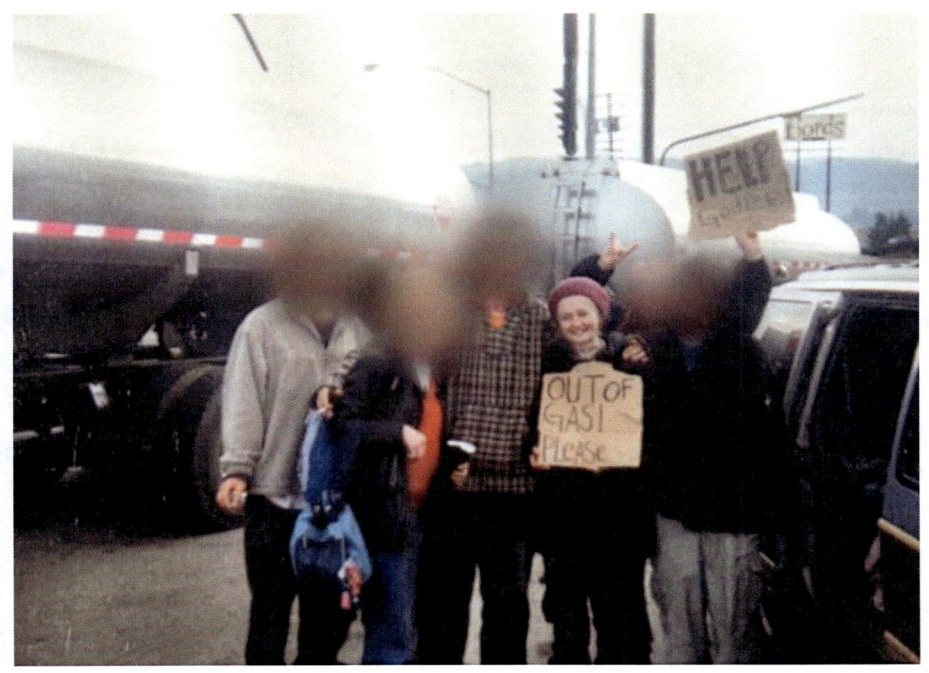

.13.

California Poppy
Eschscholzia californica

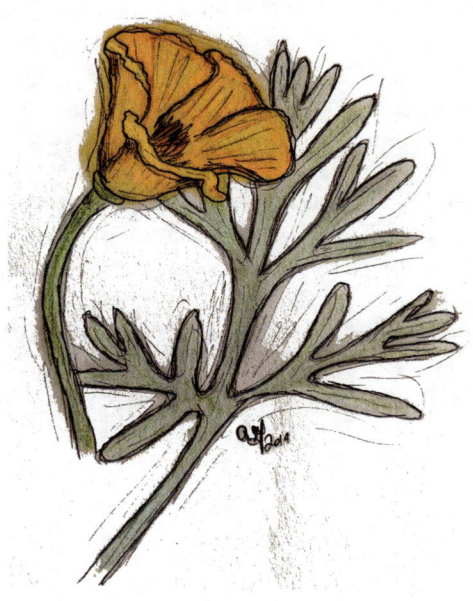

I know that was not some awe inspiring story of how I began a relationship with California Poppy, and some of you may be thinking that I am or was a monster as a child. That's okay. The most powerful relationships with plant allies are often developed through sincere pain and suffering, just like the biggest realizations about self or setting come when our actions are so drastic that we are unable to deny the fuck show (yes, fuck show) of consequences.

I suppose that's all I can really say about that.

The History of California Poppy:

While the thought of sailing on the ocean triggers a lot of bloodline trauma for me, I can't help but be swept away by the image of a coastline so thickly covered with bright orange blooms that it gives way to myths of gold and being able to navigate by their glow alone.

This is exactly what Russian naturalist Adelbert von Chamisso's ships sailing along the Californian coast in the 1800s witnessed - hundreds and hundreds of miles of coastline thick with California poppies! While this man is who gave her Latin name by no means was he the one to "discover" her as many resources will claim, this is one ally that does not have a long history of use outside of the North American continent. She has been used by many western tribes for longer than we will ever know due to genocide and violent colonization.

As the Spanish began to colonize, legends of rich gold deposits lying under any field of poppy gave rise to further exploration. While these gorgeous and giving allies had zero to do with where gold was deposited millions of years ago, it was found none the less and the legend stuck to the point that the Spanish named her 'Copa del ora', which means 'cup of gold".

Of course, this does not mean that poppy herself was only known on the American continent. Many of her species have been in use across the world since about 3400bc. Of course, a majority of this use was for opioids, and it's important to understand that California Poppy contains no opium content. California Poppy herself is actually a bit of a mystery in the way that she is so archaic we can't actually trace where she comes from. You may say, "she comes from the American continent", but the thing to know is that we can usually trace exactly where a plant began on a 'before humans took over the world' level. I'm talking, she is only even speculated to be in the Magnoliidae subclass that she's placed in. Armen Leonovich Takhtajan, a Soviet-Armenian botanist considered to be one of the most important figures in 20th century plant evolution, systematics, and biogeography, refers to California poppy as a "living fossil". Something about that makes me smile.

The many uses of California Poppy:

So how erratic are your thoughts these days, as you attempt to cope with the unbearable stress our society is facing?

How often are you feeling down and sorta hopelessness?

Are your bones screaming from a long life of toil and drudgery, or maybe it's just from that accident you got into?

How depleted do you feel? No matter how well you eat do you just feel like it's not getting you anywhere?

Is all of the above, or something entirely different keeping you from sleeping?

Maybe your kids are having a hard time with wetting the bed?

Do you find your body in a constant state of tension that eventually gives way to anxiety?

Need to support your frayed nervous system?

Got muscles spasms causing you grief?

Is your heart beating out of control?

While you may not find gold in every place this lady grows, it's clear you might find something far more valuable to those of us who are suffering - relief!

How Can California Poppy Do So Much for Us?

She's all about those alkaloids, my friends! With thousands of different alkaloids in existence in all of the plants all over the world, some which heal and more that kill, someone could write a book entirely about differing alkaloids and it'd end up being a hundred times thicker than any bible you've seen.

But I think we'll just narrow what we're gana talk about here down to some of the main ones found in our friend California Poppy, which is a ton of isoquinoline, benzylisoquinoline alkaloids and a few other things, including protopine, cryptopine, allocryptopine, sanguinarine, flavone glycosides (rutin).

When we get into talking about these really deep levels of alkaloids it's a bit harder to keep the talk from sounding...dry or overwhelming would be good words here, but I'm gana do my best to not.

Also, I think I should tell you that I am currently pretty deep into being influenced by California Poppy as I write this. I wish I could say some shit like I am doing this for a spiritual reason, so I can channel the energy of her. Truthfully, I am under insane amounts of stress and I am dosing myself with poppy in an attempt to not lose my shit and burn everything I have worked for to the fucking ground. Okay so haha, let's move on shall we?

An important thing to understand about alkaloids, beyond the fact that there are millions of them, is that they each individually can have drastically different effects on our bodies. Some can cause a violent addiction to opioids. Others can battle all sorts of cancers. Also, it's worth mentioning that the ones I am going to be talking about also have a lot of individual capabilities within each alkaloid itself, and if I ever want to finish this book I simply can't cover all of each one. So I am going to try and stick to how they relate to California Poppy's specific abilities.

Shit. This is already feeling like it sounds dry.

Okay, let's see if we can moisten it up! Keep in mind I might have an oddly dry definition of moist haha!

Protopine is a really interesting aspect of her, and is actually a huge way California poppy is such a nutritionally restorative herb. This is something that I very seldom see other folks mention. To be fair it's really not something we would know unless we deep dive into all of her little parts and how they cascade other reactions in the body. Protopine is how she helps us face down sincere depletion by increasing the availability of amino acids in our food. That may not sound like a huge deal, but amino acids are critical in nutritional uptake at a cellular level and genuinely help our bodies retain proteins.

Ready to walk into those cascading effects? Did you know that there are two categories of amino acids? Essential and nonessential. Funny enough, your body can't produce essential ones - they have to come from the food you eat. These acids play a critical role in you being alive to read these words. Just to put this out there, almost ALL of the essential amino acids are found in meat and dairy foods. You can source them from plants, but they tend to be incomplete forms and will require you to eat A LOT of different plants in large quantities to keep up safe levels of these critical acids.

So how critical are they? For the most part, amino acids are what moves nutrients into your cells. This is why she's considered a Trophorestorative - which is just a big ol fancy word meaning she gets the nutrition we consume into us on a deep cellular level. So if you eat a carrot or a turkey leg and have been using California poppy on a regular basis not only will you end up utilizing more of the nutrients in your food, you will also access more of the amino acid, putting us in a beautiful cycle of getting even more nutrition from our food into the cells that make up your body.

Okay, so we know that when we are low on amino acids we can feel pretty drained, but did you know that damn near every function in our body suffers from depleted amino acid levels as well? I'm talking your immune system crashes, your gut stops working well, you can't think clearly, your hormones become more erratic than usual (you can't "balance" hormones, folks), fertility levels drop, you suffer from insomnia, and chronic fatigue sinks her claws into us with ease.

I mean, would I rely on her solely to increase fertility levels? Nope. Would she be the only ally I use to support hormonal health? Nope. Is she a good friend for immune support? For sure, but I'd get to know some other plants too if I wanted to ward off the flu.

What about mental clarity, insomnia, and tension induced anxiety? She's currently my best friend for these issues! We know that making sure we are eating a varied healthy diet and the nutrition that comes from that will help with these issues and good amino acid levels are a big part of all of that, but is that the only way she helps with these woes? No way!

Good ol protopine joins up with cryptopine and allocryptopine to target our GABA receptors. I'm just gana acknowledge the fact that when we get into reactive plants (like nervines) it's a fucking shit show to talk about because you really have to explain the How's, What's, and Why's so much more in depth than a plant that has reactions because of food like compounds, or doesn't really rely on so many damn alkaloids. This is just me saying hold on tight while I try my best to explain what GABA receptors and GABA is and why anything that is able to affect them is gana alter us in some way.

Okay here's how a science based human would give a simple rundown of GABA receptors:

The GABA receptors are a class of receptors that respond to the neurotransmitter gamma-aminobutyric acid, the chief inhibitory compound in the mature vertebrate central nervous system.

But GABA is:

Gamma-Aminobutyric Acid, or γ-aminobutyric acid - the chief inhibitory neurotransmitter in the developmentally mature central nervous system. Its principal role is reducing neuronal excitability throughout the nervous system.

What? Listen unless you get off on learning all about neuroscience it's okay to have read those words and still not know what that exactly means. Inside of every brain skimming these words are receptors that are specifically created to release a very specific amino acid (told you amino acids are important!) that is called GABA, these acids act as a messenger to our nervous system and brain cells.

The messages being sent usually go along these lines:

"I'M FREAKING THE FUCK OUT CALM ME DOWN!"

Or

"I....can...not...function ...at ...this....slow ...pace ...can ...we ...please...speed...up..."

Meaning GABA is specifically responsible for encouraging or calming the activity of our neurons. Neurons are how our body sends information from our head to our body. Just because there's probably no real way for this not to be confusing, when your GABA is flowing excessively you are as chill as an iced cucumber, and when your GABA is sparse you are more likely to lose your shit. This is why when you take a benzo pill (they are death in a pill and an unspoken epidemic, folks. I raise my hand as a benzo survivor), you float on a cloud of "everything is gana be juuuuuuust fine". Benzos force your GABA receptors to remain wide open, which floods your brain with GABA.

Pharmaceuticals are often synthesized from alkaloids or made directly from them. So while California Poppy is NOT a benzo drug, a hand full of her alkaloids have a similar (yet much milder and far more natural) reaction when she hits our GABA receptors. When we ingest California Poppy her natural protopine, cryptopine, and allocryptopine content stimulates our GABA receptors, and we find ourselves able to gently relax. Our mind slows to a reasonable pace and our entire nervous system takes a deep relaxing breath because we say to our GABA receptors, "Hey, could I get a little help here?" versus demanding to be flooded with GABA 24/7 from pills. This naturally gives way to a restful nights sleep, an improved ability to cope with stress, and the ability to calmly evaluate if the situation we are in or facing really calls for us to be freaking out.

So often people think if something calms us it's a "depressive", and that's for sure the case for many things. How would California Poppy (especially since she's a relative to the opiate poppy, that for sure is a depressor of our bodies) be any different? Well. it comes down to the super dry scientific research that indicates an inactive and slow moving brain is more often than not a chronically depressed brain. This is usually directly related to our GABA receptors just barely crawling along. In fact, we now know that SSRIs mainly work by stimulating GABA, whereas they used to think this was a symptom of improved mood. It is important to say that depression has many, MANY different causes, both physical and emotional. Hell, usually a combo of both, so when I talk on what I talked on above please know I am in no way meaning for anything to sound cut and dry with zero nuances considered.

With all of that in mind, would I, if I was chronically depressed, forgo all help in lieu of California Poppy? No way, but I would feel comfortable leaning on her if I had gotten a handle on my depression, had some coping skills in my pocket, and just needed a little bit of support through a mildly rocky patch. I'd also like to talk about the chicken and the egg issue again for a split second (Is my anxiety causing my depression or is my depression causing my anxiety?), and remind myself in front of you all that relief from either is a way to give ourselves the room needed to heal and or cope with whichever one.

Let's pick up the pace and talk about how sometimes when we lose our shit via an anxiety attack our heart is beating out of our chest, or how when we are depleted from poor nutrient uptake or depression even walking up the slightest incline makes us feel like we're having a heart attack. There are many causes for these and, assuming you don't have an iron deficiency, California Poppy can alleviate them and support our exhausted heart!

Remember how I said one alkaloid can be responsible for many different things? Yep, here comes the allocryptopine again. She's gana join hands with sanguinarine to do some pretty amazing things for our heart health. I'm gana start this next bit off saying I never feel great reading about rats or mice or any animal being tested on, but this next one REALLY gets to me as a person with a visual-spatial mind (in other words, I imagined it vividly).There was this study done to see how botanically extracted allocryptopine might protect a heart from arrhythmia, which is where your heart beats either too quick, to slow, or off in some way. They also wanted to see how it may help protect against ischemia reperfusion heart injuries, which in human language means blood flow being somehow restricted in your body, couldn't get oxygenated, then somehow got past the obstruction and made it to your heart with no oxygen content. It really fucks you up.

So once upon a time there was a lab full of red eyed lab rabbits, and the scientists decided to restrict the blood flow on parts of the body, to the point that when they released it it damaged their hearts. Some of these unlucky and tortured bunnies were given allocryptopine before this nightmare began and some were given it after it was all said and done. The ones who had been ingesting allocryptopine on a regular basis showed not only remarkable recovery, but some showed no damage done! Shoot, even the ones who had only been given allocryptopine after showed healing beyond the ones who received nothing at all (that's how studies often work). While it is hard to know these animals suffered, it was a pretty great breakthrough learning this alkaloid has the power to save a human heart. At the same time, they also discovered that the arrhythmia that was often associated with heart damage or malfunctioning, in general, was greatly regulated. That's just what allocryptopine can do for a damaged and erratically beating heart, but what about sanguinarine?

Well, right out of the gate she is well known for being an antihypertensive alkaloid, which means your high blood pressure (whether it's from stress, hereditary, or poor diet) is gana regulate itself. This for sure takes a lot of stress off our hearts and vascular system (your veins and such), which is pretty fantastic, especially if you also have an arrhythmia. I mean, high blood pressure on top of an erratic heartbeat is just asking for a heart attack! We also know from similar studies done on whistle pigs that this alkaloid has positive inotropic effects, which basically means that our heart (a kinda sorta muscular organ) has a stronger beat, which is a great thing! They literally gave these cute little fuzz balls medicine that weakened their heartbeats to a dangerous level and then sanguinarine corrected it! Lastly, but in no way least, these same studies showed us that this powerhouse of an alkaloid reduced atherosclerosis - a type of disease that clogs up your veins and/or heart with platelets (your own blood cells). If they break free strokes can sometimes occur.

Sure California Poppy can calm an anxiety riddled heartbeat, but it's pretty shocking just how deeply she is able to support our heart health! I mean, how often do we really think of her as a heart health ally? I'd say she deserves to be given the same amount of credit that Hawthorn berries often get!

So we've talked on how this ally can calm us down and keep out heart from exploding, but how is she helping with pain if she's not filled with opiates? I mean, when we think 'poppy' we instantly think opium, and that's the one question I get asked all the time, "Does she have opium in her?" Well, no, but she does have similar alkaloids that are able to activate our opioid receptors.

Our what?

So you, me, she, he, they, and them all have these receptors in our brain that are kinda sorta like the GABA receptors we talked on, except these ones specifically create opiate-like molecules (neurotransmitters) within our body. We now know (through a pretty huge breakthrough) that these natural chemicals are responsible for some major body functions. Of course pain management is a given, but they also play a part in immune functions, emotional responses, cell health, and a healthy appetite. Shit, they're even a huge factor in every breath and heartbeat that sustains you!

They are also critical in stress management. When we are stressed these receptors send out the call that we need help coping!

We can trick them though, and that is how opioid based pain killers work. They latch onto these receptors, just like benzos do to GABA receptors, and force the door to 'stay open', so to speak. Opioids or ANYTHING that triggers these receptors floods our bodies with the opiate-like molecules. It's not that we're not in pain, it's just that we don't really have to feel it because these handy neurotransmitters block the signal being sent from our body to our brain. This is one way California Poppy helps with pain. She triggers these receptors and we feel a sense of relief. This is also how she's helping with muscle spasms, including those that make you cough for no reason, tension, and an array of other feel-like-you-got-hit-by-a-bus symptoms!

She goes a bit deeper than that though, because she also has a decent amount of flavone glycosides - rutin, to be specific. If you're reading this book in order (If not I won't judge. I jump around in books all the time.) you just got done with the Elderberry chapter that dove into how rutin is pretty powerful, but let me touch on her just a little bit here too. Rutin boasts some sincere anti-inflammatory abilities that tend to target nerve related pain. Beyond that, rutin is also a great choice for dealing with arthritic type inflammatory pain because she also helps reduce oxidative stress. That gets us right back to her powerful antioxidant and anti-inflammatory abilities. If we think of it this way, California Poppy is great for pain because her differing compounds touch on so many different types of pain it's like shooting fish in a barrel. One of her pain relief bullets is likely gana hit that one fish that's being a real asshole and causing you pain!

There's no real way to work this into the flow of things, but I can make a bad pun and say we can work on staunching the "flow" of urine that keeps soaking your child's sheets! California poppy is a really gentle ally, so much so that you'll be hard pressed to find many herbalists that won't recommend her as safe for most kids 5 or older, especially in the case of bed wetting. We have already talked on how she promotes a sense of relaxation and is great at supporting healthy nervous system functions, but when it comes to bedwetting there's no one specific alkaloid that we can link this seemingly superpower (whatever helps you stop washing piss covered things and allows your child to rest should be classified as a real life superhero, just saying.) to help our kids stop wetting the bed, but the best educated guess is that California Poppy acts more like a sleep regulator than a regular sedative.

Sleeping too deep is a common theme in kids (and adults) who wet the bed. You are so far in that you're not really able to consciously respond to your body's urges, and eventually your body says "whatever" and does its thing. So as a sleep regulator, if we sleep too deep she pulls us up a bit. The same goes for sleeping too shallow - she'll help us sleep a little deeper! I really love her for this, and although I have shamelessly wet the bed a few times in my adult life, I am more likely to suffer from some pretty legit night terrors (thanks C-PTSD) if I sleep to deep and go much further into REM than truly needed. This is why in the evening before I toss the covers over me I take a dropper full of California Poppy tincture.

Of course, there can be MANY reasons for bedwetting, both physical and emotional, so would it hurt to try her? No, but if your kiddo keeps having issues it would not be a bad idea to see a Dr, just so you know the 'Why' and from there choose a varying amount of options, be it medicines, therapies, and herbal remedies. Keeping in mind that we don't have to choose only one of these options. It can be all three!

I love California Poppy and most days (certainly those long in the past) I am not sure how I would have pulled through without her. She is genuinely my friend, and a very giving one at that!

Where Does California Poppy Grow?

While she only grows natively on the west coast of the North American continent, her stunning beauty has her planted in gardens and landscapes just about worldwide. Once you plant her she's REALLY hard to get rid of, and while this usually has to do with invasive root system, in her case it's more to do with her ability to thrive in any warm place. So each winter when the rains come she is dropping her seeds. As soon as the first thaw sets in these little seeds dive underground and begin working on taproots for weeks before her first showy leaf pops up to greet the sun! Now she's an annual, or wait, is she a perennial? Meaning her seeds need to be planted yearly, err...but not all the time. If she's happy and well established where she's at she will become a perennial and come back from taproot, but it's kinda up to her and what mood she's in during any given season!

If you do happen to live in her natural growing range of Washington, Oregon, California, Nevada, Utah, Southern Idaho, Western Texas, and the northwestern parts of Mexico you'll find her enjoying life in sunbathed fields that don't get too much moisture, sandy nutrient empty soils, rock outcroppings, and abandoned lots. She blooms from late spring well into late fall, and where it gets really hot she may dieback midsummer, only to push up again when temperatures cool, putting on one last golden petal show before the frost sets in.

Have you looked really hard with no luck? No worries, she is a horrible gardener's dream,. If you need a plant that prefers utter neglect then this is your gal! "Please forget to water me," she begs, "Oh no, don't trouble yourself feeding me fertilizer, just allow me to exist!" With that being said, she will readily take to any soil type, and even though she HATES too much watering she will adapt to most situations, and is perfect for planting in rock gardens!

When Should We Harvest California Poppy?

I begin to harvest as soon as she's set a good amount of blooms, and I usually stop just before the really intense heat of summer kicks in (late July/August where I live). I want to make sure that I have a good mix of her blooms, leaves, juicy stems, and even seed pods/buds. This is mainly because all of the alkaloids I talked on exist in different levels of different parts, so when we make sure to gather when all parts are in abundance we know we are going to be making a balanced tincture. There are some seasons where I am able to squeeze in a fall harvest if she pushes back up really well, but it will really depend on your unique bioregion.

What Cautions Should We Take?

The first thing I need you to know is that California Poppy, like other poppies, contain natural latex. In fact, it's mostly within these latexes that we find all of her alkaloids. So if you are allergic to latex, synthetic or otherwise, please proceed with caution. We don't want you dosing yourself and going into anaphylactic shock.

Also because she is coming from a place of deep alkaloids there will be a few more cautions to talk about, even though she is considered extremely gentle and often safe enough to give to kids. Remember how I said pharmaceutical medications are often made from alkaloids that have been synthesized? That can mean if you are on a lot of meds California Poppy's alkaloids may not play nice with the ones that you currently have pulsing through your bloodstream.

Some research suggests that she will interfere with MAO inhibitors.

She is considered safe for kids, but what about during pregnancy? Sadly, a few of her alkaloids have been known to cause uterine contractions, so it's best to keep our distance. It is also worth noting that she transfers through breast milk, so while I'd not personally worry about using her now and then while breastfeeding, I wouldn't use her on a regular basis until my milk was completely dried up.

Some places say to avoid her during depression, but this is the same as when some antidepressants can make us hurt ourselves by giving us just enough returned energy to go through with what we have already been thinking about doing. If you are suffering from severe depression please seek medical help. Once you have things under control California poppy may be an ally to get to know after a time.

What if we are taking antidepressants or benzos? You'll see a lot of folks yell around about the dangers of taking nervine herbs (anything that sedates us) alongside these types of medications, and while some of it is for sure founded in fact, a lot more of it is founded in a misunderstanding of how these medications or individual herbs work.

So if you're already taking copious amounts of benzo meds taking California poppy is kinda pointless. What I am supposed to say is the combo of the two may make you even drowsier and impair your motor function, but (speaking from experience, not judgment) what I am really gana say is if you are on benzos you're already more impaired than you realize, and she cant flood your brain with GABA anymore than it already is because your body is currently drowning in it.

What about SSRIs or SNRIs? The main concern here is that using a nervine alongside anything that is already amping up your serotonin levels may cause something shitty called serotonin syndrome. Yes, this is a real thing if you're taking an herb that increases serotonin levels, if you up your meds or if you come off to fast, or if you're trying SNRIs for the first time. It's kinda a crapshoot. While a handful of studies looked at her for increasing serotonin, the amounts were so negligible that you would likely be at more risk from daily exercise, which for sure increases serotonin levels.

However, if you are going through the long and brutal withdrawal of benzo meds or coming off of SSRI/SNRIs, it is best to stay far far FAR away from ANY herb that does ANYTHING to your GABA (speaking from personal experience). It is like picking a horrendously infected scab while it's trying to heal from chronic overstimulation. Please, just leave your GABA receptors alone while coming off of these types of meds, and for up to a good two years after. That is how long I had to wait to use nervines before they didn't cause withdrawal symptoms to flare back up.

I'd like to end this section by rambling a bit about the need for herbalism and herbalists alike to DRASTICALLY catch up to the 21st century, and to the new reality that a vast majority of first world humans are on one or more medications daily. While in certain situations we can not give direct medical advice and every human is ultimately liable for what they choose to put in their bodies and do their own research, it is no longer acceptable for a publically practicing herbalist that makes a living off of selling knowledge to simply say, "Be sure to check with your doctor." and feel okay with that response. We damn well know western doctors don't know anything about herbs, and we have the power to (with a small bit of effort) answer these questions. Why? Because, for example, what was once perhaps safe for all in the 1960s may no longer be something that is safe for all now, due to the new and rampant amounts of pharmaceutical based chemicals pulsing through our bodies.

In fact, if I ever write the next book in this maybe series, I'll tell the story of how a very well known and admired elderly herbalist I once deeply looked up to threw my mind and body into a horrendous death spiral with her advice due to the meds I was on, and when I approached her about it for the sake of discussion she indicated I must be mentally disabled to think x plant could have that effect, or that we could somehow ever damage GABA receptors by taking a pill. This lack of evolution with our societal changes not only could have killed me, but it became shockingly clear to me how the "Old Guard" of herbalists are doing little to nothing to understand how these medications are changing the very bodies they dedicated their lives to healing.

How Much is Too Much?

While I can't give a specific answer to this question because these aren't pharmaceuticals with huge human studies, what I can say is if you take too much California poppy you may end up feeling a bit knocked in the head the next day. I mean, not quite hungover but just not as alert as you'd normally be. This really is the case for any nervine though, and why it's best to start with really small amounts - like 1-3 drops of a tincture, then slowly work your way up from there to see how your body individually responds. It is best to do this in the evenings when you don't have anywhere to go, and hopefully the kids are asleep so you can really have the space to listen to your body.

.14.
Sometimes There's Nothing

I accept there are some things I will never truly recover from.

There are deep wounds within me that still make me collapse into my own terror-induced vomit, should I revisit them. We all, out of sheer survival's sake, from time to time forget about these festering wounds, if just for a moment's peace. We feel okay, maybe even hopeful, thinking it was all just some bad dream until a smell, a sight, a written word, a sound brings it all rushing back. In that moment our muscle memory lives it all over again. In this, we realize we can never escape the things that have been done to us. We learn to peacefully coexist, in an effort not to lose our fucking minds.

There are some cases when speaking on our traumas becomes an empowering thing. We take away their power by normalizing the event in our mind, and in doing so we regain some of what was taken - not justifying what happened, not accepting some horrendous life changing thing as 'normal' - but taking away it's ability to trigger overpowering emotional reactions. That is how we can reclaim ourselves from some of our pains.

This does not apply to the following, but I am going to tell this story one last time in my life and then bury it with every ounce of denial possible. Because if I don't I will never truly survive it.

I had never seen crawdads so large in my whole damn life! These creatures were like little lobsters - nothing like the tiny guys in my North Eastern Oregon homelands. I had been working my way up and down the coast for months now with an ever changing group of 'kids'. We often camped out in hidden places, following creeks from the beaches well into their freshwater flow, feasting off of these crawdads, miner's lettuce, wild onions I was always surprised to find, and whatever we could score from food banks.

One thing that was a constant in this group was a man who had something I wanted. Something that was mine. Something he took from me a long time back - my dog. This was the same man that told me God had given him permission to steal my fucking dog. Dogs are an important part of my life on a cultural level. They always have been and always will be, but a street kid's dog, especially for young girls, well, they are more than just a companion. This dog also came from my hometown. I picked him out from a yard I had walked passed too many times to count. This dog had survived horrors with me. This dog knew my secrets and had tasted my tears. This was my fucking dog, and he knew it. He also knew I was too small to do anything about it.

So this man, in all of his Christ like wisdom that he loved to preach suggested we share him. That we travel together, and when the time comes we would be shown who's dog he really was. As he waited for a beam of light or some shit to shine on him as the chosen one, I constantly looked for a way to dip out with my dog and get away fast enough to not be caught. In this long drawn out struggle I soon realized I was saving many younger girls from his savior complex, simply by being around to warn them. It became such an odd situation. As much as I loved that dog, I wish I would have let him go.

Up and down the coast, then up and down the coast. From the Canadian border to almost accidentally going into Mexico. The last two runs where with a girl and her boyfriend in their van. We camped a lot, went to lakes, lots of spare changing, even found someplace inland to dig crystals that we sold. I almost felt comfortable and she and I had devised a plan to get my damn dog back once and for all. Then one day while I was taking a piss in a store I came out and saw my pack on the ground and the van screeching tires, the God-Appointed Dog Thief screaming, "ONE DAY YOU WILL ACCEPT WHO YOU ARE WHORE!!!!" He then looked at me, smiled, and said God had told him their time spent around Spliffard, the God-Sent Dog had come to an end. I'm not even fucking kidding, folks.

I will never really know what happened in that van, but it's not hard to put two and two together. I'm guessing she did not accept the immaculate gift of his penis or something along those lines. Just to be clear here, I never once let this man touch me, nor did he try. In his mind, I was something from God, like a test or maybe a disciple, and he had lessons to teach me. I was well aware of his blatant insanity dipped in Christianity and if I am being honest, it was pretty common for the super Christ loving traveling kids to be a bit out of touch with reality. It was nothing I could not navigate around.

In a horrendous wave of coincidence he said we would sit there on the curb and the next people would be sent to us, and I shit you not, in less than ten minutes this old 1950s chevy truck with falling off sky blue paint pulling a tiny travel trailer from the '80s with that ugly cat shit orangish brown stripe down the center rolled up and said, "Hop in the back, we're heading up the coast and you look like you could use a ride to anywhere!" I rolled my eyes at the dog thief and hopped in the back.

We ended up outside of the Eugene area again. These folks had come from Oklahoma looking to get trim work they read about in a High Times magazine. By the time they found us those dreams had long been bust and they were beyond broke, but they were nice and had a running rig, and the knowhow to keep it that way. We showed them how to fly signs, which is not as simple as many folks think. We showed them lots of little tricks for surviving with no real money and even less food. We encountered some kids who had settled down, got a house, and set up a huge glass blowing studio. We camped out there for a week or so. I spent a lot of time in their studio and made a few decent pipes. The lady said she wanted me to stay, and that I could be her apprentice. I'd only have to pay her $100 a month for rent and food. It may as well have been a million dollars. Besides, Dog Thief was leaving and he had my dog.

Jumping in the back of the truck I asked Ron, the fellow who owned the truck, where we were heading, and he said he knew of a cool little coastal town where the locals were really nice, the beach was covered in pebbles, and there was a freshwater creek just full of crawdads on campable land. There is a name to this town, but we called it "You stop and you chat" because that's kinda what the name sounded like. But every time the real name was said during the long trip it made me have one of those power surges, where your whole body shivers with almost a heat. When we got there it was so peaceful and beautiful, a little gem along the southern coast of Oregon. The locals clearly had not been swarmed with homelessness because they where indeed very kind and that creek had the biggest crawdads I have ever seen.

One day we followed it all the way to the ocean just for fun. I remember looking at all of the lush plants and all of the colors were just so vivid it was almost too overwhelming to take it. The life on this day was all just so beautifully alive. It was as if my soul had just let go of all of the hurt and cynicism that had amassed since birth. I even slipped and called Dog Thief by his name instead of Dog Thief. He proclaimed it a miracle, and that God had finally delivered me. I just laughed and rolled my eyes as deeply as possible. That pebble beach was breathtaking, I must have picked up twenty pounds of stones, really channeling my inner magpie.

I could smell the rain coming as I stood upon the shores, and I told everyone that rain was heading our way. Soon the dark clouds rolled in to catch up with their scent and the first few drops plummeted down. We decided to walk to the parking lot off in the distance and take the road back to camp instead of getting caught in the deep brush in a downpour. It was such a warm rain for this section of the coast. A man stood in the parking lot, leaning up against a shitty little white Geo Metro. His hair was long and scraggly, just barely touching his shoulders. He was wearing almost all acid wash denim and I giggled to myself about it for some reason. He wore a baseball hat too big for his head, and his hands were holding this big beautiful carved wooden box. They all were just drawn to it like a stranger with candy, he wanted to know if we wanted to buy it or make a trade for weed.

I can't explain the energy I felt off of this man. In reality, it was more like a void of energy. His eyes had no life in them, but a darkness behind them. They seemed to not reflect light. He just kept talking and smiling at me. I'd reposition myself in the circle we were all standing in, and he would do a little shuffle and suddenly be looking me in the eye again. I said firmly we had no weed or money for his box, and we better get back to camp before it rains. At that moment he suddenly had light in his eyes, as if my words had awoken something. He said, "Oh well, I have some weed back at my house and you are welcome to stay the night out of the rain. I'll even make you some dinner!" I didn't have a chance to say fuck no before the group gave a resounding yes. The man replied, "Great, but one quick thing. Before I allow you into my home I need to hear you say that you accept Jesus Christ as your Lord and savior!" Saying 'sure' wasn't enough for him. We each individually had to say it loud and clear, all while looking him in the eye.

Every cell in my body was on fire. My stomach was in knots. A voice in my head pleaded with me not to go, but the thing is you get in the pack mentality. You believe it is safer to stick with your group, so I rationalized away the danger. I mean, there were more of us than him, right? We all piled into the car like filthy, hungry clowns. It was spotless and smelled faintly like a hospital waiting room. As he drove he told us how his mother had left him this home after her passing and he had just moved to town, but wasn't sure if he was going to sell the home or not. Suddenly, in a panic it seemed, he suggested that we just go get our truck and camper. We could park it at his house as long as we wanted to.

Pulling up to this house was not what I expected. It was for sure the nicest home I'd ever stepped my dirt stained feet into. He took us around the property, showing us his huge thriving gardens. I have never seen a garden so happy on the coast. I began to ask him what he did to keep the slugs at bay and how he managed to get his corn to grow, let alone not mold, when he snapped at me, saying it was rude to ask gardening secrets. When we stepped inside I was taken aback. This home was as void of life as his eyes were in the beginning. It was white - every fucking inch of it. White tile floors, white furniture covered in protective plastic, white walls - but like the type of walls you see in bathrooms that are waterproof, white lamps, white shelves. If it could be white it was white.

Except for one room. One room had a beige carpet and a brown wooden door. This room we would sleep in. The room that was half full of street kid packs, hoodies, a box full of dog leashes, sleeping bags, tarps, all compulsively organized. He quickly said we could have anything we wanted from this room. It was all part of a church outreach program his mother ran for the homeless youth in the area. He left us there to rummage through what looked to me like the last remnants of kids that were never heard from again. I made my fucking concern that he was gana kill us and wear our skin known loud and clear, but they all just didn't care, even though these packs would never be something a church would hand out. Many of them still had personal items in them and were all patched back together like my very own pack. You know a fellow street kids pack when you see one.

He called us out into the living room and he sat in this really regal, high backed victorian looking chair, the kind with fancy brass buttons holding the fabric in place, and lit a shittily rolled joint. He preached hard about sins and how, no matter what, only the blood of Christ could save us. Against my better judgment, I couldn't resist a religious debate. After all, I had watched my mother go through many religious phases that I always took the brunt of, so I had read plenty of the Bible and had much to say. Honestly, I was good at it and I thought maybe if I riled him up enough the others would see how dangerous he was or he'd kick us the fuck out, but I just didn't matter. Dog Thief was just drinking in his crazy-for-Christ delusions, making this man feel like he had someone on his side, I guess.

The entire time we were debating and that shitty joint went round I fully noted, out loud, that he didn't inhale, and he said it was because it was a sin, and if he did anything besides taste it he would be punished. The room went quiet and then he blurted out, loud enough to make me jump, that he would go get our dinners. I fucking hate three things in life: bologna, cheap white bread that turns to paste in your mouth, and kool aid. Fake juice drinks of any kind, really. I guess God was on my side, because this is what he proclaimed was our dinner, and I did not eat much.

I found it so odd that he had this huge thriving garden but from where I was sitting I could see through the arched doorway and into the damn near empty fridge when he opened it. There was just a pitcher of cherry red kool aid and premade sandwiches, in the exact fucking amount needed. At this point I just wanted to go to sleep at get the hell out of there in the morning, so I took two small bites of the sandwich before feeding it and the drink to Spliffard the dog. He asked us to please go into the room and try and sleep, so as not to disturb him. He had to do his evening private bible study. I felt it hit me like a warm wave.

At this point in my life, I had done plenty of drugs of various kinds. Some I did for enjoyment or escapism, whichever was clever, but a few I did because I wanted to know what it would feel like in case someone slipped them to me. In an instant, I knew I was high as fuck on ketamine, which is an animal tranquilizer often used to rape women. When I expressed what I was feeling to the group they said I was just really high and being paranoid, and to shut up and go to sleep. In a matter of moments, they were all passed out, even the dog, as he had eaten my food.

I had not eaten enough to slip into a K hole, just enough that staying awake was like drowning in air again and again, under the weight of wanting to close my eyes. It's hard to explain. I stumbled to the windows and tripped, pretty much kicking dog thief's face, and he didn't budge at all. Every single window was somehow sealed shut. I shook and slapped every person in that room, and at one point I was sure they were already dead, their breathing was so shallow. I refused to let myself sit down because I knew I would fall asleep, so I slowly paced around the room until I remembered there was a jet black phone, the only thing that was not white, in the hallway right outside the bathroom door.

I don't know how long I had been in that room, but there was no more light coming in from under the door. Turning that doorknob to this day is the most terrifying anticipation I have ever experienced. I, somehow gracefully in my deeply intoxicated state, walked right to the phone and slipped into the bathroom unseen, locking the door behind me. I made a split second choice between calling my Mother to say goodbye or 911 for help that would never get there on time. I called my mother. I just wanted to hear her voice one last time. I vaguely recall telling her that I had been drugged and I didn't know where I was, but this man was going to kill us all.

My God, Mother. I can't imagine how helpless you must have felt to hear those words. I can't really recall much of what you said other than find a way to lock the door and don't fall asleep. This is what I kept repeating in my head. I heard someone pick up on the other line - that I remember clear as day. I ran back to the room as quickly as I could. In reality, it was only a few feet away, but I could feel him make the hairs on the back of my neck stand up as I slammed the door and he screamed, "DEVILS WHORE! I KNEW YOU WERE A DEVIL'S WHORE!" The door had no lock on it and my body weight was not enough to stop anyone who wanted to come through it. I dug through my pack frantically for my knife and wedged it in the door, hoping that would keep him out, as I stood there leaning against it with my back.

The light on in the room gave the slightest bit of help staying awake, but he must have realized this. I heard a breaker flip from down the hall and everything went black. I fully expected at this point for him to just kick down the door and do whatever he was gana do. It seemed like every five minutes he would return to the door and push on it, and the second I would make a noise he would begin to berate me with bible scripture, telling me how I deserved to die for being a worthless whore that could never feel the love of God, and that only the act of dying in Jesus' name would save me.

Sometimes he would just walk by, bang on the door, and scream "GO TO SLEEP!"

I don't know how many times I screamed, "I'M STILL AWAKE" at the top of my lungs. It was clear the only realistic weapon I had against him was my consciousness, even if it was almost nonexistent.

By false dawn, I had all but lost my voice and reverted to banging on the door whenever he came. By now I had endured the longest, soul crushing beratement in my entire life. There is so much I could say here, so many little moments of sheer terror that I do not want to pass on to another human's mind. When the sun finally did rise he went quiet. I was covered in my own piss, drenched in ketamine stress sweat. Snot from crying had crusted all down my neck. Finally, they began to wake up. I frantically shook Dog Thief, saying, "We have to get out of here! He has been trying to kill us all fucking night!" They slowly got to their feet. I don't think anyone believed me until they saw Spliffard, who seemed for the most part dead.

I pulled my knife out of the door and we all readied ourselves to quietly get the hell out of there, but when we made it to the living room, I shit you not, he was standing there with a fucking breakfast tray, saying, "April had a rough night dealing with her demons, but I think you'll all feel better once you hear my bible study conclusion while eating a warm breakfast!" They all just filed past him like nothing. The goddamn second I got near him he let out a demonic wail, grabbed me by my hoodie and started screaming that I was a whore. In an instant, like some lizard shedding its tail, I slipped out of that hoodie he was clinging to, grabbed my pack and jumped in the back of the truck. His piece of shit Geo Metro was blocking the way, so we drove over his lawn and smashed down a little wooden fence. but not before he threw his bible at me with incredible fucking aim, hitting me square in the nose causing blood to explode everywhere.

I didn't really know where we were driving too. I don't think anybody did. I just laid there in the back of the truck with the wind whipping me from highway speeds, cycling between numb silence, sleep, and delirious laughter. All the while these people had no clue what had really happened. I remember crossing the state line and a man asking me if I had any fruit looking shocked when he saw my blood covered face. I remember drifting in and out of sleep. I remember Dog Thief shaking my foot to wake me up and seeing the Redwoods. He had woken me to tell me that he forgave me but hoped I had learned my lesson about not letting Jesus into my heart - that none of that would have happened if I had just accepted the love and the plan that God had in store for me. I just laid there, petting a somehow still alive dog until we came to a stop sign behind a long string of cars. Then I said goodbye to Spliffard, grabbed my pack, and hopped out without saying a word.

As they drove away that motherfucker couldn't resist screaming about how he knew God would show who the dog's true owner was.

Years have passed. I buried this deep inside of me. I just never thought of it, just blocked his face out, because that's just what you have to do to keep focusing on daily survival when you're on the streets. Until four years ago. While the TV played in the background, more noise than being watched, it all hit me again like a wave and I passed out while standing up. I had seen his face on the screen after well over a decade of refusing to recall it.

Suddenly I knew his name, and how many people he killed.

I now know, ironically, he is even housed in a maximum security prison in my proverbial back yard.

I know that the cop who didn't give a fuck about what some dirty homeless chick had to say could have stopped this from happening to others, should he have shown a single ounce of compassion.

I know he was caught a year later.

I know they say only one person ever survived an encounter with him, but they are wrong.

Five people and a dog survived this man because he wasn't brave enough to look an 86 pound girl in her face and fucking kill her in the name of Christ.

But in a way, knowing who you were freed me. My entire body unclenched as I learned of how pathetic you truly were. I say were because you will never be an 'are' again. Think about that really deeply. Your story is over. The odds are good this is the first time in a long time anyone has written of you, and I didn't even say your name.

So why are you reading these ripped out pages of a book? I wanted you to know I'm still out here - the cunt that ruined it all for you that night. I am your failure, because I know you. It's not the dead ones that haunt your dreams in that isolation cell. No, it's those of us that got away and in this, you now hold all the pain, because I am done with it.

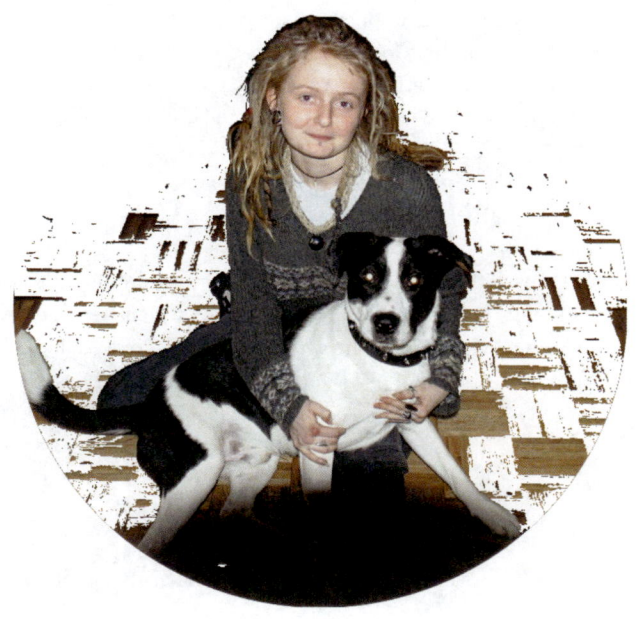

.15.
My name is Hidden

I closed my eyes and asked of myself to see a part of myself unknown. This part of me could show itself however she saw fit. It could be a human, a plant, a talking fucking rock. Anything. I told myself when I showed myself to me I would name this thing and in that, I would have no choice but to see its existence in myself.

Names, after all, speak things into our consciousness.

I sat in the early morning cold in my horribly drafty home with my eyes closed. Nothing came. I could only see the darkness of my eyelids.

As a person who lives with imaginational abilities that would drive a sane man the other way this was incredibly frustrating. When I opened my eyes a lightning bolt of thought struck, and I closed them again.

I was not seeing nothing. I was seeing the darkness of me. I asked her to share her name and my own voice said, "I am hidden." Hidden did not mean some imagined aspect of myself that wouldn't jump out and tell me what part of me she was.

I am hidden was the name of the darkness that I was seeing.

"Why do you call yourself Hidden?" I asked, waiting for an answer that did not come from my own conscious thoughts.

Eventually a small quivering voice said, "Because I don't want to be with anyone."

"Why, Hidden? Why don't you want to be with anyone?"

I sat there waiting in silence.

She replied, "They won't understand me."

"Why won't they understand you Hidden?"

This time an answer came with no hesitation.

"I am different."

In an instant my mind raced back through childhood moments, like some old film reel being rewound much too quickly to truly see each picture within a frame. What was clear as day is how I felt through my entire childhood, through my teen years, through it all.

Vastly and chronically misunderstood, treated as broken, weird, odd, as needing fixing, as not accepted, as couldn't be played with, as felt too much, as to blame, too emotional, as unable to accept things for how they are, for thinking too much, too often, too different...

The girl you have read this woman write about spent her entire life...hidden for the sake of acceptance, for the sake of survival. For the sake of anyone's comfort beside my own.

I am Hidden.

This time I closed my eyes to calm the flow of tears. It was too early in the morning for this as I thought about all of the things needing to be achieved today.

An image had come through Hidden's darkness. A little square piece of paper cut from a notebook I had very long ago fashioned into a pass of sorts. A thing I could surely show the kids in the field, including my older sister. A thing that would show them that no matter what they said I did belong in their club under that massive locust tree.

This image drifted down in my mind, floating like a fall leaf dances to the frosted grass and becomes caught on what looks to be a piece of bare copper wire, all soft from the heat that it bends just enough. It began to flow downward as if it had become a fluid, but it never slipped off of this wire.

I asked "What is holding you, Hidden? Why can't you slip away?"

No reply. I felt silly so I opened my eyes and intended to get out of my head.

Within a split second of opening them, I lost my breath when a voice so calm it somehow was all consuming said,

"You are."

This is why I tell these stories. This is why I began to scream, to cry. To publicly talk about all of the hard things that a vast majority would prefer we keep tucked away and surely should give trigger warnings before we discuss.

I refuse to be Hidden.

The very things that so often mean even as an adult I will be chronically misunderstood, as people who don't share my levels of trauma can't grasp how this affects every word I ever form. When they have a hard time relating they often respond with a violent emotional outlash that leaves no chance of understanding, let alone space for compassion.

Treated as broken by every human who thrives in their current spiritual bypassing state, as they tell me I asked for these traumas before I was born, that my suffering came from lack of a positive mindset, or that I was a horrible person in my past life and that I have to pay for my bad karma with rape, abuse, and pain.

Treated as weird for feeling my traumas are like the child I never got to be. A thing that needs to be protected from the outside world that would try and strip these sacred parts of self away. Nourished instead of left in a dark space to become the Hidden, seen as something worthy just the way they are.

Seen as odd for thinking differently about my pain than the norm dictates, for having the idea that my traumas make me stronger than the untouched. That they helped rip the ego we are all born with to shreds so I could begin to grow in ways an untouched ego would never allow.

As needing fixed from those who believe if I can just cough up a few hundred bucks for their course or some course they have taken that I'm sure to reach enlightenment. That they or this thing they swear by is somehow powerful enough to reach into my psyche and remove the very things that played a huge role in shaping me into the woman I am today. These are the same people who will read these pages and offer unasked for advice as to how I should go about "removing" my traumas.

As someone who certainly can't be played with, as it is uncomfortable to ever have discussions that don't end up making us feel all better. That are not always spoken with a soft spiritual voice, that allows vulgarity to act as a beautiful release for tension. Someone who can laugh at the painful, the tragic, the humanity that is supposed to leave us in silence and should not be played with.

It is tragic and sad how easily I and likely you could keep this list going.

Can I tell you a secret?

The only way we can survive our traumas is to understand that we already have, and the pain we feel now is from Hidden being born. The pain I ran to and from for all of those years was caused by my inability to look at her, at me, at it, and say I accept you wholey for who you are and how that feels.

Only when I stopped allowing myself to be told by the outside world that these parts of myself are broken and need to be healed was I able to understand that it was, in fact, the drive to "fix" myself that was causing me pain.

It is painful to rip a part of who you are out of your chest, and it leaves quite a hole that a majority will tell you shoving "live, laugh, love" level spirituality will fill.

It won't. You will become ravenous. You will begin feeding the Hidden. It will never be satiated.

You will dance from one thing to the next, to things created often by another human who is striving to find a way to reach enlightenment, without ever thinking there is something damaging about dividing experience and feeling into worthy and whole from unworthy and broken.

There is no wholeness of self without wholeness of self, and that damn well fucking includes the painful parts that so many are trying to remove.

There is another truth for me though. I could not hold Hidden all on my own, so I had to find a place to put her. Places that in ways existed just for her.

I put Hidden in these pages. In that Instagram post. Into that tincture.

I weave her into my prayers of gratitude left upon the land.

In this, I found another something hidden. Power.

The power to turn my pains into the very things that saved me. Into the things that give me the knowing I am strong enough to endure when others think about laying down under the weight of any given thing. The very ability that allows me to help others no longer feel alone or ashamed with their all consuming Hidden, just from the simple act of no longer remaining hidden for others false comforts.

Our pains are not something to be removed. It's our relationship with them that must shift if we ever wish to do more than simply survive.

You are not broken. I am not broken.

We are more powerful than they could ever imagine, let alone hope to be.

I am no longer hidden, and in this I am free.

.16.

How to Avoid Making Things Full of Piss & Pesticides

Always look into the legality of where you are or are not allowed to gather in your unique area.

This is a very real issue. I can't tell you how many beautifully taken pictures of someone gathering herbs I've seen plastered all over social media where it's obvious that basket full of Dandelion blooms came from a park well used by humans and dogs alike.

Does this mean that all parks are hands off for gathering?

No, we just need to have some critical thinking skills and talk on some nuances to individual situations.

"If weeds are growing they clearly haven't used any herbicides!"

Bullshit. Yeah, I really did need to come out of the gate hard like that. This is the biggest load of bullshit I hear folks proclaim when giving safe gathering advice.

Do you think the herbicide industry became a multi-billion dollar industry because they killed off all the Dandelions and Thistles forever with one single application? No way! The thing is that plants - like people - who have undergone a lot of trauma often end up being creatures of adaptation. So while there are some signs we can look for to see if a plant has been recently sprayed, it's really dangerous to think that just because you see "weeds" growing that the area is free of herbicides. Just to put this out there - herbicides are developed to target specific species of plants, so something that kills Dandelions may not touch Plantain. That's how it doesn't kill the grass when they spray.

So how can we tell if a park has been sprayed? Is it manicured? Does the grass grow all the way up to the base of the trees, or is there a grass free bare dirt/wood chip/roots showing? This means they are paying someone to regularly maintain that park and spray powerful herbicide that kills the grass around the tree, because it's a pain in the ass to try and mow around trees.

That last bit is your second hint - Is the grass in the park nicely green and mowed on a regular basis all summer long? Are the pathways clear of any grass or weeds growing along the edges? How often do you see a crew of workers there? Is there a public bathroom that's maintained well?

Do you live in a nice area - I don't mean are the people pleasant, I mean are you living somewhere that poverty isn't really a thing and there's no low income housing on your block?

All of that means you are likely at a place that the city's parks and rec department has a yearly budget in place to take care of the park, and this includes spraying for both "weeds" and insects.

So how can we ever gather from parks? Well, you're gana need to find out of the way spots. The parks that are not kept up all that well, the ones no one is having to reserve picnic tables for a birthday party in and the swing set looks sketchy as fuck. These parks at best are mowed every now and then. These types of places are honey holes for urban crafting!

Just to slip this in here - although for some of us it's taboo, cemeteries can be great to gather from, especially abandoned ones. These are almost never mowed or sprayed, and often have trees with herbal uses planted in them from long gone superstitious beliefs, such as Hewthron and Elderberry (if you live in an area where there was a large Irish settlement).

While we can't use the presence of "weeds" as an indicator of lack of spraying, if the plants are there in legions - like if the grass is more Narrow Leaf Plantain than it is grass - the odds are more in your favor of not being recently sprayed. Note that bit where I said recent? The thing to know is that just because a park has not been sprayed in a year or two does not mean there are no harmful chemicals in the soil.

Would I pick any of that Plantain? Sure, it will make a great infused oil! Would I dry that Plantain leaf and make a nourishing herbal infusion to drink it? Hell no! A perfect example of this kinda sorta 'external use only' rule for park like areas is Dandelion. Did you know that she is an expert at repairing soil? She often pulls up excess chemicals out of the ground like Roundup, pesticides, and all the body damaging heavy metals that go along with such things. So while the blooms are probably fine in an oil infusion, the roots may contain a lot of heavy metals.

Okay, so what about piss? There is SO MUCH PISS in your park, and if it's a park that has bushes I'd bet that it's not just dog piss but human too, especially if you have a homeless population. How do we avoid this, or at least decrease our odds of gathering something contaminated? Go to the park every day for a week before you gather anything, if possible. Sit there for an hour or so. How often do you see dogs? Are they on their leash or off?

Dogs that can run around will piss any ol' place, but if they have to be on their leash they are restricted to pissing where the human walks. Pay attention to the migrating paths of humans. We are in fact animals who subconsciously follow trails just like other animals.

Not that people won't go off the beaten path but we conform more than most feel comfortable admitting to themselves. Okay, so that one lady walks her dog every day along that path. Figure for every person you see with a dog there are 5 to 10 more you're not seeing walking that same path the same day, which equates to that pass being absolutely covered in dog and a no go for gathering. These well walked areas and 10-20 feet off of the path into the bushes will be where the human piss is happening. Guys can piss really easy outside!

So if it's a park where dogs are off leash more often than not, you'll either need to come to terms with the fact that what your gathering below knee level will quite possibly have urine on it, or find somewhere else to gather from. If this is not the case you can begin paying attention to where people and their dogs don't go too often - where it's inconvenient.

Really wana find a "clean" place to gather in a park? Bush through the fucking brambles, where no sane human would try to get to when there is a perfect path going around it. In there nobody is spraying or taking a piss. Plus, when you come busting out of there it's sorta fun to have someone look at you like you're a danger to them or their kid. (Haha, but as a very tiny woman that might just be something I enjoy. Who knows?)

As far as telling when a plant has actively been sprayed, the hard rule needs to be that if it's looking droopy, walk away - especially if you're not in the middle of a drought and the other plants of different species don't look the same. For example, if there's a stand of really wilted, puckered, or limp, dead and dying bull thistle, but the other plants near it look fine, that area has been sprayed.

Another good indicator is if a plant is growing oddly. Let's use Mullein as an example. Sure, it is common for her to have 1-4 or so bloom stocks, but if they're growing all contorted, oddly shaped (I once saw one that grew like a whale's tail at the top, I'm not even kidding), or real gnarly looking, there's a good possibility that they are mutated from the area having been sprayed heavily over the years.

Please know these things are not meant to scare you off from gathering if you only have access to town centered land, but it's important to be aware and to be honest with yourself and others about where you gathered what from.

Think of urban crafting along the lines of a large scale vegetable farm that is not organic and kinda has some sketchy practices. You can never really say for sure how clean that tomato you're about to buy is.

Let's start talking about in rural America, where we can see crop fields as far as the horizon. Oh boy, the plant allies on the edge of those fields and irrigation ditches grow HUGE, don't they?!

Yeah, commercial fertilizers such as anhydrous have a tendency to grow some monster plants!

I personally would rather get herbs from a park than near agricultural fields, especially if these fields are of the grain/livestock fodder growing variety. The herbicides potentially found in parks are clean pure spring water compared to the very serious herbicides, pesticides, fungicides, and chemical fertilizers used in big AG crop production.

A funny but sad story - my husband as a child used to be terrified of Mullein. He said it looked like huge dead alien monsters. I kinda laughed and it took a moment for us to realize what he was actually afraid of (and still as a grown ass man creeped out by) was the Mullein that grows in the agricultural ditches and at the edge of the millions of acres of wheat fields surrounding us. They scare me too, if I'm being honest.

They are often 10-20 feet tall, with the better part of 10-12 bloom stocks - all out of whack and producing very little leaves. This is a direct result of the many chemicals washing into her roots.

Those streams,creeks, or little canals - whatever your area calls them - that moves the water around to farms and fields are not natural, and often full of these chemicals from field runoff. Gathering near these should also be off limits.

The only time I will gather near or within a crop-based field is if I know the farmer and what practices they follow (most are all gone, as big AG buys up farm ground and ships in their own workers and multi-million dollar machines). Along that line of thought, if you still have small family farms in your area, it is a blessing. Consider making friends with them and offering to "weed" their property of any plants you may be on the hunt for! This is a good way to source herbs and support your local farms.

So what about roads? These are kinda tricky but also pretty cut and dry. Can you look up from a plant and see cars speeding by on the highway? Get the hell out of there - you can't even make topical herbal medicines with that!

Why? They're full of petroleum byproducts and dangerous levels of heavy metal. These will be very sick plants.

I would be no less than 1000 yards (half a mile) from a major highway with 4+ lanes of constant heavy traffic before I even started to consider gathering anything.

What about a two lane highway? Again all of this will depend on how busy the road is. Try to be at least 500 yards away if it's crazy busy, but I wouldn't gather any closer than probably about 300 yards.

How about busy town roads? Ask yourself how busy. Busy all day? If you can, 200 yards away would be ideal, and I would not try and push any closer than 100 yards.

Then there are neighborhood roads? Always ask the "how busy" question when making your choice, but 50-25 yards is my usual limit, unless you live in a tiny one horse town where maybe 3 cars drive by on a busy day. These are the nuances and critical thinking skills that you will have to use to make the decision for yourself.

Here is a real life example as to why we have to be careful. I live in NE Oregon and we have a lot of Morel mushrooms. Also like many places we use wood chips to decorate the medians separating roads, and since we have a logging industry here the cities often utilize the excess wood chips from lumber mills. These are the trees that grow symbiotically alongside our Morel mushrooms. So sure enough come spring mushrooms often pop up in the medians.

My home town of Pendleton, Oregon happens to be the home of one of the biggest rodeos in the world. This means come September for about one week out of the year the population (and cars) booms by nearly 50,000 people - all gridlocked, drunk, and pissing in the bushes (or right out in the road). It's a crazy event.

In fall these cars - along with all the other year round traffic - are shooting out exhaust. It gets all over the road and you'd better believe into those medians. I told his dumb ass that will remain unnamed to not gather and eat those mushrooms because they will be full of heavy metals. He ignored me and began to feast over the next week, picking them each day walking to and from work. At the end of the week he had a slight headache and two days later he was in the ER with severe heavy metal poisoning. The mushrooms he ate were full of the toxins they absorbed from the soil and woodchips. Mushrooms might be really great at pulling these things out of the soil, but plants are good at it too!

This is exactly why we need to be careful when and where we gather, and even more so if we are making things to give out or sell - I can't stress this enough!

Now let's have a discussion about some cleaner and safer land to gather from that is closer than you think:

National forest

BLM

State parks (though you usually can't gather here without a permit)

Private logging lands that give public access as a show of good faith to the nearby community

I can't tell you how many times I've had someone online scream around at me about how it's a privilege to have access to public lands. Not in the sense that we all have this privilege, and if we damage it or don't use it we can all jointly lose access to the places that some of our state and federal taxes fund the upkeep on.

I'm talking they feel that because I was born into a rural and moderately impoverished area of NE Oregon that happens to be next to the Blue Mountain range that I have a privilege that they do not. Privilege is the wrong word here. It's called an advantage to a geographical location. People in cities have more advantages in the way of shopping, schools, hospitals, and transportation, and I can drive to the mountains a bit quicker.

Privilege is something that a white skinned person has just because they have been born with white skin and they live in a systematically fucked up country founded on genocide and slavery.

Any person of any color, sexual identity, or gender has the ability to connect with the land they live near. There are no direct societal systems of oppression in place keeping you from visiting a national forest or anything similar.

There may be some shitty traffic on the way and we may have to scrape up gas money or find a ride, but these are things not many humans have the privilege to bypass.

Sure enough, most of these folks that are yelling about it (it's almost always a well-off white woman - had to say it) simply have never taken the time to see what public lands are around them. They make vast assumptions that these lands are somehow off limits to anyone who is marginalized. Because if they "don't have access", how could someone they perceive as below them - even if they don't realize it - have access to it?

This also stems from a romanticized nature of what "land" should look like. If you go by the pictures on your Instagram feed you'll think the land should be atop of some untouched mountain range that will take thousands of miles to reach and hundreds of dollars in gas.

But what if you could reach land in a day, a few hours, a few miles, the park down the road, a river walkway, a local swimming hole, a nature preserve, a state park, a hiking trail?

Did you say "but I live in New York City"? Cool, there's 842 acres of public land called Central Park.

Now, can we gather from all of these places? Nope!

But should we only go to the land if we get something tangible in return? No way! This is the same damaging mindset that has our world in a climate crisis - only taking from the land and never just being with her.

Let me break down how much land in our county is public the best I can so you get a better picture of what I am talking about.

There are **188,336,179 million acres** of national forest. These lands are overwhelmingly **free to access** and camp on. They belong to you. You can typically gather one gallon of plants or mushrooms off of these lands a day at no cost. Above one gallon a day (per person) you may need a permit. If you are gathering to sell you will absolutely need a permit no matter how little you gather, but these are usually a once a year payment and covers most "forest products". You can also hunt these lands and cut firewood to heat your home or sell with a permit.

There are **247.3 million acres** of Bureau of Land Management (BLM) that are open to the public. In general the same national forest rules apply to gathering. Most of these lands are open to camping and free to access.

There are **10,234 state parks** in the United States, and while we often can't gather here and some of the more popular ones require you to pay admission, they often have reduced income entry and free summer passes for kids. They also often have great camping grounds, bathrooms, waste disposal, clean water, rangers, and even cabins to rent. These are great places to start saving up your coffee and smoke money to take a yearly vacation to. They often have extensive well maintained trails, lakes, swimming holes and lots of things for families to do!

There are also **61 national parks,** and state+national equals about **14 million acres** of land that literally exists specifically for you to visit!

So just from these public lands alone, there are **188,346,674.300 million acres** of public land in our country, and the odds are good if you hop online and do a bit of research you will find some of it is closer to you than you realize - even if you live in a city! Also, the US National Forest website has a badass "public land near me" search feature that includes state and national parks. The BLM has one too!

I have no way of knowing how many acres of logging land is open to the public in the US, but you can easily search what logging companies possibly function in your area, and at times their website highlights public land. You can even give them a call or shoot them an email and ask!

The land is there waiting for you no matter who you are, where your ancestors came from, and no matter how much hurt you carry. Sure it may take some effort to get there at times, but the things that are truly important in life usually do.

Don't be an Asshole for the Sake of Making Remedies: A Blunt Discussion on Gathering Ethics.

I truly mean it - having a lack of ethics in your gathering practices makes you not just an asshole, but a greedy one at that. Sure we can't do better until we know better, but in the case of overharvesting I'm not so sure that most folks aren't simply ignoring that inner voice that says, "this is too much" because another voice is saying "look at how much I am getting!" Of course, if we're being honest there are two types of folks who more often than not fall into these realms - those who have just began harvesting so the excitement causes them to harvest way more than is ethical and the person who makes a living off selling herbal medicines.

The more you take, the more you can create, and the more money you make, right? It can be an easy slope to slip down, especially if you are following clean gathering rules. It can be a hard pill to swallow if you spent hours and miles getting to somewhere prestine to gather from and realize that if you follow Gathering Ethics 101 you may not even get enough to make up for the gas you just burned. That sucks!

It is a common thing though, and it's important that we talk on this often.

So let's take a moment to do just that - talk about gathering ethics for some of the plant allies in this book. It'll be easy to see how we can apply these standards to other things we harvest.

Yarrow~

When it comes to ethically harvesting Yarrow, or any plant, really understanding how she grows is the first step. She drops seed and produces new plants from her roots. In fact, in a good year a patch sends out enough root runners to double, or even triple its size. Plants that are able to increase their patch size via rhizomes can be touched "a little harder", because when we cut Yarrow we have not actually killed her. How so? Next spring she will happily come back from her roots, although the particular bloom(s) you take won't make seed to be spread.

Does this mean we can harvest all we want? Not by any means! Some folks will throw specific percentage amounts out at you, but that can be a bit hard to figure out for most so I break it down differently, and I'll go into this deeper in a bit. For Yarrow though, let's say there are 100 blooms in a field. It would not stress her out if you harvested about 50, however you have to be mindful to be cutting them in an every-other-plant pattern so you are not preventing the root structure that any one given plant is connected to.

Let me fill out this picture a bit more.

So if you have 100 Yarrow plants in a field and they somehow magically grew in clumps of 25 and each clump is let's say 10 feet apart, each one of these groups of Yarrow would kinda sorta be the same plant. I'm not gana ask you to solve a math problem at the end of this I swear!

If you fully harvest two of these patches until no plants are left you have kinda sorta killed that patch, because with no more leaves for her to bask in the sun she can't exactly save up the important sugars and starches she needs to make it through the winter. Sure she may come back so-so come spring, but if what we do causes a plant to struggle then that is unethical harvesting.

Continuing down this rabbit hole, if we only took half of each small patch we are leaving behind more than enough for the roots to not only still be nourished in prep for winter, but also for the roots to trail out another 2-3 feet in the season. The patch can come back even stronger next year.

Yarrow does not grow in patches like that though, so much as she is like an army that in the right conditions will take over an entire field, if we harvest every other bloom as we walk through the field we are not taking enough off of any one root structure to cause damage to the plant.

This is why knowing how a plant spreads herself is important. If Yarrow solely relied on seeds to spread and come back each year it would be unethical as hell to harvest 50 out of 100 plants. Nuances are important, and this is why I don't follow a cut and dry system.

The next thing that is important to know about Yarrow (and to consider about any plant) is how much wildlife relies on the plant and in what stage? This also kinda sorta can't be a blanket statement, because it will really depend on your unique bioregion, how prolific she grows, and what wildlife you do or don't have. Here in NE Oregon, we have A LOT of deer, elk, wild sheep, antelopes, and a moose population slowly gaining ground. Most of these, in particular the elk and deer, rely on Yarrow as late season food. Here our fields and meadows dry out fiercely since we are high mountain desert, but because Yarrow thrives in drought come late summer when the whole place is a tinderbox from no rain to speak of the Yarrow is doing just fine and becomes a delicacy for the deer!

This is why we stop harvesting Yarrow come midsummer, making sure that she has time to regenerate and push up lots of fat leaves from her first year's seed growth. This is a part that will require you to really do the work to get in touch with your land and know what other animal relations besides you she is busy supporting.

You might be thinking "but I took 50 plants and the animals are going to eat the rest!" This could be an issue if I was a dick about how I took 50 plants. A lot of herbalists will tell you to cut Yarrow off at the base since you are "killing" that plant, but this just stems from a misunderstanding of how she grows back from root, and can actually lead to some damaging practices.

Okay so if you happen to be harvesting a Yarrow friend and she has grown from seed and her first year of blooming and you cut the whole stem, including all of her leaves at the bottom, she will likely die. If this Yarrow did not come from seed and grew from a spreading root (which is most common in large patches), she will not likely die. However, if you cut her to the bare soil that particular part of the patch will likely die. Because of this, when I cut I mimic the natural grazers in my area. I only cut at best halfway down the stock. Now she won't put up another bloom that season (it may happen, I've just never seen it), but she will begin focusing on pushing out bottom leaves again, like she did in spring before her bloom was taking up all of her attention! From what I have seen over the years the deer usually eat a balanced amount of blooms and leaves versus wiping out just one part of any patch.

When we harvest like our animal relations we minimize our impact on the land and actually help them thrive!

Of course I am talking about Yarrow here, but this is generally how I am harvesting any plant ally that spreads semi aggressively through root and seed. Scale back when you get to a different plant that grows through root, but a bit slower.

California Poppy~

These ladies' roots are rather fragile and somewhat finicky, and while in her chapter we learned that if she really feels like it she can come back the next growing season from her roots, we really should not act like she will when gathering.

So here is a harvesting rule I follow for plant allies that don't often come back from root, and it may make some people unhappy to hear. If there is not enough to fill up a standard sized basket in the theoretical event that you were to harvest her, there is not enough for you to cut a single stock, bloom, or leaf.

That patch of California poppy has not been there long, or she is struggling to take hold in her environment. We do her no favors playing out the "10% rule" - this is the rule where most herbalists say it's ethical to take 10% of anything you come across.

This 10% rule would give you "permission" to gather hundreds and hundreds of pounds of plants if there were a few hundred acres, and that's not very ethical. It also wipes out all nuances and allows people to get around building relationships with each individual plant.

A quick story to show how lack of nuances and blindly following the 10% rule can hurt the land:

Sweetgrass is slowly disappearing from nature, both in North America and parts of Northern Europe where she is native. Many speculated it was due to overharvesting since, like white sage, she became a thing that every spiritually enlightened person needed to be smudging with. A hands off call was put in place amongst many indigenous communities of both North America and Northern Europe, but her wild stands continued to be harder and harder to find. Then a discovery was made - this amazing plant ally deeply depends on being harvested to thrive! Harvesting a large amount of even a small patch made her roots explode with growth and now the patches are again beginning to spread. She was not dying because we were taking too much, she was dying because we were not taking enough. A beautiful account of this can be read in Robin Wall Kimmerer's book Braiding Sweetgrass: Indigenous Wisdom, Scientific Knowledge, and the Teachings of Plants.

Without the beauty of nuances, this sacred plant ally would likely die off.

Like if we decided it was okay to take 10% or 5% or even 1% of a small patch of California Poppy or any other plant ally that does not grow back from root or depend on being harvested to expand.

This is why I often ask those who do these cut and dry harvest percentage ethics truly benefit?

The answer I come to more often than not is the person needing a way to harvest unethically while still being able to brag about all their ethical harvesting practices.

To my admittedly odd mind this is like me saying "I see your newborn kid is struggling to grow due to lack of nutrients, or maybe it's an unhealthy environment. Whatever, so long as I only take 10% of their food and other resources what I am doing is ethical," While that may seem like an extreme example, the land is who allows us to live. Even if you live in a concrete covered city the only reason you ate today is because of the land. If we do not treat her and her resources as something that matters beyond coming up with rules that allow us to feel good about not so good practices we are playing a part in her destruction, not her health.

Whew, that was quite a rant, huh? Must have struck a nerve!

So with California Poppy - and other plants that come back from seed every year - be sure the patch you are gathering from is well established, and while that may seem an odd thing for a plant that only comes back from seed, it's really not. The first year a plant takes root she will be all alone. She will drop seeds, and another plant or two will sprout up next season. This cycle will continue, and after many years you will find a well established patch that filling a few baskets worth of blooms, stems, and leaves will be less than even 1% of what is growing.

Another way to think of it - If you harvest from that tiny patch you have just found, you will very likely be preventing or stunting the big and beautiful patch I just spoke on from ever existing. There are no ethics to be found in those practices.

Dandelion~

You're not likely starving if you're reading this book in the spring, but the bees are. You can wait to harvest her blooms!

Seriously, even though Dandelion is an invasive species in the US and many other areas of the world she is also a main source of food for the also invasive honey bee and many other wild native bees (Honey bees come from Europe, in case you didn't know). This means each time you fill a little basket full of Dandelion blooms when the spring rays have them coming up from their deep slumber you are kinda sorta making a bee starve. I know that after a long winter it is in our instinct to go after these beautifully sunny blooms. I mean, it makes us feel like we have survived yet another winter, but the thing is that while these blooms are not going anywhere, honey bees are dying off in droves, and we must do any little thing we can to protect them!

Even if this means you can only feast on her tender little green leaves and wait for the soon to come second or third bloom head to be sent up in another week or so. A good rule to consider is that if you do not have thousands of Dandelions in your yard or wherever you are wanting to harvest from, wait until you see the surrounding trees and bushes blooming.

This lets you know that the bees now have another food source besides the Dandelion, as other blooms are now pushing up that will keep the bees well fed! If you do have metric tons of Dandelions be a browser, not a grazer. This is where you take a bloom here and there all across the area until you have the amount you're wanting versus creating spots bare of flowers. Bees and other buggies like to hop from one bloom to the next, and if we can make that hop less of an effort we owe it to them to do so. - they pollinate all of our food, after all.

On the subject of Dandelion let's talk about invasive plants for a moment.

A plant that is not from the country you are living in is considered invasive. Wild mustard (not related to mustard) is a perfect example. She is basically impossible to kill, and yearly she take's over thousands of acres of land, choking out less aggressive native plants.

However, a plant can start invasive and then after many years be classified as "naturalized". Mullein is a good example of this. No matter what you have heard, she is not native to North America, but because she does not take over undisturbed land in a way that puts pressure on native plant species she is considered naturalized.

Then - to add some spice to the mix - a plant can be from one part of a landmass and wind up getting transplanted to a different part and become an invasive species or considered naturalized to the area.

Invasive plants give us a chance to kinda sorta throw our harvesting ethics out the window, while still doing amazing work to support our bioregion. Let's dig in.

I want you to go out and harvest as much wild mustard (Sinapis arvensis) as you possibly can. I'll personally fucking pat you on the back for picking every single plant within a mile radius, even if you end up wasting a good amount of what you harvested! Why? She is murdering the land and wiping out other plant allies because most environments she finds herself in allow her to explode with unchecked growth, unlike her native habitats .

When we have an invasive species that is both aggressive and has medicinal/food uses in our environment,it is downright our responsibility as herbalists or wild food crafters to utilize this unfortunate resource in every way possible before focusing on plants native to the area. It becomes a One Two Three Punch if an invasive plant is taking over the environment and we are harvesting the native plants that are already having to fight for space. When we favor native plants over invasive ones we end up making more room for the invasive species to take hold.

This is how I can make gallons and gallons of tincture a year and still practice extremely ethical gathering. I look to the invasive plants and I make an important dent, especially since sooooooo many of the invasive plants that are here tend to have been brought here on purpose as food and medicines from varying cultures.

What about naturalized?

I have some thoughts on this that kinda go along the lines that if a plant is considered naturalized and is doing no harm to the bioregion, it should at some point in time just be considered a native plant. Plants are not people who acknowledge borders, ethnicity, or culture. That, and plants have been hopping from one landmass to the next long, long, looooong before humans even made up these borders, but that's just what I think.

Anyhow, here is where nuances come into play with naturalized plants. Let's say there is a year where Mullein does not do so great, like this year in my neck of the woods. There was not many second year plants that would create bloom stocks which, in turn, create seed. On years like this I am pretty hands off because what I harvest this season will directly affect the next two years worth of Mullein that will (or won't) be growing.

On the flip side, if I let a patch be for a few years and I get up on that mountain to discover a field of Mullein so thick that she is beginning to choke out the sunlight to the native plants below her, the situation calls for something different. While in a natural setting of undisturbed ground she almost never gets this aggressive, if the land has been recently disturbed from logging she will move in much quicker than the less aggressive native allies. At this point I will fill the back of my truck with her, and even snap bloom stocks of what I can't take to make sure metric tons of seed aren't going to drop, making an entire field of first year plants the next growing season. We will also have to return the next season and do the same thing if we notice just as many first year plants planning to bloom next year.

This corrects two years of overgrowth, and in two seasons we can throw the next two years worth of growth back into balance. The same thing should be done with native plants that become invasive. A great example we have here is our wild Roses. While they are native, as other native plants die back they fill in these gaps with severe aggression, and in doing so they become invasive - to the point that it is affecting the grazing lands of many wildlife. So while we love her, value her, and want her here, it's still important that we cut back a large amount of her.

Dandelion we will never get rid of, and she does not really pose a threat to any habitat, beyond the artificial, water-sucking, land killing, perfectly manicured home lawns. Knowing when to go hands off and when we can honestly gather as much as we want comes down to understanding the nuances of the land and her rhythms. I suppose this is why I find most percentage based gathering rules deeply misguided.

Elderberry~

"I am always having to fight the birds for my Elderberries!" This is what I see talked on again and again come fall. Yet what I never see truly discussed is the fact that if your Elderberry trees are picked clean before fall sets in you are living in a stressed bioregion. Yes, a lot of different birds rely on Elderberry as a small part of their diet in the fall and early winter, but it is not a main food source - at least it shouldn't be!

This means that if those berries get eaten up by the birds in your area the second they turn any shade besides green, those birds are having to fight for scant resources. I first noticed this about a decade ago when I was walking down a river walkway in my hometown and the elderberries had been stripped from top to bottom on the better part of 20 different trees, all down the river. I'd have maybe blamed it on humans if it wasn't July and the berries were just beginning to ripen, or if the trees were not too big for a human to reach the top. The next week I went up in elevation, away from town where nature was ample. There the berries were not stripped by the birds. A week later and the berries are still just fine. Come fall harvest, at best part of a cluster or two would be eaten, way up at the top. Please know there is no lack of birds in our mountains. In fact, birdwatchers from all over the country come here because we have such an impressive array of wild birds in one little bioregion.

I have watched this again and again over the years, and even began watching other small towns in the area. In/near town trees are always picked clean, but find some nearby nature and the picking was always far less aggressive, even not visible. This really shouldn't be a surprise though, considering that in towns and cities we have covered up all of the land with asphalt, concrete, and lawns. There is no more wild habitat for the natural berries, seeds, nuts, and bugs. In most areas birds are having to eat anything they can - ripe or otherwise - to get by.

This is why I feel a good rule to consider is this: If you are having to fight the birds for wild Elderberries you should consider bowing out of the battle because these birds are hungry. You can likely find a healthier area to harvest from, or grow your own trees and net them. If we find some nice Elder trees or bushes that the birds are not eating does this mean we can just take as many as we can reach? I'm pretty sure you can guess what I'm gana say to that -nope!

Just because birds don't overly rely on Elders in the summer does not mean they are not an important food source in the winter. In fact, grouse really rely on the berries that fall out of the tree, the same as quail and little field mice (and deer, although they like them more in the fall). I generally have an every other cluster rule on what I can reasonably reach for any tree I come across. This ensures every other lower cluster is left behind for the browsers like deer. And my short ass straight up can't reach a single berry on the top, so the birds will be able to feast just the same, leaving plenty to fall to the ground for the other creatures come winter.

What about her blooms? I mean, we know we can make some pretty amazing things - including delicious fritters - from them, but if you take the blooms from one tree you damn well better not take berries from the same tree that year! It's important to remember that any plant (yes, a tree is a plant. Don't laugh, a lot of folks don't put that together as fast as you'd think.) that puts our berries, hips, haws, and fruit like thingies in general does so by creating a bloom, and when we choose to take blooms we actively prevent the setting of those berries, hips, haws, and fruit like thingies.

With Elderberry though, we are given the gift of late season blooms. If most of the tree has already set berries we can gather all of these late season blooms and still return for berries from the same tree. Why? These late blooms 99.99% of the time will not have the chance to become viable berries before winter slams, so in taking them we are doing no harm. While I for sure gather blooms in the spring, these little gifts allow me to gather blooms from trees I did not touch in spring (and even some that I did) without putting pressure on her or taking away from the resources the animal folk will need in fall and winter.

With other plants - like Rose, for example -we can (if mindful) harvest both bloom and berry from the same plant. Roses are a great example of this. If we are sure to leave behind 2-3 petals the bees will still land and pollinate the bloom, and the bloom will still make a rosehip. Of course, this does not mean we can fully strip as many blooms as we want and then come back and do the same to her hips. I'll remind you to always be a browser, not a grazer, and to spread out your harvest as wide as possible.

Damn nuances though, making me keep writing. What if the plant that's blooming is super invasive and you want her blooms or whatever the blooms may have turned into? Be a grazer and strip her clean for the sake of your bioregion!

That Guy Seems Kinda Sketchy to Me, Just Saying~

Are you sure you want to take them with you? Beyond the obvious advice of please do not go deep into the woods or whatever with a person you don't really know, another important thing to ask yourself is Do they have respect? Will they continue to? It is really important to understand that we (as in each individual human reading this) are not the only ones after these resources. This means that even if WE are being ethical, the next human that shows up - and this could quite possibly be the one we take with us - may not be.

Mushroom pickers know this code well, albeit it mostly for money related reasons. Go ahead and ask a person who's serious about harvesting mushrooms to tell you where they go to do so. Good luck. Any self respecting mushroom forager is not gana tell you, and it may even take a few years for them to show a loved one their spots!

This has to do with protecting a resource's whereabouts, and it is something you should seriously considering anywhere you gather from.

This might sound kinda greedy to some or like I am asking you to withhold the land from people, but I'm not. It's just that we are a society so accustomed to having things handed to us with ease that we seldom hold reverence for much anymore, especially nature. So, for example, when you casually show someone where you ethically gather Reishi mushrooms once every four years, you may have unknowingly handed over the keys to a theif of sorts, who may find out how much Reshi are worth and slaughter the whole area. It also may not even be your "friend" who does it, because there is an R factor to consider. For every person you tell or show they will tell one or two people, and those two people tell two people and BOOM! Your once well respected gathering grounds are decimated.

What can we do instead? We can be encouraging in the way that we guide them to learn about the delicate nature of these resources. We can talk with them about a plant's healing nature and why it's important to touch her gently. We can redirect their brand new foraging excitement to invasive plants. In all of this, a person is made to actually learn and work towards their first harvest, and when things are not simply handed to us we are far more likely to value them.

Does this mean we can never take friends and family with us to gather things? No way! But it does mean that we need to be bold enough to say directly to their faces that you expect - should they return to an area - to follow the same ethics you practice. If you do return to find it stripped and you find they have been there via a social media post or whatever, be passionate enough to call them out on their fucked up actions.

Planting Back~

This is a really important aspect to ethical wildcrafting for our medicines. If you are harvesting from a plant that relies on its seeds to come back yearly, you best hike your ass back out there when what you have left behind goes to seed so you can encourage her to come back in numbers beyond what you have taken (so long as she is not invasive).

Some plants that we harvest the roots from make this a bit easier. Since most roots need to be dug in the fall (if we want them to have any medicinal use), after we dig then we put her seeds in the hole and kick the dirt over with our foot. Tada! We just planted back what we took!

If a plant comes back from root don't dig up the whole root! This is another great example of why we need to learn the nuances of each plant we are going out to harvest.

Be Hands Off~

It is really important to let the land rest from your hands every few seasons. Many usually think I mean don't go out and gather for an entire spring, summer, fall, and winter, and they are right! It's just that they don't think of the door this opens. I mean, if you have been going to the same patch of land in your area again and again over the season, consider exploring somewhere else while you let that section rest! This is how I have made so many amazing discoveries in the vast amounts of public land in my area - by having to find new lands so I can let others rest!

Keeping a foraging journal will help you know exactly where you have gone, how often you are putting pressure on that land, what it is you are getting, how much you are taking, and what time of year you are finding these plant allies.

This journal will also help you watch the cycles of the land, and even though you need to find new places you will, for the most part, know around what time of any given season you might find the plant you are after in a new spot!

Expectations of the Land Foster Greed~

So you're spending your day off going after a plant ally that you have really been thinking on. You blew off some event with your friends or a loved one that sounded fun, filled up your tank, and bought snacks. Even dressed great for your imagined selfies with a beautifully full basket of herbs in the woods!

These types of expectations of the land and what we will be gifted often leads to a heavy gathering hand that subconsciously, or even consciously, justifies unethical harvesting practices. Because dammit, we gave up our day off to be here! We blew off our friends and loved ones. We paid money for food and gas. The reality is not matching up with what we fantasized about and now you're saying even though I found the plant I was looking for there is not enough for me to harvest?

Fuck that, I am taking some anyways.

Think this doesn't happen? If I had 10 bucks for every time I have heard someone make this or a similar justification to gathering unethically, I'd damn near have enough money to follow behind them and plant back to help offset the damage they cause yearly to the land.

It is important to drop ALL EXPECTATIONS of what you will find - let alone be given - from the land BEFORE you even head out the door.

If you carry around what I like to call this "empty basket syndrome", you carry around a sense of self entitlement, and this will skew your gathering ethics every...single...time, no matter how ethical you think you are being.

Just to say, if I also had 10 bucks for every time I went out to the land and came back with nothing, I'd not even put a dent in the gas money I have spent on trips that end up with an empty basket.

My basket gets filled up with something that is far more important in the long run!

It gets filled up with the experience of knowing when what I was hoping for is not awake yet, or it was too late in the season for her.

Now not only do I know when I should be present next year, but where.

To know when a plant is just now taking hold, and if I should not burn gas looking there for her again for a few more years.

The beautiful blessing of simply being able to exist with the land and to admire the stunning life that is there, even if it's not meant for me to touch!

Drop all of your expectations before you go home to the land and you will always leave with exactly what she knows you truly need.

.18.

In Regards to Building Relationships With Plants, the Land, and Forgotten Knowledge.

If you were to take just one section to heart out of all the words I have put on these pages, please make it this one.

You do not need my permission to foster a relationship with the land or her plants, or to begin creating medicines. You do not need her permission either, and that guy over there is for sure talking out of his ass.

When we prop up people like they are the gatekeepers to the land and the knowledge she offers freely we are often left standing out in the cold, waiting for something that they don't have the right to withhold - especially if we do not have the financial privilege often required to pay for some course that will "grant us access" to the other side of the gate.

This is not me saying that people should not be allowed to earn a living as herbalists,which is the most common response to my firm stance against knowledge being held hostage for profit. Not at all. It's just that the vast majority of herbalist who earn a living off of selling knowledge do much less than they think to make their teachings accessible - or even understandable - to the very people who need this knowledge the most.

The ones who can't afford your course, let alone quality health insurance.

So yes, we all deserve to earn a living but we all also deserve to have a relationship with the land. If the way an herbalist goes about earning a living is to spread even an inkling of the notion that a person needs to pay for a grossly overpriced course or five (that cannot qualify or certify a person in any way, as there is no such thing as a certified herbalist in America) before they can gather a plant or make a tincture, then they are a part of the problem that continues to feed the mass disconnection that is killing our planet. It's unethical as hell to get paid for that.

This also has a ripple effect, and fosters what I like to call the "I Paid, You pay" mindset. When a person learns about herbalism through expensive courses that often reward them with worthless and fake certifications, their egos have a hard time letting go of knowledge for free. Since they paid for it, so you should pay for it too. In payment they feel validation and worth, above the lowly self-taught who didn't do the work that earns the printer paper they have hanging on their wall.

It gets worse. The I Paid, You Pay mindset then gives birth to the gross belief that only herbal knowledge that has been paid for is somehow valid, or as if money spent is what makes the human mind retain trustworthy knowhow. In this, other herbalists see money as a validator, and if you don't have it you can't even consider joining the ranks of a "taken serious" herbalist. Suddenly a vast amount of herbalists and the courses they sell are only making themselves accessible to the financially privileged.

As I love to say, it's like one big, well-to-do, financially privileged circle jerk, and those always end up messy and making folks feel dirty. I think instead of joining I'll keep talking on the need to change this, even as hateful messages from other herbalists continue to roll in.

A moment of hard truth, though? If we as a species don't learn to give more than we take - in all areas of life - there really is no hope for the future of this planet, let alone humanity.

There is another type of payment gateway often entangled with herbalism. Many will try to sell you a connection with the land along their particular brand of spirituality. They will tell you you must have these things to be a worthwhile herbalist. It triggers my gag response often, and violently.

The very fact that many of these gatekeepers think they can sell a connection to the land in the first place speaks volumes to what little, if any, connection they have.

You can not buy a connection to the land, and anyone who attempts to sell you one in any form in the way of course, video, or even a book is of the egotistical and self entitled mindset that somehow thinks they have the right to claim ownership of this thing so sacred. This thing that is a birthright to every creature born to this planet. This is the disturbingly deep mindset linked to worldwide colonization.

Can we give guidance by allowing people to witness our own connection to the land? Absolutely. Is there ever a point where it is ethical to sell what is sacred to us or - all too often - another culture being appropriated from?

No. Full stop.

We have to ask ourselves this question - If this connection means so much to us why would we choose to turn it into a commodity? If we are really as passionate about our connection to the land as these people often say in their sales pitch, why would we not want to spread this knowledge for free? To share this joy -this thing that saved us?

This is just as unethical as the herbalist who swears they can somehow help you cure cancer - just buy their course and you will be well on your way!

I guess my heart just doesn't understand that level of cruelty, especially from people who proclaim to have dedicated their lives to the land and helping the suffering humans who walk upon her.

I really need you to not just understand but **FEEL** that no matter who you are, no matter what culture you or your ancestors come from, no matter how much money you don't have in the bank, no matter what landmass you are living upon, you have not just a right but an outright responsibility to make a genuine effort to reconnect with the land and her healing ways. You don't need anyone's permission or acceptance to do so.

I know you are smart enough to do these things, to feel these things, to walk on the land with integrity, and to withstand the million screaming defensive voices who demand you need to pay.

It is simply a matter of allowing yourself to tap into the one thing that makes humans so unique - your ability to be curious. To wonder how and why something is. To put down your phone and step outside your door and see what plant allies are living near you. They are simply waiting for you to remember what the marrow in your bones has never forgotten. This knowledge, this land, the spiritual connection so many of us long for has not been lost to us for more than a blink of an eye in humanity's long history, and I assure you it will take more than a blink for our bodies and souls to forget what our ancestors have embedded into our DNA.

I know, truly I know that learning about one safe and simple plant ally at a time is not fast enough for many, but I would ask you to consider the fact that it took humanity more years than we will ever comprehend to learn these things. All you have to do is remember. I'll also say that when I see people being impatient and looking to pay for shortcuts I'll often ask them to consider that this feeling of frustration is a symptom of our society's need for instant gratification. If we don't learn how to let this go we will never truly enjoy anything real in life.

Real things take time, and the time they take has an immeasurable worth, my friends. That simply is not something we can rush or buy our way into.

A Hard-Swallowed Note on Your Worth, the Plants' Worth, & Honoring Wholeness.

This will not likely be a comfortable thing to read for many, and some of you might have read parts of this before. I have talked about the issue many times. So much so, in fact, that I have a dedicated page on my website just for it. This is really important to me, and it should be to you as well. It for sure is to the plants, so I'm going to talk on it again.

You are worth using the whole of the plant that you gather.

The plant is worth using her whole body that you gathered.

When we cast aside aspects of ourselves or the plants we are not honoring wholeness.

Let's talk about the dangers of refined "essential oils", and the damage they are doing to our health and planet alike.

So what are "essential oils"? First, I'd like to start off by saying "essential oil" is a term used to greenwash the real name of something.

They are volatile organic compounds (VOCs) that are found in minuscule amounts of every plant in existence, and their function is still debated. However, amongst that debate there are three common scientific beliefs, all of which likely hold merit.

The most disturbing of the three (when you consider that humans are slathering these on their skin and feeding them to their children) is that these compounds are being produced by plants to act as a defense mechanism against insects. In other words, pesticides! The idea is that these oils injure the rasping mechanism of insect's mouth, as well as using their scent to tell other animals, "DANGER! Don't eat me! I'll make you sick!"

Just to answer the question of what the other two beliefs are - a waste buildup or to attract pollinators. Again, it's likely all three.

Wait, but these are natural.I only have to use a tiny amount and it's made from plants so it's safe, right? I mean, I put it in a carrier oil?

Recall how I talked a lot about terpenes in the Yarrow chapter? How even these naturally occurring levels of VOCs can really do some damage to our organs, and how in naturally occurring levels they're a really powerful antibacterial, microbial, viral and fungal?

Now imagine you have refined these, and I don't mean you forgot your tea simmering on the stove refined. I'm talking one little 5ml bottle (on average for most very fragrant plants) takes about 60 pounds of plant matter to create! So in one little bottle is enough concentrated plant matter to fill the back of a pickup truck up if it was fresh, but because most industries (and even "artisanal makers") often use dried plant matter (and because plants get lighter as they dry), to get 60 pounds of dry plant you'll have to harvest a few hundred pounds worth of plants. All for that little bottle you can fit in your pocket!

So now you have this supercharged version of nothing but the plant's most volatile and dangerous compounds, and all other aspects of the plant have been discarded, literally. We look at this plant (woman) and say, "Hey, you don't know what you're doing. Let me show you how you should be. Hey, you're not strong enough as you are. Let me fix that for you. You are too much of a hassle in your whole state. Let me make you more convenient for me to work with."

And just like that we are playing with dangerous chemicals. Don't kid yourself, these are no longer "herbs" - these are extracted and refined chemical compounds. They are extremely powerful pharmaceuticals. These are things that should be regulated and have sincere FDA oversight.

Oh, you thought they did? Nope. The FDA is pretty hands off at the moment, and this multi-trillion dollar industry even gets away with rampant medical claims, while little ol me has to test every tincture I make to verify the herb I tinctured is what I say it is or I'm making an "unfounded medical claim" that can get me shut down.

These are not things we should be using to make a room smell good or your child sleep better, and I don't want to hear a fucking word about how they are safe as long as you dilute them, so let's do some fun math!

Would you sit down and willfully consume 63 pounds of Peppermint leaf? What? That's crazy to think about, right? Now consider that it takes 63 pounds of Peppermint leaf to make one 5ML bottle of "essential oil".

I know math is a pain in the ass, but I am gana break this down for you!

There are 20 drops in a milliliter, so 20 x 5ml = 100 drops. Just for fun, let's see how much Peppermint you would have to consume in one individual setting to match up to one singular drop of Peppermint "essential oil".

63 pounds divided by 100 = 0.63 pounds.

How does sitting down and eating over half a pound of Peppermint sound - still crazy? Because that's how much you would have to consume in a signal setting to ever NATURALLY encounter one drop's worth of Peppermint "essential oil".

And just because I'm on a roll, lets see how many cups of tea you would have to drink to match that amount!

The average Peppermint tea bag has 2 grams of dried plant matter in it, and most directions on store bought boxes say to use one tea bag per cup of water.

Are you ready for this?

There are 285.76 grams in 0.63 pounds.

285.76 divided by 2 = 142.88

So ONE DROP of Peppermint "essential oil" is equivalent to drinking 142 cups of Peppermint tea in a single setting.

So to really drive this home to the one random person that's thinking, "that's not very much":

There are 16 cups in a gallon of water... 142 cups divided by 16 = 8.87

Did I lose ya? Here we go - you would need to drink **9 fucking gallons** of Peppermint tea to naturally encounter **one drop's worth** of Peppermint "essential oil".

Think I'm pulling these numbers out of my ass? Nope. These come straight off of the buried Doterra essential oil page, where they tell you how much of what goes into a 5ml bottle of oil. Also, this does not change per company, no matter how "ethical" or "small" the company is. The amounts needed to make these oils are concrete.

That's why I don't want to hear about how cutting down refined volatile oils in a small amount of a carrier oil somehow makes it less refined? Unless, of course, you're using nine gallons of oil!

When I talk about this a lot of people get really defensive - like write me ten page angry letters and demand I stop speaking against "essential oils" defensive. Many of these letters will tell me up and down and back again about how effective "essential oils" are at helping them with xyz condition, but this is how I know they are not hearing what I'm saying because defensiveness and emotions have shut down critical thinking skills.

I never said they don't work - I said they're fucking dangerous.

I usually ask people if they would be chill with taking a high dose antibiotic every day? Or how would you feel if your babysitter gave your kid antibiotics every single day without your consent? That's dangerous as hell, right? It kills off all of the good bacteria in our body, makes our immune system weak, and contributes to superbugs!

If you agree with any of the above then you may want to consider that all essential oils are basically antibiotics, and because each one is made from a different plant that has differing compounds every single one will more than likely have untold long term ramifications. But thank God the gal at the farmers market put lemon "essential oils" in her scones so we can all get dosed with high grade antibiotics!

That may have been a bit of a rant, but it factual and it's an epidemic. Do you know how hard it is to buy handmade herbal products without them having been made exclusively from "essential oils", or at the very least they are added to them? I live in Oregon right next to the Washington border and both of these states have recreational Marijuana. In my area alone there are 8 different stores that anyone over the age of 21 can walk into. Out of the 8 different stores there was not a single CBD tincture that did not have "essential oils" added to the blend, even the ones for digestive aid (which is true irony since these refined volatile compounds kill off all of your gut bacteria. Weird way to support healthy digestion, if you ask me).

We know the dangerous effects of the individual compounds within these "essential oils", and while many MLM sales reps and herbalists will tell you there have been no studies that prove these oils are dangerous, that's flat out willful ignorance of what exact compounds are actually in that bottle. I can damn well tell you that the individual compounds that make up these "essential oils" have more than been studied - they have done extensive animal testing on them.

For fun, let's talk about one.

Thujone is this little killer is found in quite a few "essential oils", including the Oregano oil folks swear by, and thujone can fuck you up so bad you literally go crazy. I talked about it some in the Yarrow cautions section, but basically thujone messes with your GABA receptors. Even a singular toxic dose can cause epileptic seizures, but it doesn't end there.

When they kept feeding lab rats scaled down doses per body weight to what we as humans would be able to withstand long term use 6 times a week for 14 weeks (3 months and 2 weeks), the females rats began to drop like flies, and the males didn't fare much better. Because of the low casual doses they were all dying from neurotoxicity in the brain that came out as hyperactivity, tremors, and tonic seizures.

Thujone keeps on giving too, because when they lowered the dose and went with a long term 2 year study on rats (which would be about 45 years old in human years), they discovered the seizures of course, but also (here's a fun surprise!) increased incidences of nonneoplastic lesions (fancy talk for tumors in the brain, spleen, kidneys, and the pituitary gland) in female rats. The pituitary gland is the "master gland" that sends signals to every gland in our body, including those related to hormone control.

This is just the danger of one singular compound found in a good amount of differing "essential oils". One out of thousands. Still feel like these should be freely used in balms, salves, tinctures, and food? Still think it's chill to just have these diffusing in a daycare center or a waiting room? You may be thinking, "Well, I'm not going to take the same "essential oil" for 45 years." You may not, but your kids are well on their way because they are in everything and on everyone.

They are in the soap you bought from the store or the farmers market. They are in the toothpaste you put in your mouth. They are what you taste in line at the store because that person is wearing too much perfume. They are in your lotion, that breast massage oil, that cleaner, that handcrafted candle, that room-freshening spray you made off of a Pinterest recipe. By the time I'm in my 60's (I'm 34 now), I honestly believe we will begin to truly start seeing the damages of long term chronic toxic exposure to these refined compounds. This could all be resolved if we just had the respect and patience it takes to work with whole plant matter that we gather or order. If you don't think you are worth it, I sure hope you think your kids are.

"But I would never use essential oils internally. That's dangerous!" It sure is, and you definitely are. You just don't realize it.

I'm not even talking about the issue of them being added to foods on an increasingly disturbing level, but that if you can **smell** the oil you are **ingesting** the oil! What? You know how when you take a breath air enters your body? That's internal use, my friends! So much so that we know even by just breathing in these compounds our whole body is affected. They even kill off out gut bacteria. Think of it like secondhand smoke. You know how dangerous that is, why would breathing in airborne antibiotics and dangerous compounds be any different? Also, let's not overlook transdermal use. When you rub these refined oils onto the largest organ you have (your skin), you are absorbing the oil into your body. There is no such thing as not using "essential oils" internally - just different ways of it entering your body.

To switch gears, I'd now like to talk on the fact that I firmly believe "essential oils" are the death of hands-on herbalism.

Do me a favor and take a moment to look on Etsy. Go look at your favorite herbalist's accounts on Instagram, Facebook, or whatever future platform is ruling us - you can even pick up their recently published books.
Now tell me how many of their products are made with essential oils? How many of their recipes call for them? In the current "herbalism" trend - yes, trend - there are thousands upon thousands of people putting a drop of this, a drop of that, into some oil and beeswax and ta da, a cure all has been made, and it smells great!!

You might be thinking this is an amazing thing. More herbal medicine to go around! More people practicing herbalism!

But can I ask you something?

Where are the herbs in your herbalism?

All of the dangers that we talked on set aside, what are you trading for this instant gratification mindset? I mean, I get it. It sucks to have to wait weeks - shit, even entire months - for a properly infused oil or tincture to be ready...

...but at what cost does this convenience come?

The price is a rampant loss of connection to the land, respect for the plant nations, respect for our environment, the further loss of ancestral knowledge of plant based healing, the loss of honing a craft and the beautiful time it takes to become truly capable.

I mean, why mess with the actual plant and having to step foot upon the land when you can just order it's most toxic compounds online, put a few drops of it in a thing, and call yourself an herbalist?

All of this upsets me, but the following is what makes me angry enough to keep talking about it.

In America alone there are millions and millions and millions of bottles of these oils produced yearly. Remember how one little bottle of a fragrant plant takes about 63 pound to make? It is even more if the plant has a weak smell.

Okay, let's pretend we made a million bottles of Peppermint oil. Ready to have your mind blown?

To make one million bottles of Peppermint "essential oil" it would take 630 thousand pounds of plant matter - over half a million pounds!

How we can say we love the Earth and are concerned about her welfare, while in the same breath advocating for the use of these refined oils that are using millions of pounds of plant matter - only to extract her most volatile compounds and toss the rest of her aside as worthless? "The Big Guys" don't even use the hydrosol they create, so every single part of the plant is cast aside. The big hitting companies are contributing to endangered plants and trees going extinct (Sandalwood, anyone?), as they harvest to keep up with the ever growing demand that convenience feeds.

I have seen this happen before. I see the ramifications of this type of convenience disconnect daily, and so do you.

As a young girl I loved thumbing through my grandmother's (and even my mother's) cookbooks. Seeing all of the intricate and whole ingredient recipes with all of the intricate notes. To me it was magic that these simple, whole things could be arranged in such a way to make a beautiful and delicious meal. - that simply moving flavors and ingredients in one way or another created a whole new experience of nourishment!

Now in my mid 30's when I pick up a cookbook or click on a blog recipe, 90% of the time the ingredients listed are "a box of", "a can of", or "a packet of". Very rarely are the ingredients whole, let alone anything that our grandmothers would recognize.

Now ask yourself how well that shift has treated our bodies, our cultures, our lands?

This is what "essential oils" are to herbalism.

The death of knowledge and health go hand in hand, and both die under the heel of one thing, and one thing alone.

Convenience.

This is why I will never use them in any of my offerings. I do not allow them in my home, and rarely call medicines home from other makers. Why should I, when I can infuse an oil of my choice with the herbs I am wanting to use?
Why should I when I can make a safe, simple, and easy tincture? Why should I when I can drink a nourishing herbal infusion or have a nice relaxing cup of tea made from whole plant matter?

What is the difference, really? Why does whole plant matter mean that much?

Because refined volatile oils - for all of their strength - only carry a minimal amount of the plant's healing abilities. When we choose to infuse whole plant matter into oil and make this into salves, lotions, creams, and balms, we are actually creating a well rounded offering that has ALL of the plant's healing properties, not only her most refined ones.

Many will say that they don't have access to whole plant matter, and that these oils are great for people who live in the city. Everyone assumes you need access to great untouched swaths of land to work with whole real plant matter.

This is absurd. If you are thinking that it is important that you understand you have the ability to order whole plant matter online (since you likely bought this copy of my book online). There is no shortage of any herb you could ever want online and hundreds of reputable sellers. If you buy in bulk they are usually very cheap. You can even start a buying club to buy less but still get bulk savings!

The next thing people will say is that "essential oils" give them a way to comfortably begin working with herbs.

What I am about to say is important, and I need you to hear this and deeply consider it. To allow this message past your emotions and through your defensiveness. **If you don't feel confident in working with the plant as a whole, you have no business working with the plant's most toxic aspects.** Not only are "essential oils" the plant's most toxic aspect, they have been refined greatly and often behave entirely differently in and on our bodies than whole plant matters do.

You will hurt yourself. You will hurt others. But it does not have to be this way.

If you are still reading, I want you to hear another message that is just as important.

You are smart enough to work with these plants in their whole state.

You are worth enough to work with these plants in their whole state.

You are capable of making beautiful healing creations the slow and whole way in which your ancestors did.

These last words I have to say may very well be the most important.

These plants deserve our respect. You see, it is they who are the real healers, not the humans who wield them. Yet when millions of pounds of plant matter are boiled and cast aside, having only deemed the most volatile compound of any worth, what message do you suppose that sends to the land on our behalf? At what volume does that speak to our lack of reverence?

I'd say it's pretty deafening.

.20.
Harvesting Tips & Tricks for the Plants in Discussion

Yarrow ~

With this gal, if you intend to gather a fair amount and you'll be touching her for more than an hour, I would consider wearing gloves. While I personally have never had a photosensitive or dermatitis reaction, it does really suck to have her oils all over your hands and rub your eyes!

Plus, if your body does have a reaction to her, gloves will be a must when harvesting. Please know that most folks who get a slight rash while harvesting with bare hands don't tend to have reactions to her when, for example, she's made into an infused oil.

When harvesting, attempt to mimic wild grazing and foraging animals, and never cut her all the way to the base. Instead, cut about halfway down the bloom stock at most. This encourages her to push new base leaf up and provides important feed for wildlife. Be sure you are taking plants in a scattered every-other-few-plants fashion versus concentrating on one are until all of the blooms are gone.

With how pungent she is, I prefer to harvest in the morning before the sun gets too high and the heat gets the fragrance of large patches burning our eyes or making our nose run!

If you plan on curing her (like drying, but better), strip her leaves from her stem, cut off her bloom, then chop up her stems into small pieces. This helps the differing parts cure a bit easier/more evenly. Once her steams are cured, you'll dull the hell out of your sharpest pair of scissors trying to cut through them, but if we don't do this more often than not what happens is you'll think she's dry enough to put away and come back a few weeks or months later to find she still had moisture in her stems and now it has caused the whole bag to mold.

Comfrey~

Are you sure that's where you want to plant her? Like, SO sure you accept that she will always be there? Because once you stick this lady in the ground, you're not getting rid of her! Oh, you'll just dig her up? Cool, 5 more plants will take her place, because when we disturb her roots she spreads!

Seriously though, once we plant her we have a friend for life - and if you want more friends just break up a root. Each tiny piece of root will become a new plant.

We can kinda sorta find Comfrey in the wild that has not been planted by human hands, but this is the wild variety and - while she is amazing for external use - she needs to be hands off internally. With that being said, only wild Comfrey can grow from seed. The hybrid variety has sterile seeds and must be started from root.

Have a good pair of gloves! For all of the soothing she offers us, I always joke it's just because she feels bad about how mad her fresh leaves and scratchy little hairs can rip our skin up! I often wear gloves and a long sleeve shirt if I am harvesting a good amount from the garden.

Most folks wait for her to bloom and then cut the whole plant. That is for sure an option, but here are a few different methods to try and find which you like the results of best.

If I am growing Comfrey for internal use I allow her to go past blooming before I harvest her largest leaves. I simply cut back and discard, take the biggest leaves, and allow her to keep growing. I can repeat this a few times in a season, and each time we cut back her big leaf the little ones work on getting bigger.

Not planning to use her internally? Consider not allowing her to bloom. Cut off any bloom stock that pops up and you will be overwhelmed by the amount of leaves she throws up. My patch this last season went 5 feet wide with just one row of plants!

Curing her is a bit tricky. She has a really moist stem down her leaf, so when the leaf itself is bone dry the stem will still be flexible. If you put her in a bag or container she will rot on you. Some say to split the stems long ways, and while you could do this it would be a lot of work if you have more than a small basket full. I prefer to chop her up - not super crazy small pieces, but small enough that once she is cured I can use her as is and don't have to get all itchy again. This means the stems are all cut up and the moisture can be pulled out evenly. I'll talk more about the difference between curing and drying at the end of this chapter.

Dandelion~

We need to wait until spring is in full bloom before we harvest her so we don't starve the bees, but after that it's time to start plucking blooms and feasting on leaves!

It's best to gather her blooms in the middle of the day when it's nice and warm out because her dense flowers really hold onto moisture - not a big deal if you plan on tincturing or fermenting her, but if you want to cure them for an oil infusion you want her as dry as possible when gathering.

Also, be prepared to find puffballs in your curing cabinet! Meaning, if you gather a bloom and she was on the verge of closing up and turning into the seed puffs we all love to make wishes with, she will still do this as she cures. This is just a thing that happens, and while you could compulsively watch for new blooms to open and only harvest those, it's honestly not really that big of a deal.

When it comes to harvesting her leaves for spring eating, pick the new tender growth. The older leaves will be tough and much more bitter. Some folks eat these greens raw. I simmer them in water, toss the water off, then saute them in butter and whatever herbs I'm in the mood for.

Some will say you can dig her roots in spring because this time of year she's good for prostate health, but that's a funny statement since in fall she is also good for prostate health.

The thing worth discussing again is that a root is a plant's "root cellar" - the place where a plant works all summer to store up sugars, starches, vitamins, minerals and all of her healing compounds that we are after for our own health. Each plant relies on what she has stored up all summer to eat during the winter This is how they survive with no sun. Shoot, even plants that don't come back from the root each year still do this. So when we dig a root in the spring we are basically raiding someone's empty root cellar or food pantry and expecting to find some big bountiful healing meal. That's just not going to happen.

However ,when we dig a root in the fall - especially after the first frost or week of consistently cool weather - we get a summer's worth of sugars, starches, vitamins, minerals and all of her healing compounds, and that makes the effort of digging a root (and likely killing the plant) worth it.

Are there roots that we do dig in the spring? For sure, but these tend to be the seriously potent ones really high in volatile oils. Balsamroot is a good example. She is so potent that spring digging before she's been too long above ground is ideal because come fall she is way too powerful an expectorant (makes us cough and such). I have seen fall dug root make a dude break his fucking ribs from the coughing fit it induced. I wasn't there to stop him from tincture of fall dug root, but I was able to help him recover from the aftermath.

This brings us back to the importance of nuances. While I can say that most roots need to be dug in the fall, I would never set this rule in stone. Instead I would say to get to know each plant you are working with and see for yourself if she's better off dug in the fall, or if she is too powerful and needs to be dug in the spring when she is depleted.

Since the world of manicured lawns wages war on her, when it comes to digging Dandelion you will find no shortage of awesomely effective tools to uproot her with ease!

After you have gathered a nice pile be sure to chop her up while still fresh, then allow her to cure for a week before jarring up. After curing she can also be roasted at 350*F in the oven until she's a deep golden brown color. If you're wanting to make tea, roasting brings out a deep nutty flavor that the plain cured root will not have.

Plantain~

If there is one plant I know you can find it's this gal, since she literally thrives under the pressure of being walked on!

Beyond this, she is just about the easiest plant to harvest, and even easier to cure. When you find a patch (no matter her variety), take the biggest leaves and leave the little ones. In a week go back and do this again. In another week go back and do this again. In another week go back and...well, you get the point.

If you live in a place where the temps never really drop below 40*F you can keep going back weekly all year round, and she will keep giving and giving. She is a really aggressive invasive plant, yet she does not really hurt native plants of a region. She's aggressive in the way that the more we harvest the more she makes. The more we walk on her the more she spreads. She likes to be touched!

While she does have a thick main stem, it seems to cure evenly alongside the leaf. Usually I know she is ready to be stored when her stem breaks with minimal resistance.

Got stung by a bee and want to chew up some fresh to spit on it? If you have that option, I really suggest using the smallest, most recently pushed out leaves. The older ones have a very tough and dirty texture that will make you never try chewing them again. The smaller ones, however, have a smoother texture with a very "plant" like taste. They aren't great, but also aren't bad - just kinda "meh" in flavor and texture.

Elderberry~

Are you sure they're ripe, or are you just excited to start gathering? When I see folks start offering Elderberry syrups or tinctures in August, it's a pretty sure bet there was a fair amount of under ripe berries in your basket. I think a lot of this has to do with them trying to beat the birds instead of waiting for when true ripeness comes, around September. The best way to be sure what your gathering is fully ripe (beyond checking for any signs of green berries left on the tree (or shrub, depending on what variety grows near you)) is to do the squeeze test. A truly ripe and ready to go Elderberry should not be firm, but feel like a squishy little sack of water! You should be able to shoot the inside/seed out of the skin with barely any pressure.

Of course, when she is ripe can depend on your bioregion (and even Elder species), but as a person who lives in the north - with a short growing season and both blue and black varieties - our trees adapt to the short summers and still are not really ripe until September. I don't really see any reason why trees in a longer growing season would drastically speed up when they ripen. If anything, you might not find truly ripe berries until early October!

If I have the chance I will wait even longer, past the first stage of ripeness, when she gets kissed by frost and the birds are acting a bit drunk from eating her now boozy and fermenting berries. These make amazing tincture, the tree having had pushed her all into those berries just before going to sleep for the winter.

When you harvest your berries, don't worry about leaf ending up on the stems. You'll want to cure these leaves for an infused oil that makes a great bruise remedy. this I am always making sure to harvest extra leaf!

No matter when you decide to harvest, every year I feel horrible watching people face the struggle of processing their Elderberries. I mean, you spent hours picking off each individual berry just to have maybe a bowl full of kinda mashed berries to show for it. And you have HOW MANY more to do?

Want to get all of the berries off of their stems in a few moments?

Right after you gather them, cut off all of the leaves and get them curing. Then pop your berries into the freezer for 24-72 hours, until they are fully frozen. When you are ready, just brush your hand against the frozen berries and watch them cascade off of the stems! However, this will only work if you have a really cold freezer, so turn your freezer down to it's coldest setting at least a day before you head out to harvest. Also, only pull out one bag at a time when you process them. As soon as they begin to thaw they will no longer effortlessly fall off.

We drive many miles in our area, hopping from one mountain top to the next and putting away a huge amount of Elderberries every fall. Just the other day my husband, daughter, and I destemmed 3 gallons worth of finished berries in about 20 mins. Because I am a wimp I put on some cheap cotton gloves and then slip plastic gloves over those. The cold berries will freeze your hands good!

You can use these frozen berries the same as you would fresh to make tinctures, jellies, or syrups. Use them up within a year if they are being stored in a deep freezer, in six months in a normal refrigerator freezer.

Don't have access to a freezer or have no freezer space to spare? That's okay! If you are mainly wanting dried berries for making a delicious tea all winter, you can cure them right on the stem. This takes a little while, and you need to be sure that each clump you hang has good space between the next, but once they are fully cured you will be able to brush these berries off of the stems with your fingers. While there will be more tiny bits of stems still attached compared to the frozen ones, this won't hurt you any since you'll be simmering them for a tea.

Speaking of simmering, remember it is important to always cook your Elderberry in some way to get rid of the glycosides. Beyond that, raw Elderberries can make folks feel really nauseated when eaten in more than tasting amounts .

California Poppy~

Take a breath and wait for her to bloom for a good bit before you get to gathering! I know when we see her first cheerful and golden glowing little orange bloom it's so easy to dive right in, but resist the urge if you want to make a tincture (or even infused oil) worth making.

When we wait until we see a really good amount of blooms, buds, and even seed pods, we can be sure we are getting all aspects of her. She is a complex lady, and all of her alkaloids I talked on are not all found evenly throughout. Some are in her blooms, some are in her leaves, and some are in her seed pods. I suspect this is why I at times people say they tried a California Poppy tincture and It did nothing for them. It was likely made with leaf more than anything else.

While we can never be exactly precise when gathering (if we did we would lose all joy in the act) I always make an effort to have about 70% leaves, 20% blooms/buds, and 10% early developed seed pod in my basket by the end of a harvest.

I like to harvest her in the evening after her blooms have closed for the day. Then they are nice and compact, and as I gather I don't end up with broken petals all over the bottom of my basket. She remains whole and relatively undisturbed besides. This is 100% just a personal preference I have, and even I do not always follow it.

After harvesting she loses her vigor pretty quickly, and while some plant allies can hang out in the fridge for a day or so waiting to be tinctured, California Poppy cannot. Before you go out and harvest her be prepared to get her put up with vodka or whatever your plans are before you head out the door. If a plant wilts quickly after harvest in normal outdoor - not left in hot car conditions -you know she needs to be put up fast because her medicinal properties are fleeting!

Curing Versus Drying~

When we dry something we are depending on evaporation to occur, and we often use heat to speed this process up in the way of a dehydrator - you know, that thing you got to make your own jerky or dried fruit that you used maybe once before it ended up gathering dust somewhere.

This is how a majority of folks go about processing their herbs. They either hang them up to dry or pop them in a dehydrator.

The main reason I don't prefer this method is because the plants lose all of their vibrancy, and become very dull looking. At some point you will forget about hanging it, and when you remember it will be covered in dust and unusable. Heat during the drying phase is also how we kill off a lot of the medicinal properties of a plant.

When we cure something we are actively pulling moisture out of the plant in a cool dark setting, instead of relying on heat and evaporation. Our plant materials end up remaining vibrant in color, ready for storage in half the time, and has all of her healing properties intact.

How do we cure our plants? We buy a cheap dehumidifier that pulls the moisture out of anything it's near (including the air) and we designate a closet (or a cheap little free-standing clothes closet) to put in with our herbs. We can make shelves out of mesh material, wire fencing, or just hang them in there and turn the dehumidifier on. By the next morning, you will already be able to see the water in the tank that has been pulled out of the plants! Usually by the 2nd-4th day - depending on how much you have in there and the thickness of the plants stem - it is ready to be stored! When we dry something it can take up to two weeks before enough evaporation has occurred that we can store it away for later use.

If you are a Marijuana smoker, the herb you get that has a nice smooth taste and doesn't burn your throat when you smoke it has been cured. Most serious growers have legit curing setups because anyone can grow good weed, but it will only stay that way if you know how to cure it well. This is the same for the herbs we gather and use for different things. Anyone can gather high quality and healthy herbs, but if you don't treat them well after harvesting the quality is nowhere to be found.

Sound like it's gana be really expensive? Nah, you can get a little dehumidifier online for less than the cost of this book, and if you gut that closet of stuff you don't even realize you still have, setting up a curing cabinet will at best cost you $30 bucks.

One thing I like to do for roots and thicker stems is laying them in my cabinet on top of cardboard. It helps pull the moisture out even quicker. If you can only afford the dehumidifier and not making shelving, consider simply laying out cardboard until you can afford to fix it up a better. When I am done curing my herbs I use vacuum seal bags to store them. Some folks like to use jars, and that's fine. I prefer the bags since I harvest a lot and often, and I can suck the air out of them. This makes my harvest keep longer than if I had jarred them.

Just a heads up - If you really get going on your herbal journey you will find jars take up a lot of space. Even the biggest half gallon canning jars won't fit as much as you think they will.

If you do use jars, resist the urge to display them somewhere that sun hits them or it's really warm. The sun and prolonged warmth are the death of both nutritional and medicinal values in plant matter - seriously, folks. One of the Sun's jobs is to trigger decomposition in dead things, and when we expose our dead plant matter to her we waste all of our hard work (and the life of the plant).

You'll never see me buying herbs out of jars that are displayed near a window for customers to buy, and you'll never see me placing my infused oil (or anything similar) out in the sun for "solar infusing".

.21.

The Utter Simplicity of Making Tinctures

This is ridiculous. This will be outright absurd. This might even make you a touch skeptical.

It can't really be that easy to make a tincture, can it?

Ready to find out? Let's make a tincture!

Lightly chop up enough **fresh** plant matter to fill a jar of your choice to the top.

Dump 100 proof vodka over the plant matter until you hit the rim of the jar.

Put a cap on the jar, then slap a label on it that says what's in it and the date you made it.

Set it in a cool dark place for 6-8 weeks.

When the wait time is up, strain the plant matter out of the vodka.

The vodka has now been transformed into a tincture, to be taken in drop amounts at a time.

A quart jar worth of tincture could be enough to last you a decade!

For those who may be skeptical, my guess is you're been diving deeply into tincture making via western herbalism. You're thinking, "What about the ratios? What about the potency? What about the dilution math? What about all of the confusing hours of study I've done or that course I paid for to sorta understand how to make tinctures?"

Let's break this all down.

A solid 90+% of herbalists make their tinctures out of dried plant matter and high proof medical grade alcohol.

This is also how every book they sell, every article they write, and every course they teach will tell you it must be done.

If you read the section where I ranted about the danger of refined volatile oils ("essential oils") you may remember how I said the companies that make tinctures tend to use dried plant material. To get 63 pounds of dried Yarrow they would likely need to harvest and dry a few hundred pounds of fresh Yarrow.

So when we are making tinctures out of dried plant matter you have to follow specific ratios, where you figure out how much fresh plant went into making how much dried plant so you don't accidentally put too much into your jar. Confusing? It gets worse from here.

Okay, so let's say they figure out that one cup of dried Yarrow in a quart jar would be equal to four cups of fresh Yarrow. Cool, one cup of dried yarrow can make one quart of tincture. That wasn't hard! *Insert maniacal laugh he* That would only be the case if you weren't using 190 proof pure, kill-you-dead-alcohol. Now you have to do the math and say, "Okay, how much dried plant matter can I add to 190 proof alcohol and then dilute when done with distilled water to get to a safe ingestion ratio of 1:1?

The amounts of wet to dry Yarrow that I have given is theoretical, because I don't care to do needlessly complicated work just to get to the same result I can in 5 minutes.

The hilarious irony here is that they usually do all of this to get a 50% alcohol ratio and have enough of the dried Yarrow's medicinal properties present that it equals the same as if they used fresh plant matter.

Don't see the irony yet? Gimme a sec!

When I put fresh Yarrow in a jar and dump 100 proof vodka (50% alcohol 50% water) over top, I have already gotten the end result that they are getting with their dried plant matter, high proof alcohol, distilled water, and math. When I strain my tincture there is automatically a one part plant to one part alcohol ratio, and each drop is already 50% water and 50% alcohol.

Yet these two types of tinctures could not be more different.

A tincture made out of dried plant matter and high proof alcohol - even once diluted - is as volatile as the word 'fuck' is towards a stranger. Why? Well, there are a few issues to talk on. When we use dried plant matter, in general, the only things left after curing or drying are the plant's most volatile properties. All of its water soluble properties, for the most part, have dissipated during the drying or curing - especially if there was heat involved in the drying process, and there often is. This, on top of the fact that 190 proof alcohol is extremely caustic (able to erode/break down/eat away) towards anything it touches, means it ruthlessly extracts dangerous levels of the most volatile parts of any plant that it comes into contact with.

This level of extraction ends up making a tincture that is extremely potent, which is great if you're wanting your herbs to act like pharmaceutical medicines. That is what they are when made this way. You have, much like "essential oils", only extracted the plants most potent and dangerous aspects, casting the rest of her aside.

Wana see something crazy? Go get some pitch or sap - whatever you like to call it - off of a pine tree. Get a good amount. Put one clump in a jar you don't care about and the other clump in another jar of equally meaningless value. Fill jar A up with 100 proof vodka (which has 50% alcohol content) and fill jar B up with 190 proof alcohol (if you can legally buy it in your state that is...). Put the lids on and walk away for a few hours. In that short amount of time the vodka will have barely changed color, but the one with 190 proof in it will be damn near, if not all the way, dissolved already. Now imagine that action on something that is not hard as hell to dissolve like pitch is. Something like oh, I don't know, plant matter maybe.

When we make a tincture out of fresh plant matter we are not just getting her most volatile aspects, but also her water soluble properties. Maybe you're thinking, "Cool, I'll just use fresh plant matter in my 190 proof alcohol!" Nope, there's no water in the alcohol to extract them! When we use 100 proof vodka our jar is filled up with 50% alcohol and 50% water. This allows for a well balanced and well rounded tincture that does not act like a pharmaceutical drug, but instead like the plant we are trying to get to know in her whole worthy state.

So why in the world would folks choose to make tinctures with dried plant matter and 190 proof alcohol?

There are a few reasons. They may not know any different, or if they do they tend to end up feeling defensive when someone brings it up - especially if they paid to learn that way. It's not uncommon for these types of herbalists to put people like me down as "folk herbalists", which is really demeaning if you think about the context it's being used in. They are saying "Oh, she just doesn't have the training that I do." I run into this shit all the time.

Another reason is that they don't really want to be an herbalist, so much as they want to play at being a green coated homeopathic doctor and using herbs like pharmaceuticals gets them to that place. There is nothing wrong with this, it's just important that we call it out for what it is - people who equate reactions with health. As a pharmaceutically dependent society we all do this. We say things like, "My stomach was messed up, but an antacid healed it." Can you stop taking it? If not, then it didn't heal anything. It just caused a change in your body and you equated that with being healed. Tinctures made out of dried plant matter and high proof alcohol are basically the same, and these folks who practice this way often lean towards very reactive and borderline poisonous plants because these will for sure give their patients instant reactions.

Then there's the pesky reason of convenience, profit, and instant gratification. It's not exactly convenient to have to go out and harvest the plant when its fresh whenever you want to make a tincture. There is no guarantee that you will even find it, and what happens if you can't make enough to sell all year long? I mean, if you can't make a new batch since it's now the dead of winter, you're going to miss out on sales! AND it's going to take me between 6-8 weeks for the tincture to be ready? That's crazy! With 190 proof I can proclaim my tincture done in as little as a week!

I am not attacking anyone specific here. There are many different ways we can prefer to do things, and that's perfectly okay! There is just such a disconnect from the land in herbalism these days, and I firmly believe this comes from treating plants like they are nothing more than pharmaceuticals. There are so many long term (as well as up and coming) herbalists who seldom, if ever, lay hands on fresh plant matter in their practices that it would shock you. While I know it's harder for some of us to get out to the land and gather, grow a garden, or source fresh herbs, it is by no means impossible. It is just less convenient.

This does not mean that we always have to make tinctures out of fresh plant matter. It is just really important to understand the vast difference. For Example, a catnip tincture made from fresh herb and 100 proof vodka may have you feeling nice and relaxed, but one made with dried herbs and high proof alcohol might make you violently vomit because there is far too much nepetalactone in it. I see a lot of folks get injured by high proof dried plant matter tinctures and then become gun shy towards all herbs. This is a huge blow to people taking their healing into their own hands and wanting to reconnect with the land underfoot.

"Come on, woman, tell us when we can use dried plant matter!" I will forgo having a tincture of any leafy plant if I can't find her to make a fresh tincture. However, here are the things that I - if I really want and can't access or find an alternative plant that I can make fresh - will use dried with 100 proof vodka:

Roots~

Nonvolatile roots. Volatile? If the root you are wanting to use has no real scent, such as Dandelion, I would feel okay using her dried in a tincture. If a root has a strong odor she has high volatile oil levels, and remember these refine as the root dries. That aside, roots are literally meant to hold onto their medicinal properties. In all begrudgingly offered honesty, there is not the biggest difference between a fresh root and a dried root.

Berries~

Like roots, berries are engineered by nature to hold onto their medicinal properties. They are basically a little womb for the seed within, meant to nourish its life should it sprout come spring. Just like with roots, only fill your jar up halfway.

Woody Mushrooms~

Most really rigid mushrooms in the Polyporaceae Family, turkey tail mushroom being a good example. While most mushrooms wither away and shrink up vastly when dried, these woods mushrooms pretty much stay the same size. They do lose a bit of water content but, nowhere near the 90% like a Lion's mane mushroom would. Because of this, and the fact that they - just like roots and berries - hold onto their medicinal properties really well when dried, making them also fine to tincture dried.

A note on mushroom - most need heat to extract their PSK levels (Polysaccharide K), amongst other things, so it won't be as simple as a standard tincture. You'll have to make a decoction, do some dilution math, and then add this to your tincture.

If you decide that you are going to make some sort of dried root or berry tincture, be mindful to only fill your jar halfway with the dried plant, because a.) if it was fresh, it would take up more space - too much dried can lead to too strong - and b.) the roots or berries will expand as they absorb the vodka, bursting your jar. Most dried woody mushrooms won't expand because they can't really shrink up, and the dried volume that would fill a jar is the same as the fresh volume that would fill a jar.

Making a tincture really is as easy as dumping vodka over fresh plant matter, but that does not mean there isn't an art to it, and this art goes by the name of Nuance! Let's jabber on them while talking about some of the plant allies from earlier chapters we can make tinctures out of.

Yarrow~

Some say they prefer a Yarrow tincture made out of leaves, yet others say she's best when only made from the bloom. I say if you can harvest bloom, leaf, and stem, it'd probably be a good idea to tincture it all too! The debate usually comes from the idea that one seems to work better for ABC issue, and the other seems to work better for XYZ issue. I want the whole damn alphabet present, so I am not going to break her out into sections. The funny thing is that I have people compliment me in droves for how great my Yarrow tincture is. I am not doing anything all that special. I'm simply using all of her!

With that in mind, I like to make sure I have about equal parts bloom, stem, and leaf, which is usually how it works out naturally. One thing to know about Yarrow is that if you let her steep for more than 6 weeks you can get this really weird looking "black stuff" in your tincture. I don't even want to think about how much perfectly fine tincture has probably been dumped out because of this!

This is simply some of her volatile oils separating out of the water content, and a sign that she has been sitting there a while. It tends to settle to the bottom and you can strain off the tincture from above. Would I willfully ingest these oils? Nah, just separate it off from your tincture before bottling. I mainly notice it happen when we have had a cooler summer and, if I had to guess, this is because the heat really gets her flaunting her smell. In doing so, she loses some of these oils. When it's cool there is just extra build up, so to speak.

Comfrey~

I am just including Comfrey in this section so I can tell you to never use a Comfrey tincture internally - even from the hybrid variety - or the alkaloids will fuck your liver up! However, she is a great addition to external healing sprays! She is a pretty straight forward tincture to make. Just chop her up and pour vodka over top.

Elderberry~

If you have not used the freezer method to liberate yourself from hours of painstakingly picking each individual berry off its stem, I know it will be easy to tell yourself that a half a jar full of berries is enough, but you really do need to fill whatever jar you use all the way to the top with berries if you want to make more than Elderberry flavored vodka!

This means that if you don't want to pick any more you need to choose a jar small enough that what you did pick will fill to the top.

I also like to put my Elderberry tincture in a dark, warm place while she is extracting. I find it makes a really potent (like, no light is getting through thick) extract, and that heat is going to help kill off those glycosides that are in her berries and little stem pieces. To warm her up I love to use seed starting mats, and in the infused oil section I'll jabber about how to make a heat.
If you're working with the common black Elderberry, consider adding some honey and turning your tincture into an elixir. Beyond getting more of her water soluble properties from the honey's ability to extract them, it will help take the edge off of her somewhat bitter flavor. I usually add about ¼ cup per quart jar (4 cups in a quart), so you can scale up or down from there to make a nice elixir.

California Poppy~

I'm just gana be real here. The difference between a shitty, ineffective California Poppy tincture and one that will likely give a good amount of relief comes down to three things:

1.) Make sure there are leaves, stems, blooms/buds, and seed pods.
2.) Pack your jar pretty well. No need to ramrod it ,but you should not be able to fit much more in the jar if you did.
3.) Get alcohol poured over her within no more than an hour of gathering - maybe two if you gather in the evening when its cooler out.

You may see black spots show up on her leaves as she tinctures. This is just her cellular structure breaking down some from the alcohol contact, and it does not always happen. Sometimes they go beautifully translucent. It reminds me of a mermaid or an underwater kelp forest, as off as that sounds. Plants, even if the same species, are still individual beings, and will react differently to the same thing depending on the season, the weather, or I'd even dare to say their mood!

Is there a whitish green "sludge" on the bottom of your jar after she sat for a really long time? It's not mold. It's a combination of inulin (which is a type of fiber) and a bit of her pollen mixed with the parts of her the alcohol degraded away. Just shake it back in.

Remember, she does have natural latex content, so proceed with caution if you or loved ones have latex allergies.

Dandelion~

Roots, blooms, leaves, whatever you want to tincture of her is just fine, but her roots are the most common thing to dig into (shitty pun intended). I really love digging her fall roots to make a simple digestive aid for the coming heavy winter foods I know I am going to be existing on soon enough.

You should know though, root tinctures - from freshly dug roots, anyhow - are a real labor of love, and while I know you think you have dug a lot, by the time you get her cleaned up a bit, dead leaf taken off, then chopped up, it condenses really quickly. I do my best to dig enough root to fill the jar up loosely. This means when you pour the vodka over top the amount will kinda sorta magically shrink a bit, usually to a little over half a jar packed well.

You could keep on digging and keep on digging to really pack the jar full, but it's best not to if you want any real amount of tincture for your efforts. In other words, roots tend to take up space more than other plant parts, and when it comes time to strain you'll only get at best half of what you're expecting That can be a bummer if you only made a pint's worth!

All roots contain inulin, which is a digestive resistant fiber. This is a good thing, and the more stressed out a plant is the more she will release into your tincture. Because we can't digest it, this fiber makes it all the way through us, delivering the medicinal benefits of the plant as she goes on her merry way.

This white, powdery looking substance scares the hell out of out of folks new to tincturing. It can be really thick on the bottom of a jar or pile up on the plant matter, and it looks like mold or something we did wrong! Nope, it's just inulin, which is in too many plants to count, especially their roots.

What if we didn't know these nuances?

I mean, if you stick to safe simple plants that have been in use since the dawn of time, fresh plant matter, and some good ol' vodka, you won't likely end up hurting yourself as you learn them. It really is pretty hard to mess up a straight forward tincture. I'd just give the advice of starting small in terms of how big of a batch you make, so you're not out a ton of money or plant allies if you somehow find a way to mess up making a tincture, or if you end up not liking how it does or does not make your feel.

But let's talk about some things that will help you nail your first batch or your hundredth batch!

Ewwwww!~

Oh no there's a bug in my tincture! Is it ruined?!

This is the required sacrifice to make any tincture. You have never made, they have never made, and we will never make a tincture that does not have a little bit of bug in it! Bugs live on plants. This is just a fact!

Should we use plants that are covered in hundreds of bugs? No.

Should we let our plant allies lay out for a little bit to let bugs escape? Yep.

Can we take a little bit of time to go over the plants to get off any bugs that are hiding? You probably should.

Will you die from a bug or two being tinctured? Probably not.

Does using dried plant matter get us around this? No, it just means you're tincturing chopped up bug bits.

Bugs and tinctures are just a thing.

Beyond the Pouring~

So one reason it is really important to pick a jar that you can fill up all the way with your chopped up plant matter is that you also need to fill it all the way up with alcohol to prevent oxidation. Here is a visualization to help you understand what I am talking about. You take a bite of an apple, set it down, and come back two hours later. What happened to the flesh of the apple when it was exposed to air? It turned brown, right? This is oxidation, and it's slowly degrading the nutritional value of your next bite.

Okay, so tinctures don't have any real nutritional value to speak of, but the plants that are being tinctured do, and they also contain the medicinal value that will be degraded by oxidation - the same way nutrients will. If you have space for air in your jar you will also have oxidation. While this will always slowly occur as we open jars, fill bottles, and all around use our tinctures, the most damaging time for it do so is when the tincture is being made.

So when I, for example, strain out my Yarrow tincture she's usually a lovely golden color, but as I draw from the jar over time she turns a darker golden color from oxidation. If I leave air in the jar while the plant matter is there, when I strain her she will be a really dark brown color because the plant matter is more susceptible to oxidation than alcohol is.

It probably didn't go bad~

I mean, it's been sitting capped in that jar for like three years. It's gana kill me, right? Nope, tinctures (even with plant matter left in them) are extremely shelf stable. Have you ever found a capped bottle of vodka and been like, "Damn, it spoiled!"? Not all of us will be able to relate to that question, but the answer is no. Noone has ever really found a spoiled bottle of liquor. In fact, with scotch or whiskey the older it is the more it costs!

However, this does not mean tinctures can't go bad! Here are a few guidance rules:

1.) If it's in a tightly capped jar with a metal lid, has been in a cool dark place, and is 50% alcohol content, it's perfectly safe to use for about a decade, even if it still has plant matter in it. After that I'd see if the lid was corroding, and if not I'd say you maybe even have another 5 years before the potency begins to drop off. If it's been in a hot place or in direct sun for that long I would not use it. It probably won't kill ya, but probably won't do you any good either.

2.) If it's tightly capped in a tincture dropper bottle and kept in a cool dark place ,you've got about 5 years to use it up. After that, the water content will have slowly evaporated off since the dropper cap is not airtight, and it can be dangerous to use as it's now concentrated. If, on the flip side, you keep it in a really hot place, the alcohol content can evaporate off much quicker than the water and bacteria can grow. This is uncommon considering alcohol evaporates off at a lower temp than water does, but it does happen.

This is why I only bottle tinctures for myself as I need them. When I take them out of a jar and put them into a dropper bottle the 10 year countdown instantly jumps to 5 or less. You can get lids that fit the tops of dropper bottles though, and then you're back up to the 10 year range. This is also why it's really important to put what and when you made it on ANY bottle you fill up. You won't likely remember what's in it otherwise, let alone when you made it!

Straining Means to Strain It~

I don't mean to be a smartass, but I get asked this question a lot! What does straining mean? It's so hard for me not to be like, "It means to strain it..." However, when I step back and remember that in our current culture the average human that is in their mid 30s or younger has never cooked a whole fucking chicken or anything beyond basic meals (since we are all so dependent on convenient, quick, and cheap take out food), it's very likely the people who ask this question have just never really done the type of cooking that requires them to use a strainer. So I'm gana bust out some options while I elaborate!

When the 6-8 week extracting time is up or whenever we get around to it, the next step is to separate the plant matter from the vodka. All of the plant's medicinal values have now been absorbed into the vodka. Here are some options and tools we can use to do this with:

1.) My favorite thing to use is a fine micron, food grade, nylon mesh nut milk bag. That name always makes me laugh like a 16 year old boy who thinks dicks are hilarious! No joke, those these things are incredibly durable, easily hand washed, don't really stain, and can be sanitized with ease.

2.) If you don't want to use nylon you can get these in cotton or other fabrics but please know if you plan on selling things to people cross contamination is a big issue here as they are hard to sanitize.

3.) If you don't mind teeny tiny bits of plant matter in your tincture you can use a metal mesh type strainer. They usually sell a 5-pack with cascading sizes in any cooking isle of wally world or the like. These are a good choice for beginners, as you can use them for so many different things and are easily washed and sanitized.

4.) Cheesecloth. A lot of people swear by it, but I fucking hate the stuff. Even with a tight weave be prepared to get cotton strings in your tincture, and for it to utterly fall apart when you are washing it. Wana know the truth? I would rather buy a brand new white colored cotton bandana and use that than cheesecloth!

The next step is to find something to strain into. The first time I suggest using a wide bowl until you get a feel for how your set up works. If not you are likely to spill all over the place, and that is always a bummer! Here is how I usually do it for small batches with the nut milk (haha) bag.

1.) Slip the bag into a clean, empty jar the same size as your tincture jar. Now pull it up just over the edge and cinch the string tight.

2.) Pop a canning funnel into the top of the empty jar ,over the nut milk bag.

3.) Slowly begin to pour your tincture, plant matter and all, into the funnel - and I mean slowly!

4.) Once it's all in there take off the funnel and tie the bag closed.

5.) Begin to pull the bag out of the jar. The pressure of it fitting out of the opening will press some of the tincture out for you.

6.) Pop the funnel back in the jar and begin to squeeze. The plant matter and tincture will begin falling down into the funnel/jar. Squeeze as much as you can. You can even twist the bag to help.

7.) Tada! You just strained your tincture and it is all ready to use!

There is no wrong way to strain something, though. You just need to get the plant matter out of the vodka in any way that works for you!

What do we do with the plant now that we have tinctured it? Most of the time I add her to my compost pile, but if it's something like Elderberry or Yarrow I may pop it in my freezer for the sake of making a "tincture tea". This is where we use spent tinctured plant matter to make a weak tea. It will be like taking a good dose of tincture though, and the hot water tends to evaporate off most (if not all) of the alcohol.

How Much to Take~

I actually really dislike giving people advice on what dosage they should take. These are not pharmaceuticals with a ton of studies to tell us how much any given person of any given body weight can tolerate, and I don't know you or any of your bodies quirks.

I am, however, cGMP/FDA compliant with my herbal business, which means I have to not only have my tinctures lab tested (I am actually really proud of this. So few take this step), I also have to state a suggested use on every bottle.

In fact, the suggested use amount on each bottle is the amount of tincture that the lab tests for things like dangerous levels of heavy metal and or microbes. Like how many parts per million are present in each suggested dose.

I generally suggest if a plant is more or less considered okay to use on a daily basis between 5-15 drops as needed. This is a really common dose for most commonly made tinctures. It is best to start at the lower dose of 5 drops (like a single drop that comes out of the dropper) and see how that makes you feel or how your individual body responds. For example, if you know your body is really sensitive to things consider only taking two drops, maybe even a singular drop.

Whatever dose you start with, you can slowly and gently work your way up until you:

a.) Find what works for you.
b.) Find the level where your body says, "Too much!" and scale back.

If the plant is a bit stronger I may suggest not taking her for more than three times a day, or for more than a week in a row. This will apply to whatever dose from the 0-x number of drops you end up feeling is right for your body.
I feel like I really need you to understand that I primarily work with safe, simple plant allies, many food based. When you get into the more dangerous realms like Poke Root, for example, a huge grown-ass man may, at best, be able to handle one singular drop. Two might make him sick as hell. This is why it's important to take some time to get to know what we have tinctured. Of course, doing this before we gather her is ideal, but you will have 6-8 weeks to decide which dose commonly used for that specific plant feels right to you.

I suppose the main bit of info I need to get across here is that even with guidelines that allow me - or anyone else - to paint with general strokes, we need to take a moment to get to know each plant, to listen to our body, and always start on the 'barely any' side of the scale, then work our way up to 'more'.

The next question I often get asked is how to take the dose you have decided on?

90% of the time I take my tincture in a little bit of water or juice. Just put your dose into the water or juice and drink it down.

The only time I take a tincture straight is if I need her to hit my bloodstream NOW. Then I will take her sublingually under my tongue. When does this apply? Usually only with herbs that sedate. If you are having an anxiety attack or tension headache, I would put the poppy tincture under your tongue, count to 30, and then drink something. We should not do this constantly, as the tissue under our tongue is so sensitive even 100 proof vodka is kinda rough on it!

Are you alcohol free?

No biggie, just drop you dose into a cup of really warm water - but not so hot we wouldn't want to take a drink of it. In about 35-45 minutes the absolutely minuscule amount of alcohol will have evaporated off, leaving behind the medicinal content of the plant ally.

Just to put the truly minuscule amount of alcohol into perspective - if your tincture is made from 100 proof vodka, each drop is 50% water and 50% alcohol. If you take 10 drops of tincture, that's only 5 drops of alcohol. There is more alcohol in your toothpaste, a ripe banana, or the vanilla you make cookies with.

I think tinctures are actually a really good way to recover from alcoholism, if this is what causes your aversion. We learn to associate alcohol as a tool to bring us health and connection to plants versus it being a destructive, all consuming force that disconnects us from the people and places around us.

A Friend to All is a Friend to None~

I like my friends just as they are. I have never had the urge to smash two people into one person.

I also know that If I am hopping from one person to the next and never giving myself enough time to truly get to know said person I won't actually have friends, just a bunch of kinda sorta acquaintances.

I don't see tinctures as any different, but let me do like I usually do and elaborate some!

I will never make, let alone hand you, a tincture that has more than one herb in her, and I really want you to think about why. If you take a combination of herbs that have been tinctured together or mixed afterward you have absolutely no way of knowing what herb caused what if you have a reaction - whether for the good or bad. I don't care how good of an herbalist you are. Full stop.

What if the reaction was pretty bad? What if you broke out in hives? Couldn't breathe? Shit yourself violently for hours? Vomited for days?

Do you feel like after that you're gana be up to taking each and every one of those plants individually, until finally you find the one that is going to throw you into the same hell again? Yeah, I didn't think so.

Combination tinctures have the power to break our relationship with a bunch of plants all at once. We become gun shy as fuck to take ANY herb that was in the blend we made or bought. However, if you took a tincture that was made out of just one plant ally and had that reaction, you would know that you and her couldn't be friends. No hard feelings, see ya around, Chick! But we all know deep down we ain't gana talk to her again. We most likely are gana dip into a different isle if we see her in the store, hahaha!

What if we had a good reaction though, and something in this blend we made or bought made us feel really great? Like, this has finally lifted the weight of something going on with our body! What would the problem be with that?

Well, the first issue is that you don't know who is helping you. Now you'll either have to take this exact blend for the rest of your life (consuming other herbs that you body really doesn't need, pushing your body more than is healthy), or you do a process of elimination. Take one at a time until you finally find the one that was helping, potentially sliding back into feeling whatever sorta way until you hit the nail on the head.

Some unethical shit slips into this too. What if this super awesome anxiety tincture blend you bought for yourself ends up being a huge help - like, gives you your life back? That's great, right? Sure, but what happens when you/they run out and it was a very specific blend that you don't know how to recreate, let alone which herbs in it actually helped Aren't you kinda held hostage? Made to be dependant? I mean, if we know a California poppy tincture really knocks our anxiety the fuck out, when the person who makes it runs out can't we just make it ourselves with ease? We don't even have to try and figure out what plant it was that helps us? Even if the person can't make it themselves, I'd bet my last dollar that with the help of the almighty Google search engine they find it for sale somewhere!

Now, in no way does this mean we can't take more than one tincture at a time. It is just best to let ourselves get to know one plant friend at a time. I will take a new tincture all by itself for a week or more to see what she does to my body, and to really understand her. Then, once I am comfortable with her, I will slowly begin taking her alongside another plant ally I think might compliment. For the next week, I will see how they play together, how it makes me feel, what together they do that apart they could not.

Even then I won't blend them together. Nope, I just put my doses as needed into a bit of water, but I never combine them in a bottle together. It is just really important that we give ourselves time to see who does what, how long that takes to happen, and what kinda gross it might make us feel before we bring in anyone else. In this, you will actually be able to know who caused what, and what bad reaction might come from two plants combined that may be just fine for you taken individually.

Tinctures are a really amazing way to step into a meaningful and ethical relationship with both the land and her plant allies. They are cheap, easy to make, and a little goes a long way. It takes such a tiny amount to fill up a quart jar, no matter the plant ally, and they will last forever. Most importantly of all, you are beyond smart enough to do this!

.22.

A Nuanced Dance of Making Herbal Infused Oils

"This chick uses the word 'nuanced' way too much!" I'm not even going to argue it. I will also say another time or five that that word seems to be lost on humanity as a whole, and the ramifications lead to hostility. When we apply it to the world of herbalism we can suddenly see what a vastly complex dance it is with every step each of us takes. We can have discussions without getting angry. We can self evaluate and reflect on the "why" of the different choice ourselves and others make in any given situation.

It might be funny to think that something as simple as a few herbs soaking in oil would be a place to explore this, but that's the thing to understand in life - there is not a single place, thing, situation, or act of creating that would not deeply benefit from considering nuance.

So there's this kinda sorta not so quietly raging debate about how herbal infused oils should be made in the herbalism world.

Team A says they should always be made with freshly wilted plant matter for the most potent oil.

Team B says they should always be made with dried plant matter to prevent our oils from going rancid.

I have seen extremely hostile arguments over this in comment sections. I have seen people denounce someone as a knowledgeable herbalist for being on the other side of the debate. I have had people lose their shit on me for simply saying there's probably a time and place for both options.

So let's dance through some of these differences and see when one way or the other may be the best choice for whatever we are trying our hand at making. We'll start by breaking apart the differences and thought processes behind them.

When team A gets to screaming (or even quietly whispering) that freshly wilted plants make a higher quality infused oil, they are not wrong, but only during certain circumstances. Yes, if we put wilted plant matter (meaning most, but not all, water content has been evaporated) into oil and then stick it in a dark cool place for no more than 6 weeks that oil WILL be more deeply infused - I'll even use the word potent - than dry plant matter put into oil and set in a cool dark place for 6 weeks.

There's no arguing to be done about that.

We even know that using the dried forms of some plant allies to make an infused oil, such as the blooms of Saint John's Wort, is downright useless. THIS is a perfect example of how an infused oil made with freshly wilted plant matter will make a higher quality oil.

In comes team B with some aggression, saying using freshly wilted plant matter in oil more often than not ends up makes an infused oil go rancid, either during the infusion process or soon after the process is over. They are not wrong. We must accept the fact that when we introduce water to oil we make the perfect conditions for bacterial, fungal, and yeast explosions.

Just like we know Saint John's Wort needs to be made out of freshly wilted plant matter, we also know that Comfrey is notorious at making oil go violently rancid with sincere speeds if we leave even the slightest amount of moisture in her. Even if we pop our oil in the fridge and don't let it go past 4 weeks of infusing, 99% of the time you will vomit from the smell when you open the jar.

Oka,y so we know that a 6 week infused oil with freshly wilted plant matter is stronger and some plants must be used this way, but at the same time we know that when we follow this method there's a chance of having to dump out all of our hard work and that some plants will make our oil go rancid, no matter how hard we try. How in the hell are we supposed to work with this knowledge? Seems like we would really have to join either team A or B, right?

Fucking nuances, people!

Sure, that Plantain oil you made out of freshly wilted leaves is amazing after 6 weeks of infusing compared to the one someone else made with dried plant, but what if the only reason this way is "better" is the more constraining rules we have to follow for freshly wilted plants? Stick with me here for a second, folks! When we make an infused oil with kinda wet plants these are the "rules" that most herbalists will agree on:

1.) Wilt the plant for 2-4 days, making sure to split the stems so excess moisture can escape - but be sure it does not get to dry. It should still be flexible without breaking.

2.) Pour your oil of choice over the wilted plants all the way to the top of the jar, as air will increase your odds of spoiling and oxidation.

3.) Label and place your jar in a cool dark place (55*F-65*F) for no more than 6 weeks to infuse. Check weekly or even daily for mold, rancidity, and other signs of spoilage.

I legit just showed you how easy an infused oil is to make with wilted plant matter, so there's that, but let's look at a few things here.

When we work with kinda fresh plant matter we are:

a.) Constrained by a 6 week infusing time frame before the plant matter begins to rot.

b.) Have the issue of oxidation and spoilage.

c.) Can't use any heat whatsoever.

None of these constraints are an issue when working with dried plant matter because:

a.) With no moisture content present there is no need for a time limit, as the dry plant matter does not rot.

b.) Since the dried plant matter is not fresh, oxidation is minimal and spoilage from mold, yeast, and fungus can not happen.

c.) We can use heat to extract the oil soluble properties of the plant.

Still with me? No? Gimme a sec to pull this all together.

So an oil made with wilted plant matter is only of "higher quality" compared to one with dried plant matter because folks are still making the dried ones like they do the wet ones! They are trapped in the idea that the side they choose is the only way to do something, yet when we remove these self imposed constraints and look at the types of infused oils differently, a whole new level of understanding infused oils will open up to us!

The last debate I had about this, a lady got so defensive to my constant ability to say "what about ____?" that she told me to die. The thing she thought she got from the wilted plant matter is the water soluble properties, which you hear me say is really important when we are making tinctures, but really hear me out, folks...

Water soluble properties are pretty much only soluble in water. That's why we call them "water soluble". In no way, shape, or form are you extracting specific water soluble properties into your oil. Are their things that can be soluble in both water and oil? Well yeah, but they are not coming from the moisture you leave behind in your plant. It's a well known scientific fact that water and oil do not mix without the use of emulsification chemicals of some sort.

So any medicinal properties that are solely residing within the water content of a plant is not, I repeat, **is not** extracting into your oil, and you **are not** getting any added medicinal benefits from using wilted plant matter. We also know that many oil soluble properties release much better if there is heat involved. The heat helps break down the cellular structure of a plant and the cells are what hold all the good we are after!

This is why we don't want to store our herbs in hot conditions. Wait, was that a bit hypocritical sounding, or at least confusing?

Here's the thing, IF our plants are just in a ziplock bag or mason jar getting hot day in and day out, they are rapidly losing their ability to heal and nourish us, but when we add oil we **WANT** to make this happen and we use the oil to **CATCH** these dissipating properties. Also, the oil itself degrades the cellular structure of the plant material. So yeah, if we put some dried Plantain in oil and stick it somewhere cool, in 6 weeks there won't be much in that oil to heal us since the plant matter is not degrading much when dry without the help of heat.

On that note, wilted plant matter infused oils are stronger at 6 weeks because the plant is literally rotting. Her cellular structure breaks down, releasing her oil soluble medicinal - and even some nutritional properties - into the oil.

I swear to God all of that is just leading me to this:

These are just TWO different methods for breaking down the cellular structure of the plant to release her bits and pieces we are after. Each of these two options are just that - options. But like any other option in life, they can be suited to specific situations or come with drawbacks. Currently I seem to be enjoying doing a,b,c, or 1,2,3 breakdowns so I am gana stick with it for the sake of enjoying the work I am doing. Let's look at a few drawbacks and benefits for fresh and dried infused oils.

Wilted Plant Matter Infused Oil Benefits:

1.) The first benefit that most will notice and appreciate right off the bat is that these are ready to be used much sooner. These oils can only sit for 6 weeks max, but depending on the plant and how rapid she decays can be ready to use in as little as 2-3 weeks.

2.) The next benefit is, in my opinion, the biggest. This the only way we can make a worthwhile infused herbal oil for some plants. Some properties of plants are oil and water soluble, but dissipate as the plant dries. Such as Hypericin, which is what's in Saint John's wort that makes her fresh infused oil turn red - but ONLY if we use freshly wilted blooms.

3.) We are given the gift of having a hands-on relationship with our local plant allies and the land that carries us when we learn to seek these plants out in their particular season and unique environment. This often leads to a deeper sense of understanding and connection.

Wilted Plant Matter Infused Oil Drawbacks:

1.) These oils can only sit for 6 weeks max before the plant matter has rotted to the point that mold, yeast, fungus, or rancidity will set in. It is easy to forget about something hidden away for 6 weeks and find it 10+ weeks later, unusable.

2.) With a 6 week timeframe we are not always able to end up with a fully infused oil, and the risk of an oil becoming off places a set time limit on infusing.

3.) It is not a matter of if an oil goes bad, it's a matter of when. Eventually at some point we will waste both oil and plant allies that we have spent time harvesting.

4.) If we live in a very warm climate we may not have realistic access to a cool enough place to stash our jars of oil.

5.) The shelf life of most herbal infused oils is one year, but wilted plant matter oils have a tendency to go rancid in 6 months if not stored in perfectly cool temps.

6.) We should not use these oils to make water/oil based emulsification creations, such as creams, lotions, or body butters. Without testing we do not know if mold, bacteria, and or fungus is present. Remember, by the time you see mold, fungus, and some bacterial colonies it has already been there for a good while, invisible to our eyes.

7.) We can only make these oils within particular seasons and if a plant ally grows near us. How much we make or what plant ally we are using we may end up putting too much pressure on the land by wildcrafting herbs that we can just as easily - and at times more ethically - obtain from an herb farm.

8.) Accessing the land to harvest may not be as realistic to folks living in cities or to those who have physical limitations.

9.) We can not press the plant matter after infusing with oil because the water content will be squeezed out into the oil. This means we will waste a fair amount of the oil we used to infuse with.

Dried Plant Matter Infused Oil Benefits:

1.) We do not run the risk of water content causing mold, bacteria, or fungus, which means it is extremely unlikely that we are ever going to end up wasting our time, oil, and plant allies from any oil gone bad.

2.) We have no 6 week time limit that prevents us from infusing a plant to her full extent, which in my experience leads to a much more potently infused oil, especially if the plant is not aromatic.

3.) We can make these oils any time of the year with any plants we are able to order, and we may be able to prevent undue pressure that wildcrafting herbs creates in our unique environment by choosing to support ethically ran herb farms instead.

4.) They are a more realistically accessible option to folks who live in cities or have physical limitations that keep them from accessing the land.

5.) They are very shelf stable and rancidity is rather uncommon.

6.) We can expose these oils to heat.

7.) These are the only herbal oils that should be used in water/oil based emulsification creations such as creams, lotions, and body butters since there is no moisture present which mold, bacteria, and fungus generally require to live.

8.) We can press these to reclaim all of the oil we infuse, meaning we will waste less.

Dried Plant Matter Infused Oil Drawbacks:

1.) These oils really do need a full 6-8 weeks of infusing with low and steady heat (75*F-80*f) for the plant allies' cellular structure to break down well, and this will often require the use of electricity - especially in the winter months.

2.) There are certain plants, such as Saint John's Wort, that no matter how long we infuse are useless - and at times dangerous - to use in a fully dried state.

3.) We often have to gather double or even triple amounts of wildcrafted plant matter to end up with enough to make a dried plant oil infusion, and this can put pressure on our plant allies and the land.

4.) We run the risk of becoming what I like to call a Brown Box Herbalist. This is an herbalist who only works with herbs that get delivered in brown cardboard boxes, never stepping foot out on the land. This often leads to a damaging disconnect from the land.

5.) No matter how hard we try, we may not know how well the plants were treated. The same goes for the human that harvested them when we order from other humans.

It's probably bold for me to say this, but when I see someone adamantly debate that we must make herbal infused oils with fresh or dried plant allies across the board it kinda seems like to me they haven't taken the time to really think about the big picture nuances of each different method and how each option will be uniquely suited at one time or another to whatever specific thing we are doing our other humans individual experiences.

Okay, are we ready to talk about making infused oils out of a few plant allies in the book?

Yarrow~

When it comes to highly scented plant allies such as Yarrow, I chose to do a wilted plant matter infusion when I am able. Why?

Well, the parts of her I am after are really potent, so we don't exactly need heat or extended infusing times to get these to transfer into the oil. In fact, I never let something that has a lot of Yarrow in it go past 4 weeks of infusing (for external use. Tinctures are different.), because I don't want to irritate my skin.

To wilt your Yarrow after gathering, pluck off her leaves, cut off her blooms, then chop her stems into small manageable pieces. Now you can pop these into a curing cabinet for about 1-2 days, or you can lay them out in a dark place on cardboard for 2-3 days. The trick is to get a fair amount of moisture out, but no so much that they are actually dry. Be checking daily.

When the time comes, fill any jar you like halfway up with her leaves, blooms, and stems. You could fill the jar up all the way but she is a pretty powerful ally, so there is no real reason to for an infused oil. You do, however, need to fill the jar all the way up with oil and wait 10-15 mins before you cap it, to give all of the air bubbles a chance to rise to the top. Add more oil as the level drops.

Cap and then label what plant ally she is, what oil was used, what day you made it, and what date 4 weeks from then will be.

Now set your jar somewhere cool and dark, like a basement or a bedroom closet. Avoid stashing it in your kitchen. It's not as cool as you think in that bottom panty cupboard.

I have never personally had a Yarrow infused oil go bad on me. If I had to guess it's from her strong ability to kill mold, bacteria, and fungus. It is still a good idea to check her once a week for any signs of spoilage, and if all looks well just give the jar a shake and tuck her away again.

When the 4 weeks is up, strain her to separate the plant from the oil. Check out the tincture section of the book for tips and tricks. One really important thing to know is that we never want to press or squeeze wilted plants, because this will release water. If that water gets into the oil you carefully infused it will go bad, even with Yarrow's amazing ability to kill off yuck.

This oil can now be put back into a jar and tucked away in a cool dark place until you need her - or you can turn her into any number of things!

Here is a step by step list of all the stuff I just jabbered about for those who like them:

1.) Gather fresh Yarrow. Pluck off her leaves, cut off her blooms, then chop up her stems into small manageable pieces.

2.) Place these into a curing cabinet for about 1-2 days, or you can lay them out in a dark place on cardboard for 2-3 days.

3.) Check daily for dryness level. You want to get out a fair amount of moisture, but no so much she is actually dry. You should still be able to bend her leaves, stems, and blooms without them crumbling.

4.) After wilting, choose a jar that you can fill halfway up with her leaves, blooms, and stems. Keep in mind, you will also need enough oil to fill this jar all the way to the top.

5.) Fill the jar all the way up with oil of your choosing and wait 10-15 mins before capping, giving all the air bubbles a chance to rise to the top. Add more oil as the level drops from escaping air.

6.) Cap. Label with who she is, what oil was used, what day you made it, and what date 4 weeks from then will be.

7.) Set your jar somewhere cool and dark, like a basement or a bedroom closet. Avoid your kitchen - it not as cool in that bottom panty cupboard as you think, especially if you use your oven often.

8.) When 4 weeks is up, strain her to separate the plant from the oil. No matter what, **do not** squeeze or press the plant matter in any way. You can allow excess oil to drip off for an hour or so, but resist the urge to squeeze more out.

9.) Your infused oil is now ready to use in just about any way you would like!

Want to make a dried Yarrow infusion or use dried Yarrow alongside other infused herbs? Be sure to read the 'Fresh? Dry? How do We do These Things, Again?' section further on.

Plantain~

This gal is kinda slimy, which means she is kinda on the "wet" side for plant friend. In fact, some varieties of her can even grow in the water. If I am needing her ASAP, I will do a very well wilted oil infusion and not let her go more than two weeks. Past that is when she really tends to spoil.

I think and I am just thinking out loud here, but some plant allies spoil quicker as wilted oil because they have different rates of cellular degradation (they rot faster) when they die and are exposed to oil. A really rigid plant may be able to infuse longer, but something like rose petals will spoil oil in a snap! Of course, this also has to do with how much water is in any given plant.

So Plantain is both really full of water and breaks down easily, so two weeks of infusing seems to be about the max. Now sure, maybe you got some to go to four, or even six weeks, but how long did the oil last after straining? That's important to consider when we are infusing.

Wanting to make a wilted Plantain infused oil? Follow the same basic steps above for Yarrow, but if you want to make a dried Plantain oil, here is what we are gana do:

1.) After harvesting your Plantain, chop her up well. No need to pulverize her - a few passes with a kitchen knife or scissors will do.

2.) Place her into a curing cabinet for about 4-6 days, or you can lay her on cardboard out in a dark place for 6-8 days.

3.) The goal is to fully dry her. We don't need her to be so dry that she collapses into a powder, but you should be able to crush a piece of her in your hand pretty easy.

4.) Choose a jar that you can fill all the way up with her leaves. Remember, you will also need enough oil to fill this jar all the way to the top.

5.) Fill the jar all the way up with oil of your choosing and wait 10-15 mins before capping, giving the oil time to fully get into all of the nooks and crannies. Add more oil if the level drops from soaking in.

6.) Cap. Label with who she is, what oil was used, what day you made it, and what date 6-8 weeks from then will be.

7.) Set your jar somewhere warm and dark. You can check out my suggestions for these places in the 'How to Get That Heat' section at the end of this chapter.

8.) When the 6-8 weeks is up, strain her to separate the plant from the oil. Try to squeeze or press the plant matter in any way you can to get back as much oil as possible.

9.) Your infused oil is now ready to use in just about any way you would like!

Dandelion~

Both the blooms and roots of any plant are super easy to spoil oil with, because both hold so much moisture! Dandelion blooms in particular are really hard to wilt well, because her base will be fresh while her blooms are fully dried.

Roots tend to be the same way and - unless they are chopped up really fine - may seem dry on the outside but still waterlogged on the inside. For roots - especially those with no real scent - it's a real shame not to go past the 6 week mark on infusing. It really takes some time to break down her tough and rigid cell walls!

This is why for Dandelion (and most other) roots, I won't go less than 8 weeks with heat before I strain! If the root has a really strong scent, 4 weeks is usually what I feel comfortable with for a dried root infusion as well as wilted.

Because the Dandelion blooms break down so easily - even fully dried - you will have a really nice infused oil in as little as 2-3 weeks if kept in a warm, dark place. There is no need to chop up the blooms when drying, but do go at the roots pretty well. I like to make sure they are no bigger than ½ inch pieces, but don't worry about busting out a ruler. I just eye it.

You can follow the same directions for the Plantain leaf infusion, but here are a few tips to know:

1.) With roots you only need to fill up about half the jar. These are potent parts of our plant ally, and it would take A LOT to fill a jar all the way up.

2.) The blooms are pure fluff! You will want to pack them a bit so when you pour oil over top you won't watch them shrink into barely 1/4th of the jar once its filled.

Comfrey~

I cannot stress enough - If you are harvesting and drying your own Comfrey, **your Comfrey needs to be DRY to make an oil infusion that does not go rancid!** It's always a heartbreaking moment when someone tries to make their first infused oil and they choose to try with wilted Comfrey. I am not saying there aren't success stories out there. I'm just saying they sure as hell don't outweigh the failure stories!

If you are using dried, store bought Comfrey, you're good to go. Simply follow these instructions:

1.) Choose a jar that you can fill all the way up with her leaves. Remember, you will also need enough oil to fill the jar all the way to the top.

2.) Fill the jar with the oil of your choosing and wait 10-15 mins before capping, giving the oil time to fully soak into all of the nooks and crannies. Add more oil if the level drops from soaking in.

3.) Cap. Label with who she is, what oil was used, what day you made it, and what date 6-8 weeks from then will be.

4.) Set your jar somewhere warm and dark. Check out my suggestions for these places in the 'How to Get That Heat' section at the end of this chapter.

5.) When the 6-8 weeks is up, strain her to separate the plant from the oil. Try to squeeze or press the plant matter in any way you can to get back as much oil as possible.

6.) Your infused oil is now ready to use in just about any way you would like!

If you are using **freshly harvested Comfrey**, do these steps first:

1.) Curing or drying her is a bit tricky. She has a really moist stem down her leaf, so while the leaf itself is bone dry the stem will still be flexible, and if you pour oil over this stem she will likely make your oil go rancid.

2.) Wear gloves. She's itchy.

3.) If you don't have a lot to process, split the stems long ways. Then chop the entire leaf into pretty small pieces.

4.) If you have a lot, splitting all of the stems is not realistic - but chop her up **really well**.

5.) Place her into a curing cabinet for about 8-10 days, or you can lay her out on cardboard in a dark place for 13-15 days.

6.) The goal is to fully dry her. We want her to be so dry that she crumbles. Check many pieces of her stem before declaring her ready to use.

7.) Now you can follow the infusing steps above and not end up with a rancid oil!

Elderberry Blooms~

I'm going to be straight forward, if you are working with black Elderberry (Sambucus nigra) blooms, your infused oil is possibly going to smell like cat piss. This is not because she has cat piss in her, but she does contain butyric acid. This kinda has a natural lovely scent of urine and vomit. This will make you think your oil has gone rancid. While it likely hasn't, ain't no one trying to rub THAT all over their skin!

Most Elders have butyric acid in their blooms, but the common black variety really seems to pack a wallop! Thankfully this acid does not transfer her scent over into wines or the like, but I'll tell you what - oil really holds onto the scent!

If you are lucky enough to have the common blue variety in your neck of the woods (Sambucus cerulea), the rest of this bit is for you! Elder blossoms that don't smell like piss-filled vomit are great for skincare, but only if her blooms bone dry. In fact, if you still want to give black Elder blooms a try, you'll like what I am about to say!

Butyric acid evaporates off at 68*F. this means as we heat infuse we are breaking down that pissy smell maybe one weird human might pay good money for, haha. For those of us who aren't into that kinda thing, the good news is we have a few options here. Let's talk about the When, What, and How, then address the piss in the room:

1.) When you harvest your blooms, be sure that the whole cluster is in full bloom.

2.) Be mindful not to gather blooms that have been doing their thing for very long. If they are turning a darker color or have tiny little berries formed under them, you have missed your chance with that bunch.

3.) Instead of trying to hand pluck these tiny little blooms, cut away the thickest stems. This allows the big cluster to turn into many small clusters.

4.) Put these bloom clusters on cardboard in your curing cabinet or laid out to dry.

5.) Let these cure for about 4-6 days or dry for 7-9 days. They are ready when barely touching the blooms causes them to drop off.

6.) You have two options here: a.) Carefully put your bloom clusters into a big sealable clear bag and shake the living hell out of it. All of the blooms will fall off and then you can use a pasta colander to separate the blooms from the stem by shaking it back and forth. This is ideal if you have a lot. b.) With your hands over a bowl slowly begin knocking off the blooms, collecting them into the bowl.

7.) No matter which step you choose, next sift your blooms back and forth into a fine mesh strainer. This will cut back on the huge amount of pollen you have also collected, as it will fall through as the blooms stay.

8.) Choose a jar that you can fill halfway up with her tiny blooms. Remember you will also need enough oil to fill this jar all the way to the top.

9.) Fill the jar with the oil of your choosing and wait 10-15 mins before capping it to give the oil time to completely get into all of the nooks and crannies. Add more oil if the level drops.

10.) Cap. Label with who she is, what oil was used, what day you made it, and what date 6-8 weeks from then will be.

11.) Now set your jar somewhere warm and dark. You can check out my suggestions for these places in the 'How to Get That Heat' section at the end of this chapter.

12.) When the 6-8 weeks is up, strain her to separate the plant from the oil. Try to squeeze or press the plant matter any way you can to get back as much oil as possible.

That's the basic how to, but what can we do to help keep our oil from smelling like a house with too many cats? A few things:

a.) Use a really wide jar so there is a lot of surface space, then leave about ¼ inch of headspace for an air gap. Now poke a bunch of small holes in the lid of the jar. This (if your heated area gets warm enough) will allow the surface space needed for the butyric acid to evaporate, and the holes in your lid will give it a way to escape.

b.) If after infusing you notice your oil still has that back ally funk that so many bars are famous for, you can put your oil in a double boiler and bring the temperature up to about 80*F and hold for 3-4 hours - you'll need a thermometer. This will destroy and evaporate off the butyric acid and once it cools down you should really notice a scent difference. This might not work well if you've chosen an oil with a really low smoking point to infuse with.

c.) Infuse your blooms with another really fragrant plant ally of your choosing. This can at least help bury that smell if it's not super overwhelming. This will not work for someone like me who has a super nose, so if you are selling this humbly offer a refund when the person says it smells like piss. Because it does.

This is actually a perfect example of when the nuances between a wilted infused oil and dried hot infused oil come into play. When these blooms are moist and cold her butyric acid is gana smell even worse!

There are so many oils to choose from~

Let me start by saying these are just a very small handful of oils to consider. Don't be afraid to try others or blend these oils to match the end result you're dreaming of when creating an herbal infused oil!

Avocado Oil ~

This oil is hands down my favorite to work with. In fact, it's just about all I use. I am mindful to source it organically and from orchards grown within the US, as there is a lot of suffering involved with Avocados grown in Mexico, both for the people and the land.

This oil is extracted from her seed and is amazing for all skin types (but especially sensitive), absorbs quickly, and is packed with healthy fatty acids and Vitamin A, B, D, and E!

If you are wanting to make something for eczema, psoriasis, or other skin conditions, she is once again my first choice. She is also going to help increase the collagen in your skin, fade age spots, and is pretty damn great for scar tissue.

She has a really high smoke point, which also means she is heat stable. I almost never have freshly wilted infused oils go rancid when using her.

Now imagine what she can do with plant allies infused into her. It's easy to see why I swoon over her!

Coconut Oil~

We all know Coconut oil and with all of the absurd health claims floating around, who knows, maybe this oil will cure your herpes. (That was a joke. She won't.)

However, she is not a horrible choice to work with since she does have good fatty acids and decent vitamin levels - in particular vitamin K, which makes her good for things like dark rings under our eyes, dark spots, and bruising.

To work with her in a cold state you will have to get the refined form that does not go solid at room temperature, so she's kinda a no go for wilted oil infusion. Keep in mind that allergies to coconut are really common. In fact, this is why I personally no longer work with her.

She has a mild scent of coconut when she's not refined, and no scent when she is. I think she is best at is catching smell. I am not entirely sure why (and believe me I have tried to find out, to no avail), but compared to all other oils she really holds onto scents. This can be a good thing for good smelling plant allies, but a not so great thing if the plant is rather pungent.

She is a good moisturizer, but does leave some folks' skin feeling a bit on the greasy side. With how mild she is, coconut oil is a great option for sensitive skin.

Grapeseed Oil~

This gal is a great choice for an infused oil you are wanting to use for a body massage or breast massage oil because she has a real knack for sinking in quick and deep into the skin.

She is super moisturizing and has great polyunsaturated fats levels, while also having higher linoleic acid than many other oils. That is how she's such a great moisturizer. Llinoleic acid creates a barrier on our skin that holds in moisture.

She truly does have a smooth and silky texture, and does not leave a greasy film. She is also kinda hypo-allergenic, and a pretty affordable option to try out.

I have never used her to do a wilted plant infused oil, but she works really great with heat infused oils. Depending on the herb the end result is usually so dark that light tends to not pass through. This tells me she is doing a great job at breaking down the dried plant matter's cellular structure!

Olive Oil~

Chances are if you have bought a balm, lotion, or body oil, olive oil was what she was made out of. At the very least, she was included.

She is a great emollient, which means she moisturizes by trapping a thin layer of oil on your skin, but this is also why she's not super ideal for skin that is not dry. She will take forever to absorb in, and you will for sure look shiny.

I'm going to be totally honest here - people use her because she is cheap and plentiful. However, a small amount of research will show you that when she is cheap and plentiful you are almost never getting pure olive oil. If you are, it's not going to be cheap. It is cut with all sorts of other unlisted oils and not that long ago they even discovered a company out of China was buying it cheap and then cutting it petroleum byproducts before they flipped it again.

I also notice she goes rancid easily on her own, and even faster if we introduce plants, whether dried or wilted. She is an economical option for beginners, but I'm warning you now - don't go making gallons of things with her until you really get the feel for infused oils and the specific brand of olive oil you will be working with, or you'll end up dumping out a ton of your infusions when they go rancid.

First thing I ask when someone reaches as to why their oil infusion when rancid is, "Did you use olive oil?" 80% of the time their answer is yes.

Sunflower Oil~

She's cheap, got a ton of vitamins A, D, E, and there are many types of her available to suit individual skin needs!

She is also really easily absorbed into the skin, and her high antioxidant levels make her great for dry, aged, and weathered skin. While she is not the fanciest oil, she is a really good starter oil. While you want to check the expiration date on the bottle you buy, she is not super likely to go rancid if it's freshly made.

Safflower Oil~

Speaking of different types of Sunflower oil, this lady is a cousin of hers and another great and affordable option to begin working with for herbal infused oils! She is great for dry and acne prone skin, and has the ability to help combat irritations such as rashes and inflammation.

She is loaded with Oleic, Linoleic, Palmitic, Stearic, Linolenic, and Palmitoleic acids, which means she also is great for increasing collagen which tightens and tones. Because she is packed with antioxidants, she encourages a youthful appearance and is pretty good for dark spots and scarring.

She takes a bit longer to soak into skin that is not dry, so I would probably not solely use her for face oils, but she infuses well and I have not noticed her going rancid more than usual.

Alright, let's take a quick look at how any oil you chose might be made. Don't worry, it'll say on the bottle:

Cold Pressed~ This is where little to no heat is used to smash out the oil. This creates higher end oils and is gana be seen on most top shelf oil options for cosmetics. However, you can't really do this with all oils (like Vegetable), so if you are looking and looking for an oil in cold pressed form and can't find it, they probably can't make it that way.

Expeller Pressed~ This is when real heat comes into play and they use friction and hydraulic presses to get every last drop out! These are still pretty high quality oils, and is how most oils for the cosmetic industry are made. This process won't jack the price up as much as cold pressed, so it's a good option.

Unrefined~ Think of this as just raw oil that is smashed with zero heat and is allowed to pass through a screen to catch some of the plant matter. These often have a high scent of whatever plant they smashed, and will make just about anything you infuse with wilted plant matter go rancid in a heartbeat. They have a lot of plant matter and proteins left in them from the raw pressing process. Great for super fancy cooking, not so much for making herbal creations.

Refined~ These oils have been heated to really high levels, screened, heated again, and are about as "clean" as you're gana get from an oil. They often have no scent, are lighter in color, and while this is not always a healthy oil to be eating, they are very useful and practical for anyone starting out on a budget.

Partially Refined~ These are just what they sound like - a refined oil that's not quite as refined. This is usually used for strong smelling oils so you don't have to smell them. They are a small step above refined oil in quality.

Fresh? Dry? How do We do These Things Again?~

I figure giving another good solid rundown is not a bad idea, and I know some of you want to cut through my novel worth of words and just see the How laid out step by step, so let's do just that. I will say to check out the section back a ways where I give specific info for the individual plant allies in this book, as you will find some nuances there I may not cover in this area.

Making an Herbal Infused Oil with Freshly Wilted Plant Matter:

1.) Wilt the plant you are wanting to infuse for 2-4 days, making sure to split the stems so excess moisture can escape. Be sure it does not get too dry. It should still be flexible without breaking.

2.) Pour your oil of choice over the wilted plants all the way to the top of the jar. Air will increase your odds of spoiling and oxidation.

3.) Wait about 10-15 mins for air bubbles to escape before capping. Add more oil if the level decreases.

4.) Label and place your jar in a cool dark place (55*F-65*F) for no more than 6 weeks of infusing. Check weekly (or even daily) for mold, rancidity, and other signs of spoilage.

5.) When the infusing time is done, strain her to separate the plant from the oil. No matter what, do not squeeze or press the plant matter in any way! You can allow excess oil to drip off for an hour or so, but resist the urge to squeeze more out.

6.) Your infused oil is now ready to use in just about any way you would like!

Tips:
Due to how full your jar will be, expect your oil to weep out of the lid. It's a good idea to place a plate or a towel you don't care about under your jar(s) to catch the oil.

Don't put your infusing jars or finished oil anywhere near the kitchen. It is warmer there than you think, especially if you use the oven often.

If you live somewhere hot, after straining you can keep your oil in the fridge. Some oils will go cloudy in very cold temperatures, but will go away when warmed back up.

Consider setting an automated reminder on your smartphone for the date she needs to be pressed. Freshly wilted plant infusions are not forgiving to us forgetting them.

Making an Herbal Infused Oil with Dried Plant Matter:

1.) Choose a jar that you can fill either all the way up or to whatever level you decide. Remember, you will also need enough oil to fill this jar all the way to the top.

2.) Fill the jar with the oil of your choosing and wait 10-15 mins before capping to give the oil time to fully get into all of the nooks and crannies. Add more oil if the level drops from soaking in.

3.) Cap. Label with who she is, what oil was used, what day you made it, and what date 6-8 weeks from then will be.

4.) Set your jar somewhere warm and dark. You can check out my suggestions for these places in the How to Get That Heat Section at the end of this chapter.

5.) When the 6-8 weeks is up, strain her to separate the plant from the oil. Try to squeeze or press the plant matter in any way you can to get back as much oil as possible.

6.) Your infused oil is now ready to use in just about any way you would like!

Tips:
Due to how full your jar will be and the fact that oil expands when warmed, expect your oil to weep out of the lid. It's a good idea to place a plate or a towel you don't care about under your jar(s) to catch the oil.

Making an Herbal Infused Oil with Freshly Wilted Plant Matter AND Dried Plant Matter:

Follow the same steps for the wilted plant matter infused oil, but here are some things to consider when choosing how to make these blends.

Are the dried plant bits you are wanting to use really tough and rigid, like roots and bark? The cool and short infusing time constraints for the wilted plant matter won't get you very far with rigid plant matter. Consider infusing these bits separately with heat, and then adding this oil to your wilted infused oil. You can even make your dried infused oils first, and then use this oil to make your freshly wilted oils.

If you want to infuse dried and wilted at the same time, add more dried plant matter than you think you'll need. This will get you a little bit further in the cool and short infusing times. On the other hand, if you are picking a dried plant matter that is well scented, there is no need to add more than you planned.

Truthfully, whenever possible I prefer to infuse my freshly wilted separate from my dried, mainly because if the freshly wilted oil does spoil, I only end up wasting that oil and plant ally versus that plus the dried plant ally I added.

When to Choose Fresh and When to Choose Dry~

This answer will only be found as you are getting to know any given plant ally you are working with. By this I mean you will need to use your curiosity to ask questions like:

Does this plant have properties that dissipate when she's dried, like Saint John's Wort or Skullcap? If so, are these the things I am after?

Is this a really tough plant that needs heat to truly extract the bits of her I am after?

Is this a really wet plant, and can her properties be extracted the same if dried? Is it worth risking my oil going bad?

Is this a kinda sorta rare plant? If so, is it worth the risk of wasting her if my oil goes bad?

What will I be using this oil for? Am I making a water-based emulsified creation that I can't risk adding mold, bacteria, and fungal contamination to?

Is this something that I need access to on a daily and consistent basis for my external skin health? If so, can I make enough in one season with freshly wilted plant matter to last me an entire year?

That Smells Like Death, Please Don't Church it Up~

I once watched a 2 minute video on infusing violet leaves for breast health that had over one million views. In this video the woman said in a quaint southern accent, "Now don't you worry none about your oil smelling a bit musty or sour after infusing, we can church that right up with a few drops of our favorite essential oil!"

This is how instead of healing your or someone else's skin, you give them a fucking flesh eating disease. I am not even being dramatic. If you are using freshly wilted plant matter there will be microscopic amounts of water in your oil, and if these little bits get a bit more as the infusing process goes along you have the perfect conditions for (and I have said it a million times now) mold, bacterial growth, fungus, and I'll add in rancidity. If you know your oil has gone bad, this is what you need to do:

Dump it out. There is **nothing** you can do to save it. You can't heat it. You can't strain it. You can't cool it. If you try to mask the scent with "essential oils" or in any other way you are **unethical as fuck,** and more concerned with making money or wasting money than you are with helping yourself or others.

Look, I get it. It really sucks to waste that oil, that plant, and your time, but it won't suck as much as ending up with a serious injury from rubbing any amount of dangerous molds, bacteria, or fungus on our skin. If you truly can't afford to take the risk of ending up with an oil you have to dump, stick with using dried plant matter. Does this guarantee our oil can't go rancid? No, but the odds are far less likely.

You see, rancidity is not so much due to mold, bacteria, or fungus as it is the oil itself going rotten. Oil, at its heart, is a food product after all, and they all have expiration dates. So even when the plant matter we add is completely dry, there is still a chance it will speed up this process. That's why it's best to use all herbal infused oil within a year of straining. At a year the herbal properties we have infused begin to drop off slightly, but the real risk is the likely odds of randicidity.

I remember thinking to myself, "No way are EO's gana cover up the smell of rancid oil!" Rancid oil smells like death - like someone stuck roadkill in a jar, poured oil over the top, and then set it in the sun for a week. As it gets further along the smell builds, so if at first your oil just smells a bit sour or musty, or it stinks in a way that the plant does not smell, then there is something wrong. I am a very curious creature though, and I like to see if some shit that is said is really a thing, either through compulsive research or actually experimenting.

So I made some oil go really make-you-vomit rancid on purpose with the help of fresh Comfrey and extra virgin olive oil. Then I ordered a tiny little vial of Lavender "essential oil" and added it to the rancid oil. I gave it a good shake and - I swear on my children's life - the only thing I could smell was Lavender, and that were only 5 drops her to one gallon of rancid oil! I wondered if this was because the vapors from the volatile oils were rising to the mouth of the jar, so I poured some of the oil in a cheap, secondhand pot. I expected to smell the foul rotten oil as it heated, but nope. It just smelled like an overly scented bathroom in someones grandma's house. I added a bit of beeswax to make it a salve, and poured a bit in a tin. When it cooled I put on a glove and rubbed some on warm plastic wrap covering a heating pad, kinda sorta trying to mimic warm skin. The only thing I smelled was Lavender.

This is a great way for me to touch on yet again the dangers of "essential oils" right quick. These highly refined volatile compounds have such a potent scent that if you are adding them to your infused oils, to that massage oil, to the balms you turn your oils into or whatever, **you will not smell when the oil has gone rancid!** While I know many reading this will still use "essential oils" on a regular basis in your creations, at the very least consider not using them during the infusing phase because you will have no way of smelling if your oil has gone rancid.

Here comes something scary, though. Mold, bacteria, and fungus rarely have smells, and if they do it's only because the jar is now solid mold, bacteria, and/or fungus. The main reason I rarely use freshly wilted plant matter when making something a bit complicated (like a water based emulsified creation) is because until these things fully take over all of your oil **you will not be able to see them with your naked eye**. These things are microscopic until they fruit or become large colonies. Here is a really good Gross-You-Out example - Ya know that one time you went to make a sandwich and you noticed a tiny bit of fuzzy mold on the heel, so you just tossed the heal and grabbed some bread from further back in the bag? You just ate a moldy sandwich. Mold spores had already fully spread through every inch of that loaf of bread. The fuzz finally popping up is simply the mold being far enough along in its process to bloom.

This is why if I can make my infused oil out of dried plant matter, I do. Mold, fungus and most bacteria can't grow in oil. There has to be water present.

How can we tell if there is mold or fungus?

1.) Mold needs air, so you will normally find it near the top of your jar. Even if you fill the jar all the way to the top, a little bit of air does get in through the lid.

2.) Anything that does not look like the plant and oil is likely something funky.

3.) If you are using blooms, pollen can accumulate on the plant matter and the bottom of the jar, but anything that sticks to the side of the jar is likely a fungus.

4.) Do not listen to folks who tell you you can simply remove the mold from the top surface. Remember the moldy sandwich story. The whole jar is mold you just can't see it.

5.) If it does have a funky smell that is not what the plant or oil smells like, be skeptical. If it gets worse, it's trash.

6.) Mold won't shake back in. No amount of shaking will dissipate this. The little chunks will maybe get smaller but they won't go back into the oil.

7.) If you are not sure, check it again in a week. Odds are good if it's alive, it's growing. You should see more developed.

8.) Really REALLY want to be sure? Buy yourself a little tabletop bacteria, yeast, and mold incubator, and some test strips. This will cost about $300 bucks, but it's the only way I am 100% sure my freshly wilted infused oils are safe to use. I have caught more than one batch of oil that looks fine to the naked eye with mold hiding in it.

Please don't let this kinda stuff freak you out. Instead, let it make you feel confident in what you are doing. Like you have the knowhow to damn well say to yourself and anyone else that you did your absolute best when making something, and so if something does go wrong it was not for lack of understanding, let alone effort to get it right!

How to Get That Heat~

Three words. Seed. Heating. Mat. I am serious. These fairly inexpensive things are freaking fantastic at heating our jars up, and they come in all different sizes. You can even get controllers with them to set the exact temperature you want them to heat to!

Here are some things to know and a few tips that make using them great:

1.) A mat with no heat controller box thingy (technical term folks, haha) will only get up to about 72*, and the heat radiates up through the bottom of your jar.

2.) The more jars you have on the mat the more they will act as a conduit for heat, and will push up into the 80*F-85* range. Make sure the jars are touching each other.

3.) The jars in the middle are always warmer than the jars on the outside. Be sure to rotate weekly for even heating.

4.) Don't burn your fucking house down by putting blankets or anything similar to catch more heat. I almost did, once.

5.) If you are using the heat controller option the mat will turn off when the temperature you want is hit, but a good one should click back on when the temperature drops.

6.) Remember that heat makes oil expand, so the jars will leak. No big deal. The mat is moisture proof and can be wiped down easily.

Don't want to buy a heat mat? These places in your home are likely warmer than the rest of the house:

1.) Have an electric water heater tank? The tops of these are usually in the 70*F-75*F range. Be sure to have something under your jar to catch any oil that leaks. These are usually in a kinda dark part of the house, but if yours is not just toss a towel or blanket over your jar.

2.) The tops of refrigerators are usually pretty warm, and since these are in the kitchen it will often be in the 80*F range up, especially in summer.

3.) A cupboard above or directly next to your oven is a good option in winter IF you use the oven on an almost daily basis to be generating heat.

4.) Next to floor vents that blow out heat in winter.

5.) Next to **but NOT on top of** your wood burning or pellet stove in winter.

6.) In an unvented garage during the summer months but, be mindful. The temperatures can get too high in here. You don't want to go much above 100*F.

Where we don't want to source heat from:

1.) The Sun. I know, I know. You see so many pretty pictures of beautifully colored jars infusing in the sun on a huge amount of social media posts, but here's the thing - these oils are basically useless if they were put there for more than the sake of taking a picture. The Sun is for sure THE original source for heat, but she is also the great decomposer. She has the power to not just break down plant matter, but to utterly and fully degrade the medicinal and nutritional properties of your herbal infused oil. This is why we get such fast and rapid color in our oils, or Sun Tea. No big deal for a jug of tea that only sat there for a few hours, but a real big deal for oils that have set for days, weeks, and even months at a time. This is why I say a **dark** and warm place over and over again. Light kills.

2.) A crockpot. Just stop. Unless you are leaving this thing on for weeks at a time, at best you are catching color and a bit of scent. Nothing in a crockpot for 24, 48, or 72 hours is any more healing than the plain oil is. The same goes for heating up oil and plant matter on top of the stove. In no way is this enough time to fully break down the cellular structure of the plant, let alone allow the heavy minerals and vitamin content to absorb into the oil. You are just catching color and scent. Another thing to consider - even if it is breaking down the cells, the high level of heat from the stovetop is going to destroy and degrade all of the properties we are after. Same goes for leaving the oven on low. This is not going to do much unless the jars are in there for weeks at a time.

Slow medicine is healing medicine. These shortcuts only shortchange us out of what our plant allies can truly offer, both in healing and a lesson in patience.

.23.

The humble transforming of infused oils into balms, salves, & butters.

So you've made way more oil than you need or you're not a fan of rubbing plain oil on your skin. What can we do?

Get busy making balms, salves, and butters!

The first thing I need you to know is that these are in no way as complicated as many seem to think! Does this mean I'm not going to end up talking for 10 pages about them? I make no guarantees on that! What I do know is that besides tinctures and body oils, balms, salves, and oil based butters are the easiest things I make!

Before we get to how, let's talk about the differences between these three creations and when one would be preferred over the other!

What is a Balm?

A balm is just wax thickened oil that we use a higher amount of wax in, resulting in a bit firmer of a setup. Meaning when our hot oils and melted wax cool down to room temperature, the resulting combination makes for a creation that has a really firm texture.

This firmer texture means not only will we have to use a bit of pressure to get some out of the container we poured it into, but it also takes a bit more heat for it to melt once on our skin. The higher amounts of wax make balms really rest on top of the skin, and hold these healing herbal infused oils on the surface a bit longer before soaking in. This also means they are a great choice for dry skin issues.

Their heat resistant aspects make them ideal for summer shipping, since the more wax it has the higher melting point there is.

Balms are a great choice if the issue you are trying to target with your infused oil is on the surface, if you need hydration, and if you're living in warmer climates. On the flip side, some do not like how long it takes to soak in when it's hot out, but whatever oil you end up choosing will affect this greatly.

What is a Salve?

A salve, on the other hand, has quite a bit less wax than a balm. When it cools it sets up softly. This softer texture means it scoops out easily and melts rapidly into the skin, giving way to quick absorption. Again, this can be affected by what oil you are using.

With how soft and melty they are, they are not ideal for shipping in summer or for super warm climates. Funny enough, most folks try to remedy this by adding more wax, which is fine but it's no longer a salve - it's a balm!

Salves are usually liked over balms in the summer because they absorb pretty quickly, but this also means that I will choose to make a salve when the ailment I made the oil to help with is deeper in our body, like soft tissue and muscles. A good example is anything for pain relief. We want it to deeply penetrate our skin.

What is a Butter?

A butter can be made in a lot of ways, and every way still calls it a "butter". In this space a butter is a balm that has way more wax added. Then we freeze it, chop it up, and then beat the ever living hell out of it until it whips into a nice buttery texture.

An oil and wax only butter is usually a wintertime thing. Even with the extra wax the heat makes the whipped texture collapse easy. There is nothing wrong with it if this happens. It's just pretty heavy to use afterwards.

Butters are ideal when we really need deep hydration and to seriously hold the healing properties of our infused oil in place. Although it is similar to a balm kinda, the whipping seems to both keep it on the surface and help it sink deeply in, so it's a nice balance between the two for colder months.

You can make these in summer, but it will be hard to keep them whipped, and you will need to store it in the fridge, which will give it a harder texture (from the cold). Don't even try to ship them in the heat. It won't work out, I promise.

On the upside, these butters do not need preservatives since there is no water content present, unlike most body butters. That is why I really prefer these for breast massage butters and such.

Things We Can Add:

By no means are we limited to just wax and oil in our balms, salves, or butters!

Healthy Animal Fats~

Before you cringe, acknowledge the fact that basically all infused remedies your ancestors made (no matter what culture(s) you come from) used some sort of animal fat. They did not have the massive setups required to make refined oils. If I can get away with adding an animal fat to whatever I am making I do so in a heartbeat! Why? Our skin loves real fat! Our bodies love real fat! Not only do these fats often have amazing healing properties of their own, they trick our body to pull the healing oils in deeper. So as your likely-fat-deprived skin (from daily showers in chlorinated water) pulls this fat into itself , and the herbs we have infused into the oil get pulled along for the ride!

1.) Tallow by far is my personal number one choice. Tallow is rendered down fat from red meat animals. Now don't freak out, but you are a red meat animal. Just like a cow, a deer, a goat, a bear. Anything that has red flesh is a red meat animal. This means we all have similar fats, and our bodies recognize these fats over all others. Tallow is pulled in the deepest of them all, and has the best health benefits for our skin. Make sure the tallow you source is from grass fed animals, or consider making your own out of wild game if your family actively hunts. This is one more way to use up every bit of the animals that die giving us the gift of a nourished life.

Here are the benefits of tallow for our skin:

Tallow contains the same lipids found in the healthy, supple skin of any red meat animal. That means you. Lipids are a huge part of the membrane that is present in every single cell of our bodies. They are how moisture flows in and out of our cells. Not enough lipids means dry and unhappy skin! These lipids create a semi protective barrier that prevents infection, maintains moisture, flexibility, and structure of the cell. In a nutshell, tallow can prevent dry skin at a cellular level without suffocating our skin!

As if that wasn't reason enough, tallow from grass fed animals is also packed with Vitamins A, D, K, E. This means she's got powerful antioxidant properties that makes her amazing at fighting free radicals that play a huge part in our skin aging not so gracefully!

2.) Lard is the second most common thing used as an animal fat. Lard, unlike tallow, is specifically made from pigs and pigs alone. Just like you may not have enjoyed hearing that you are a red meat animal, you may or may not enjoy knowing that you and a pig are creepily similar on a cellular level. No, that was not an underhanded fat joke - that's a fact! Because of this our skin also really gets down with lard! While tallow shares this ability too, lard is great at balancing our sebum - which is just a fancy word for the oil some glands in our skin make.

Here are the benefits of lard on its own accord for our skin:

Lard has a lot of similar lipids as tallow, so we already know she's great at offering moisture at a cellular level. Lard is also great for helping us reduce oily skin with its oil. This may sound crazy, but when your oil levels are out of control this is actually due to your skin being dry. It throws a shit fit every time you wash oil off, and before you know it you are in a vicious cycle where you are constantly trying to strip the oil your skin is working itself to death to replace. You can usually break this cycle with lard and other healthy animal fats, because your skin is getting what it needs and the lard is washing the excess oil off of your face.

One area that lard outshines tallow is that pigs are amazing at processing sunlight and storing it as Vitamin D in their fat. This makes lard particularly amazing at getting rid of dark spots, fine lines, and outright producing collagen - which is what makes youthful skin look youthful!

When sourcing lard, don't buy the junk sold in tubs for cheap. This is laden with chemicals. Instead, look for a high quality grass fed leaf lard, or something of similar quality.

While tallow and lard are the most commonly used animal fats, you can even jump into the world of poultry fats like emu, duck, and chicken. If you are really looking for a unique way to connect with your ancestors, look into what animals they hunted or farmed and the odds are good there were women rendering these fats down, to not only feed their families but to infuse herbs to heal them!

Butters~

These are in no way shape or form "butter" or even the body butter I talked on above, but what the cosmetic industry calls refined and solid parts of certain plants.

Cocoa Butter~

This "butter" is high in fatty acids, which is why it's great for hydrating, nourishing, and improving our skin's elasticity. That last bit is why folks swear by her for preventing stretch marks, and maybe even softening the appearance of the ones that do show up. The fat in cocoa butter acts similar to animal fats by forming a protective barrier over the skin to hold in moisture. Cocoa butter is also rich in natural compounds called phytochemicals, which means there are good levels of antioxidants present.

This butter when unrefined has a chocolate scent, so you will need the refined butter if you don't want that scent in what you're making. It also has a nicely smooth texture in balms, salves, and butters. However, the unrefined can have little bits in it, so melt it down separately and strain before adding to your hot oil and wax pot.

Shea Butter~

This one also has high concentrations of fatty acids and vitamins that hydrate, nourish, and are great for helping boost collagen production, but it is also a pretty powerful emollient. This just means it holds in moisture while deeply softening our skin. The thing I love her for is her high levels of vitamin K. This makes her great for dark spots, bruising, and dark rings under our eyes.

Unrefined she has a nutty smell that you will either love or hate. The refined has no smell. In small amounts she is nice and smooth in our creations, but I find that too much can make things a bit heavy feeling.

Mango Butter~

This butter is like Shea and Cocoa got together and had a supercharged baby. It not only has the ability to do all of the above things, but has twice the levels of acids, fats, vitamins, minerals, and a slew of everything else! The downfall is that it is so hard that it is difficult to work with. While we can rub the other butters into our skin as is, if we want Mango butter on our skin it really needs to be put in your creations and melted down as an ingredient.

Sadly this butter will not smell like mangoes, but unrefined it does have a slightly sweet and fatty smell.

These are just three commonly used and easily obtained butters that we can add to our balms, salves, and butters. There are for sure more out there to explore, and we by no means only have to use one at a time!

Oils~

This might seem funny since we are turning our herbal infused oils into this, but some oils we don't need much of, or a large amount will cost us our first born child so we only want to add a little bit.

Jojoba Oil~

This oil is expensive as hell, but a little goes a really long way! This means as little as a few tablespoons can really enhance our creations with is anti-inflammatory properties, which knock out chafing and chapping, reduce redness caused by drying, tackle eczema and rosacea, and keep our skin from throwing a temper tantrum. The E and B-complex Vitamins in this oil also lend a hand to skin repair and damage control from free radicals.

This oil is not great yet gives good "slip", which means rubbing something into our skin is effortless and goes a long way.

Castor Oil~

This might make you laugh or feel a bit concerned, but my other half calls this "The Devil's Oil". To be fair, this is because we are handling gallons and gallons of it and this oil is THICK and COATS everything. By the end of the day no matter how hard we try we are covered in a suffocating layer of thick Devils Oil, haha!

If you're not dealing with huge amounts of it like we are there is no need to be afraid, especially because castor oil contains crazy high levels of antioxidants that fight free radicals on our skin, a powerful antibacterial great for acne, and pulls down inflammation. It is great to add a bit (and I mean just a bit, like a tablespoon or two) to your creations if you are really wanting something that locks moisture in.

Apricot Kernel Oil~

This is a great non-greasy, enriching emollient (it helps hold in moisture and smooth out skin). Packed with vitamins, minerals, and acids, she is really loved for her ability to revitalize, soothe, and prevent acne and inflammation. With its high levels of vitamin K content, it is another great choice for creations meant to target dark spots, under eyes, and bruising.

You can add these right to your jar of infusing oil, but I like to wait until I'm at the hot spot - that way as I do cooling setup testes (I'll get to that) I can check the texture, and see if I need to add more. Doing this I can start slowly, and then add until I am happy with it. The other way won't be able to correct it if you add too much without cutting your oil with plain oil, which will make your creation weaker.

Minerals and Other Things~

While most of these next things will not absorb into oils, the oils will absorb into them.

Clays~

There are so many types of clays I am not going to dive that deep here, but most clays have the ability to help pull toxins out of our skin and pull up things like boils and ingrown hairs. They can either hold in moisture or be used to dry up an issue, and have varying different types of mineral content. There are so, so, so, sooooo many types of clays that you need to look into yourself to see what one may fit your creation the best.

Activated Charcoal~

This is going to stain anything you touch until you get it in the pot. With that in mind, don't overdo how much you put in. Activated charcoal is amazing for pulling serious things out of your skin, like deep boils, ingrown toenails, splinters and even deep infection. It is also very drying, so it is a great thing to add to anything that is meant to combat fungal infections or wet weeping skin conditions. It's also a common thing in homemade deodorants because it dries so well, but it will stain clothing and even some skin if you put too much. I can't stress enough to have a light hand!

Salts~

This is another thing we can add for drying, but it's also great if we are looking to make something that aids in healing of wounds. You will want a finely powdered sea salt or it will be rough on the skin. On the flip side that roughness can be tapped into for the creations we want to have good skin exfoliation properties.

Freshly Powdered Herbs~

I say freshly powdered here because powdered herbs lose their medicinal and nutritional properties rapidly. By the time you order and receive them they are usually worthless. However, if we powder our own with a coffee grinder we can add these to give a healing boost, and this is really ideal if we are making something for antibacterial reasons, like how powdered Yarrow would be great for a wound salve.

An important thing to know about any of these is that they will not dissolve into your balm, salve, or butter, so when you are getting ready to pour these things you will need to be constantly stirring to kick up the additions. They tend to settle on the bottom, and you want them evenly distributed when pouring you balm and salves.

Things We Can't Add:

These are things that no matter how cool we think it'd be we can't add them to oil without getting into the more complicated realms of emulsification - which is the process of using various chemicals to make molecularly force water and oil to combine. I will say it's not all that hard, but it's a whole different book for sure.

Waters~

Anything that is water based. I'm talking teas, gels (like aloe), water, milk, honey (powdered honey is usable), anything that needed water or has a high (or even low) water content can not be added to balms, salves, or butters. It will never blend together, and it will cause your oil to spoil.

Tinctures~

These are a type of water, but the alcohol in them also can't be added with any luck. Did you just have an "ah, ha!" moment where you said to yourself, "I make glycerine tinctures!"? Glycerine is, and is not, an oil. It's kinda sorta an alcohol too, but it is not oil soluble. So it also can't be added.

Preservatives~

I mean, you can add a preservative but it's pointless. It won't stop something from going rancid, and mold/fungus won't grow in your salve/balm/butter unless your freshly wilted oil was a failure and it had water content in it. If you do decide to add one, you will need to find one that is oil soluble and can handle high heat. Some European countries require them if you will be selling your creations, regardless of them actually being needed.

The Right Tools:

Just to be clear, I got by making tons of creations with very little tools, and while in some ways the poverty trauma in me feels proud of that, my worn out body sings a different song. Do we need every gadget? No, but please hear me when I say if you begin making more than a little here and a little there, buy the tools to make your work easier. Whenever possible, if you can save up to do so. Your body deserves it. Also, if this feels like a real passion you are going to follow buy equipment you can grow into, not out of . These are things I would redo if I could go back in time before my herbal business.

Double Boiler~

These come in so handy, and for more than just making balms or salves. They are also great for making syrups, simmering honeys, bringing oil up to a set temperature, and so much more.

These are just a pot that fits kinda airtight into another pot. The bottom pot holds water and the top pot holds the oils and waxes that we are wanting to combine. When we turn our stove on it boils the water below, which transfers the heat to the pot above. This is a great way to heat our oils and waxes without scorching them, and gives us pretty good control over the temperature.

I started off with a little 2 quart double boiler that I found for a few bucks at a thrift store (now I use two five gallon ones!), but even brand new they are not overly expensive. If you can't afford to buy one, no worries. Before I found one on the cheap I used a stainless steel bowl on top of my old spaghetti pot that was simmering away. As long as the bowl makes a snug fit and isn't huge this works okay to heat things up. If the bowl is too wide it never really gets evenly warm.

You can also stick your canning jar full of oil and wax in a pot with simmering water about halfway up the jar and melt it all together, but you risk blowing the bottom out of your jar from the heat and vibration of the simmering water. I've had it happen once, which was the last time I ever used that method.

I have seen folks recommend putting a jar into the microwave and making a salve this way. Please don't. It will kill all of your hard work infusing your oils since microwaves makes everything in the oil practically void, just like they do to our food. Plus, it is going to give you a really fucked up texture.

Confectionery Funnel~

For years I used glass measuring cups to pour any hot oil I created, and these are fine. Messy, but fine. After years I could pour hundreds of tins to the same level in no time flat. I will also tell you this murdered my back, neck, and my arm. Then I got this neat little thing called a confectionery funnel. This is a funnel with a handle that has a lever you can push down that lifts a little stopper at the bottom of the funnel. It is a beautiful thing, my friends. I almost never spill. I can fly through filling any size tin. I can control the flow with different sized tips for the end of the funnel and it's so easy on my body!

I have only ever seen them online, but I live in a rural area with minimal shopping resources. If you live in a bigger area you may find one. Be sure you get a metal one. They range from $30-$100+ bucks, so there are a lot of options.

Of course, glass or metal liquid measuring cups are fine, but find ones with a more pronounced pouring spout than the pyrex ones, because these things suuuuuuk for pouring oil.

Spatulas, Spoons, Bowls~

You will want a varying assortment of stirring spoons and spatulas to scrape bowls and such. Make sure that they are either silicon, solid stainless steel, or some sort of noncorrosive metal that can handle high heat. Never use anything wooden. These have a lot of bacteria in/on them, can't be sanitized, and will forever be saturated with the oil and wax. You will cross contaminate things again and again, every single time you use it.

 If you are buying new, consider getting ones that are streamlined - meaning they are made from one solid piece of metal or silicone. This makes clean up much easier, and will prevent cross contamination vastly.

Any time you get a chance to snatch up stainless steel bowls for cheap, jump on it! You will need more of these than you can ever imagine. Plus, using glass, ceramic, or plastic is problematic. Glass bowls will break at some point when you are pouring something hot into them. Ceramic often has cracks in the glaze, and that can be a big source of cross contamination. Most food safe plastic cant go above 100*F. Then it begins leaching chemicals and is never safe for food contact again. Stainless steel is where it's at, folks, and is why the commercial kitchen I designed and built is 90% stainless steel!

Mixers~

If you want to make a body butter you will need something along the lines of a KitchenAid mixer. Cheaper brands may work, but you may also burn your motor out. These are a real investment, but you can sometimes buy them used and save a lot of money. You will also need the whisk and the beater attachment for making body butters.

Now you may not like the sound of this, but if you are going to buy things specifically to begin making tinctures, infused herbal oils, balms, salves, butters and beyond, deeply consider using these things only to do that. Do not use them to make food. Cross contamination is a very real thing and if you don't have a commercial sanitizing dishwasher making sure there is no food residue left behind after washing can be harder than you think. It just takes one person with a severe allergy to something you enjoy cooking to change both their lives and yours, for the worse. Work as clean as possible, and then just a little bit cleaner. You, your friends and family, and anyone you may end up selling something to are worth clean creations.

What are We Going to Put This In?

Tins~

You can buy little tins in all different sizes from many places online, but **be sure to find out if the tins you are buying are FDA approved for cosmetic contact**. There is a real issue of tins coming over from China that are uncoated aluminum, and this is just asking for trouble. Most reputable sites will state that their tins are FDA approved for cosmetic or even food contact, and usually if you order a whole box it is also printed on the packaging.

When it comes time to fill your tins, the volume is always found at the first "line" inside of the tin, but if you aren't making a lot you can fill them pretty close to the top if you'd like. So if you have a 3 oz tin and fill it to the brim, it's about 4 oz of salve or balm. Write down how many tins you filled with any given batch you made. This will make ordering the exact amount of tins you need for the next batch of the same size a snap, no matter what it is.

Tubes~

Making lip balm? Make sure if the tubes you buy are plastic they are BPA free and rated for high heat contact. Even then, allow your salve or balm to cool off quite a bit before pouring. Consider buying a chapstick filling tray. This will make things MUCH easier.

Jars~

You can fill up any kind of jar you want, just be sure they are not colder than room temperature or your salve is gana break the, glass especially if they are something like leftover baby food jars and not canning jars. I use gallon and half gallon jars to store my unused salve or balm. Then I pop it in the oven on low for a few hours until it is fully melted down and ready to pour again. Be mindful what kind of jars you use to store solid balms or salves in, as they need to be heated and oven safe. Otherwise you will have a horrible fucking mess that will damn near ruin your oven if the jar shatters!

How to Make:

Balms~

1.) Place a plate in your freezer. This will make sense near the end.

2.) Fill the bottom portion of your double boiler with enough water that it almost comes in contact with the top pot. You'll know you have put in too much water if the top pot floats.

3.) Pour your herbal infused oil into the top of the double boiler.

4.) For every **4 cups** of oil, add **3 ½ cups** of beeswax pellets or shavings.

5.) Add any additional butters or oils at this point.

6.) Turn the burner under your double boiler on to medium high heat.

7.) Place a lid over the top of the pot to prevent the moisture from steam getting into your balm.

8.) Once the water is clearly boiling, turn down the heat to medium low. Steam will be coming out the sides of your double boiler.

9.) As the waxes and butters first begin to melt, they will all rise to the top of the pot and then harden into one big layer. This is normal. Take a spoon and slowly break through the layer, mixing it back into the hot oil. This may take a few times, and the wax will stick to your spoon. Eventually it will melt off, so no need to worry or try to scrape it off.

10.) Keep stirring occasionally until all waxes are dissolved.

11.) If you are going to add any minerals, now is the time to very slowly stir them in, a little at a time.

12.) Be sure to let this continue to heat for another 10-15 minutes **even after all waxes are dissolved** to the naked eye. They are still melting, you just can't see it happening anymore.

13.) Go get the plate from your freezer. With a spoon pour about a quarter-sized amount of your hot oil and wax onto the cold plate. After 3-5 minutes, this little bit of balm will set up fully. Do you like the texture? Want it to be firmer? Want to add more butters, oils, or wax? Is it just right? It is better to do this test now than to wait until you have filled up a ton of tins!

14.) As soon as it's how you are wanting, your balm is ready to be poured into containers of your choice! Be careful. It's hot as hell!

Salves~

1.) Place a plate in your freezer. This will make sense at the end.

2.) Fill the bottom portion of your double boiler with enough water that it almost comes in contact with the top pot. You'll know you have put in too much water if the top pot floats.

3.) Pour your herbal infused oil into the top of the double boiler.

4.) For every **4 cups** of oil add **2 cups** of beeswax pellets or shavings.

5.) Add any additional butters or oils at this point.

6.) Turn the burner under your double boiler on to medium high heat.

7.) Place a lid over the top of the pot to prevent the moisture from steam getting into your balm.

8.) Once the water is clearly boiling, turn down the heat to medium low. Steam will be coming out of the sides of your double boiler.

9.) As the waxes and butters first begin to melt they will all rise to the top of the pot and then harden into one big layer. This is normal. Simply take a spoon and slowly break through the layer, mixing it back into the hot oil. This may take a few times, and the wax will stick to your spoon. Eventually it will melt off, so no need to worry or try to scrape it off.

10.) Keep stirring occasionally until all waxes are dissolved.

11.) If you are going to add any minerals, now is the time to very slowly stir them in, a little at a time.

12.) Be sure to let this continue to heat for another 10-15 minutes, **even after all waxes are dissolved to the naked eye**. They are still melting, you just can't see it happening anymore.

13.) Go get the plate from your freezer. With a spoon pour about a quarter-sized amount of your hot oil and wax onto the cold plate. Wait about 3-5 minutes and this little bit of balm will set up fully. Do you like the texture? Want it to be firmer? Want to add more butters, oils, or wax? Is it just right? It is better to do this test now than to wait until you have filled up a ton of tins!

14.) As soon as it's how you are wanting, your balm is ready to be poured into containers of your choice! Be careful. It's hot as hell!

So yeah, that was the same recipe twice, right? The only difference between a balm and a salve is the amount of wax you add and that is the **only difference** in each of these recipes. We'll jump into the body butter in just a moment, but first let's talk about a few more things to consider for the balms and salves.

Does the "butter" or animal fat you may be adding set up firm when cool? How much are you adding? If you are adding more than a tablespoon or so per four cups of oil, you will need to adjust for this in a balm or a salve. A lot of extra butters will make a balm way to hard, and a salve more like a balm.

If the amount you are adding is ¼ cup or more in volume, remove that amount of beeswax from the wax you will be adding.

How much extra oil are you adding? Is your tallow or lard on the runny side? If adding more than two tablespoons per four cups of your herbal infused oil, you will need to add the equivalent amount of wax to a balm or a salve per four cups. If not, your balm may be too soft and your salve may be way too soft. This is also why the set up test on a frozen plate is important. You can add more wax or more oil as needed to get you to the level of firmness or softness you are wanting.

Whatever pot you choose to use for your oil portion, it is important to leave about 4 inches or so of "head room", because hot oil expands and as waxes and butters melt they become liquid. The best way to make sure you have this extra space is to add the waxes and butters to your pots **and then** your oils.

Butter~

1.) Place a plate in your freezer. This will make sense at the end.

2.) Fill the bottom portion of your double boiler with enough water that it almost comes in contact with the top pot. You'll know you have put in too much water if the top pot floats.

3.) Pour your herbal infused oil into the top of the double boiler.

4.) For every **4 cups** of oil add **4 ½ cups** of beeswax pellets or shavings.

5.) Add any additional butters or oils at this point.

6.) Turn the burner under your double boiler on to medium high heat.

7.) Place a lid over the top of the pot to prevent the moisture from steam getting into your balm.

8.) Once the water is clearly boiling, turn down the heat to medium low. Steam will be coming out of the sides of your double boiler.

9.) As the waxes and butters first begin to melt they will all rise to the top of the pot and then harden into one big layer. This is normal. Simply take a spoon and slowly break through the layer, mixing it back into the hot oil. This may take a few times, and the wax will stick to your spoon. It will melt off, so no need to worry or try to scrape it off.

10.) Keep stirring occasionally until all waxes are dissolved.

11.) If you are going to add any minerals, now is the time to very slowly stir them in, a little at a time.

12.) Be sure to let this continue to heat for another 10-15 minutes, **even after all waxes are dissolved to the naked eye**. They are still melting, you just can't see it happening anymore.

13.) Get the plate from your freezer. With a spoon pour about a quarter-sized amount of your hot oil and wax onto the cold plate. Wait about 3-5 minutes and this little bit of balm will set up fully. Here is where you really need to be sure that this is **downright hard** from all of the wax in it, or it won't whip into a good butter!

14.) Now we need to pour this into a big metal bowl or we can use big cake pans, making a ¼ inch layer on the bottom of each.

15.) After pouring ,allow to come to room temperature. Once fully cooled and set up, pop these in your freezer.

16.) After 24 hours, take it out of the freezer and chop it up into small pieces. This will not be as easy as it sounds - it's hard, frozen balm! However, the coldness is the key to it whipping well.

17.) With your beater blade in your countertop mixer, begin beating small amounts of frozen/cold balm at a time. Make sure your mixer is "locked", and don't go much above medium speed at first.

18.) As each small amount breaks down, add in a bit more. Stop every now and then to scrape down the sides of the bowl to ensure all is getting beaten. Repeat this step until everything has been added.

19.) Now you can kick up the speed of your mixer to high, but never leave it unattended. It will probably form a "cave" of stiff balm at first, but keep pushing this back into the beater. Soon the stiffness will "break", and suddenly you end up with a really creamy, but still thick body butter.

20.) Now your butter is ready to be jarred up! I pop them in the fridge for a few hours to set the texture, then they are ready to go and should keep their whip - so long as they are not kept in a really warm place.

This will take a few times of doing before you get the hang of it, and I suggest you start with small batches. Understand that frozen balm is as hard as I say it is to chop, and that if your pieces are bigger than an inch in size it is really hard to get them to break down smoothly without a big commercial blender .

Some people like to add a bit of Arrowroot powder, in an attempt to make these pure oil butters a bit less heavy. While I have never personally found a result I like with this, don't be afraid to experiment! You'll want to add a few tablespoons to the melting pot and blend it well before getting to the beating part.

Troubleshooting:

Sometimes things just don't go as we plan, but we can usually figure out how to prevent this the next time around!

Cracked or Sagged When Cooled~

Okay, so you have poured all of your salve or balm, and as it cooled you notice the middle kinda collapsed in or formed a little crack. If the surface is not smooth and even, I can tell you what happened.

It cooled down way too fast. This can be from eager folks putting it somewhere cool, like the fridge, basement, outside in the cool weather, in front of a fan, or near an opened up windows meant to let cool air in. The warm kitchen - or wherever you made these - is where you need to cool them, and as the room slowly and naturally cools down from the hot stove no longer being on, the salve or balm will slowly cool.

There is one other cause, in case you are still scratching your head since you did nothing to make it cool faster. If there are high wax levels (like in a balm) and you didn't let it melt down long enough, the wax is not fully or evenly dissolved into the hot oil. Just like in the hot pot when you first started, the wax rises to the top and cools before the hot oil and waxes below. It will all eventually set up, but the faster set time on top traps heat in below. This can cause cracks in the top, or when the bottom cools the top can drop down into a concave.

To solve these issues, always let your salves or balms cool naturally - making sure to do nothing to speed the process up, and always be sure to let you wax and oil sit in your hot pot another 10-15 mins after your wax has melted to the naked eye, and stir often to be sure all waxes and butters are fully dissolved and evenly distributed.

Too Thin or Thick~

So, you poured your salve or balm and you feel like it's just too thin and melty? Well, unless you want to individually melt down each tin in the oven and pour them bit by bit back into the pot, the best thing to do next time is follow the plate in the freezer advice! This also means you need to add more wax. Try adding ½ cup at a time, fully melt, then do the plate test. If it's firm enough you're good to go, or you can keep adding more wax ½ cup at a time. If you are making really big batches, you can add 2 cups at a time until you get the firmness you are looking for. Write down what you did!

What if we wish it was a bit thinner? Again, we really want to be testing it before we pour it, but this means next time you need to ease up on your waxes or butters. If you have done the plate test and this is how you found out it's too thick, the only way to fix this is to add more oil. Of course, more herbal infused oil would be best, but you can add plain oil too. Start with ½ cup at a time and allow it to mix and heat well. Then do the frozen plate test. Repeat until you get what you are looking for.

Feels Gritty~

This can be from a few different things:

a.) You need to let your waxes melt longer. Beyond this making our balms or salves crack, it can make for a gritty feeling when we try to rub the tiny bits of undissolved waxes and butters into our skin. I can't stress enough how important that extra 10-15 mins of heating is!

b.) You may have put too much of a plant based butter in, or you simply do not like the feel of the butter you have chosen to work with.

c.) You have added minerals or other things that cannot be dissolved. You will always feel these in your salve, balms, and even butters.

Kinda Clumpy~

Does your body butter have chunks in it? While this method means you will always find a few little pieces of unwhipped balm here and there, if you have a lot throughout the whole batch, odds are good the pieces you were beating were not small enough or you did not whip it long enough.

Be sure you are scraping down the sides of the bowl during the whole process, and if the bottom of the bowl seems lumpy rebeat it before you jar it up. You can also try scaling back on the wax if this really drives you nuts, but it will not be so much of a butter as it will be kinda sorta a cream.

Smells Funny~

If after a while you open up a jar or a tin and you notice a funky smell that was not there before, sadly this means the oil in your balm or salve has gone rancid, and there is nothing you can do but throw it out. This can happen to the perfectly made herbal infused oils, so don't beat yourself up over it.

If you have other tins or jars of the oil you used to make the balm, salve, or butter, be sure to go back and check these for rancidity. They may be fine. It is possible that just one tin went bad.

Make sure the oils you choose to work with are not close to their expiration date. Wilt any fresh plant oil infusions very well. Store your creations in a cool, dark, and dry environment. Also, always be sure to write the date of what you made on the tins or whatever you used in some way. It may have gone bad because its old as hell.

Balms and salves are truly easy to make and are extremely versatile! While the process is pretty much always the same, what you have infused into the oil you are thickening can be different every single time. This is a great place to think about how plants can interact together, and allow your curiosity to explode into reality - one little tin at a time!

.24.
Making Nourishing Herbal Infusions & When to Forgo for the Sake of Tea.

I swear to God, half of the time I have the stamina to do anything it's from the gallons of nourishing herbal infusion I drink on a weekly basis. While I'm sure the food I eat and sleep I get are part of the reason I have energy, I can for sure say if I don't drink my infusions I feel a noticeable difference!

Let's break down the differences between nourishing herbal infusions and teas and go from there.

Nourishing Herbal Infusions~

These are when we take a specific weighed out amount of dried herb, place the herb into a jar, pour boiling water over top, cap, and allow to set between 4-24 hours before we strain out the plant matter. This long timeframe and the water going from very hot to room temperature allows really high levels of nutrients and medicinal properties out of whatever herb we are working with.

Of course, the main reason folks make these is to drink, but we can also use them as ingredients in making herbal creations that contain water, like lotions or creams. We can also use them on our hair, in our bath, soaking our feet, and even to fertilize other plants.

They are absolutely packed with vitamins, minerals, and medicinal properties due to large amounts of herb used and the long set time.

Tea~

While I feel pretty sure we all know what tea is, you never really know these days. Tea is like a nourishing herbal infusion in the way that you need dried herbs and hot water to make it, but tea is usually made with a blend of different herbs, and there is a very small amount of herb(s) per one little teacup or mug. We often also add sweetener, and some of us add cream. These are often allowed to steep in hot water for 5-15 minutes, max.

The main reason for teas is because they are tasty, relaxing, and they help us feel warm. Stronger herbs give us **some** healing actions. We can cook with them, and even rinse our hair in them.

These have very little vitamins or minerals, and will only have any real worthwhile medicinal value if the herb used is very fragrant or has a lot of tannins.

When to Choose a Nourishing Herbal Infusion~

If the plant ally we are working with does not have much of a scent and heals us primarily from her nutritional content, this is an ideal choice for a nourishing herbal infusion. Take Plantain as an example. She has no real smell and is packed with a lot of really amazing vitamins and minerals. Alongside of her medicinal qualities, this makes her ideal for a nourishing herbal infusion. Whether we are going to be drinking it or using it in some other way, the bigger volume of herb and the longer wait time will ensure we get all we are wanting from her.

When to Choose a Tea~

Teas are best for the plant allies that have a really strong scent, as these plants often don't heal us in the way of nutritional content, but really high levels of different volatile oils and other compounds. This also means that a little goes a very long way. We don't need a ton of herb in our hot water, and a long brew time is actually somewhat dangerous. Yarrow is a perfect example here. She is extremely fragrant, and - while very healing in small amounts - if you made an herbal infusion out of her and drank it you could really hurt yourself.

When to Kinda Sorta Make Both~

Because there is never anything in the world that is as cut and dry as we often assume, there are other plants that kinda need to be made like an infusion, but also a tea. I mean, things like roots and mushrooms should not really be made into a full-on, set-for-24-hour infusion, but it's also pointless to just soak a tiny amount in some hot water for a handful of minutes.

Dandelion root is a good example of this. If you make a nourishing herbal infusion you'll probably vomit from drinking it, but if you just let it sit in some hot water for a moment the water won't even make it all the way to the center of the root pieces.

These herbs - anything that is really pretty firm - need to be actively simmered. Roots usually need to be simmered for 20-30 mins depending on how bitter they are, and most mushrooms need to be simmered for no less than an hour to release their highly prized PSK content (which fights cancer). This is yet another great example as to why we need to get to know each plant ally we are working with - so we can ask ourselves if she is better made in this way or another way?

You Made Broth~

I am sorry to say that if you are using fresh plant matter to try and make a nourishing herbal infusion, tea, or simmered down brew, you made none of these things. You made a weak broth. All of these things can only be made with dried herbs, and there is a really good reason for this! I want you to picture a really big uncooked potato in your mind. It's pretty firm, right? Like, it's so firm that if you threw an uncooked potato at someone as hard as you could it would not be unreasonable to assume that you could knock a mother fucker out, right? Haha, you just imagined doing that! Well, some of you did. Now imagine what would happen if you picked up a handful of mashed potatoes and lobbed it at someone's face as hard as you could. At best you'd just really piss this poor person off but hey, maybe they had it coming!

So what's the difference here? Why does one form of potato knock someone's teeth out and the other is what someone's gana have to eat now that they have no teeth?

Cooking breaks down the cellular structure. The potato is really hard in its uncooked form because like all plants it has a rigid cellular structure when raw. The mashed potatoes are really soft because cooking breaks down the tough membrane that makes the cell rigid. This is why we get almost no nutrients from eating raw vegetables. Our stomach is not capable of cooking our food.

But wouldn't boiling our fresh plant in hot water count as cooking? For sure it does, but just like with oil infusions it has limits to how much it can release, and it has to be boiled the whole time. Pouring boiling water over a fresh plant would get the process started, but it stops there, and because the plant is already wet the hot water not only can't be absorbed well into the plant, but begins to cool down as soon as you pour it into your jar or cup. Did you know that drying a plant kinda counts as cooking it? When we dry a plant its cellular membranes break down. This is just a natural part of the decaying process.

So when we pour boiling water over the top of dried herbs, a few things happen:

a.) The already weakened and broken down cells release their nutritional values with much more ease than fresh plant matter.

b.) The water is able to fully saturate the plants dried out cells, and as it cools it fully extracts a ton of the nutritional value that we would not get from fresh plant matter.

That is why when you use fresh herbs to try and make any of these things, you are basically just making a very weak broth. Also, please know I can't be held responsible for any trouble you may get in if you act out the potato experiment half drunk at some holiday dinner thing you didn't want to go to in the first place.

Let's Get to Making~

I am going to give you the quick and easy rundown of how to make nourishing herbal infusions, but before you jump in be sure to do a bit of digging into what herbal ally you are wanting to use for the sake of learning any nuances that might come into play with her!

Nourishing Herbal Infusions~

Things you will need to get started:

- A quart sized canning jar with a lid.
- Something to boil water in.
- Some sort of kitchen scale that can weigh in oz increments.
- A weighed out ounce of the herb you will be working with.
- A spoon to stir with.
- Anything fine mesh to strain with.

Ready for how hard this is gana be?

1.) Weigh out one ounce (28 grams) of your individual dried herb.

2.) Put it in your jar, or better yet use your jar as the thing you weighed it with. That cuts out the first step.

3.) Bring 4 cups of water to a rolling boil.

4.) Slowly pour the boiling water over the herb.

5.) Once it reaches the top give it a stir, which should make space for you to add a bit more water.

6.) Cap and let it sit for 4-24 hours, placing it in the fridge once it hits room temperature.

7.) After the wait time is up, strain the herb out of the now infused water.

8.) Your infusion is now ready to drink or use however you intend! Keep them in the fridge and use within 3 days max for most herbs.

Here are some tips and such:

If you are working with a kinda slimy plant ally like Comfrey, you may want to consider doing this process twice with the same plant matter. So after you strain it, you use the herb that you already infused your water with again. This often is when the good, slimy bits that heal mucous membranes are released.

If you are working with someone who has lots of fuzzy hair like Mullein leaf, it's really important that you strain this through very tightly woven cloth, or a mesh nylon nut milk ba. These hairs can often irritate our lungs and stomach lining.

Remember, if a plant has a really strong smell like mint, chamomile, or yarrow, we can't make nourishing herbal infusions out of these because we will extract far too much of their high volatile oil levels. This can really damage our bodies, and is the same as taking "essential oils" internally.

Plants that are high in proteins like Stinging Nettle and Oatstraw usually need to be used up in two days, as they spoil quickly.

When we heal ourselves using nourishment we need to be patient. It takes time for these allies to undo the often lifetime of damage we and our situations have done. Give regular use for a solid 3-6 months a chance before you decide it isn't helping you.

Try to cycle through different infusions on a regular basis, and be mindful to know what medicinal actions any one plant has. Red Clover, for example, is great for hormonal health - but she is also a blood thinner, and should not be drank for more than a few days in a row each week.

Don't think you're being clever by putting a bunch of herbs in a jar at once to make an infusion. Remember the bit in the tincture section about how you will have no idea what plant caused what reaction whether its for good or bad? Yeah that applies here too, but also you shortchange yourself because the one ounce of herb is how much you need of ANY plant to fully saturate the 4 cups of boiling water.

What do we do with the leftover plant matter? Well, if you're not going to be re-brewing it you can compost it, feed it to any chickens you may have, or dump it around the base of plants in your garden - or anywhere out on bare earth where it can begin returning to the soil. Also, if you don't have access to any of these places, I'm not gana judge you for putting it in your trashcan like any other food scraps.

Let's Take a Look at the Herbs in the Book to See Where They Fit In~

Yarrow is too potent for making nourishing herbal infusions for the sake of drinking. Please, never do this. She makes a nice strong cup of tea with a simple 5-10 min hot water over top brew. Be sure to take the plant matter out, as letting it set will rapidly extract her volatile compounds. If you see what looks like an oil slick in a parking lot after it rains that makes rainbow colors in the top of your cup, she has brewed too long.

You can, however, make these long brewed infusions (4 hours max) to add to your bath, as a cool rag for foot soaks or on the back of the neck for fevers, and as an ingredient in herbal creations.

Plantain, like talked on a bit earlier, is great for a nourishing herbal infusion - both internally for all sorts of digestive upsets and externally for just about any skin issue you have going on. I love to add her to anything I am making that is for sunburns!

Dandelion is best used roasted as a long simmered brew, but if you do decide to make a nourishing herbal infusion, don't let it set for more than 4 hours - and only put ½ an ounce into the quart jar versus a full one because roots are potent!

Elderberry can be used as a simmered tea or an herbal infusion, but like Dandelion, she should only be made with half an ounce of dried berries per quart because they pack a punch of medicinal content, and a half ounce will do just fine! I personally like making a simmered tea out of her because I think it tastes better, but that's just me. I would not make her blooms into an infusion because they are far too fragrant, but they work just fine as a steeped tea!

Comfrey is good for a nourishing herbal infusion, so long as you have the hybrid variety (S. × uplandicum), and I would not drink her more than once a week or so if you had no specific need to. Externally, it's a great option to soak sprained ankles in or to help speed up wound that can stand a little moisture on them - even as a hair rinse to strengthen and encourage growth!

California Poppy is not really fragrant, but I still would not use her as an herbal infusion - and I'll tell ya right now as a tea she does not taste pleasant! Tincture really is the way to go. I will say that you could make an infusion to help heal up wounds, as some of her alkaloids are decent at that, and this is a pretty traditional use that has recently fallen to the wayside in favor of more effective plant allies.

Nourishing herbal infusions are a really great and pretty accessible way for everyone to develop relationships with amazing plant allies, even if we can't use them internally all the time. I'd also say that in a society where all of our affordable-for-most food is void of nutrients, infusions that can be drank are a great way to fill this gap when we can't really afford to change it in other ways!

.25.

How to Make the Often Overlooked Compress, Poultice, & Sitz Baths, Because Sometimes We Need to Soak Our Ass in a Bowl of Warm Water.

You may not think to yourself, "I wish I could stick my ass in a bowl of warm water." very often, but I'm telling you the first time you try it to help heal up one thing or another you'll quickly realize how powerfully healing it can be. How shocked you will be when a compress or poultice heals something up that has been unresolved for however many years! These things have been in practice by humans for thousands and thousands of years, and it's no real surprise - considering how simple they are to do!

So what are they, and why are they so great? Let's get to talking about it. As usual, we'll start by learning what they are.

Compress~

A compress is when we take nourishing herbal infusions, tea, or any water like substance with herbs infused into it and we arm it up and soak a towel in it. We then apply this warm, wet towel to some sort of issue we have going on like a wound, skin complaint, even sprains and broken bones. Compresses are a good choice if you have a pretty big area you need to cover - like you want to wrap an entire leg, or the area needing help is somewhere awkward. They are also ideal for pulling up things like boils or even cysts.

Poultice~

A poultice is when we use a plant that has been simmered for a while in warm water, just fresh smashed, or even chewed up and apply it directly to the skin. Usually, we use a cloth or some sort of plastic wrap to hold it in place. These are pretty common for scabbed over wounds, rashes, bug bites, and things that don't cover a very large area and are not on an overly awkward part of the body. If you made an infusion for the sake of making a compress, you will also have the plant matter to make a poultice.

Sitz Bath~

A sitz bath is where you take warm herbal infused water, strain out all of the plant matter, dump it into something like a wide bowl, and stick your ass into the warm water. These are pretty standard after giving birth, but are also really great for hemorrhoids, boils and cysts, anal fissure (ouch), ingrown hairs, infections, and I don't know maybe you just feel cold down there, haha!

Here Comes the How To:

Compresses~

1.) If using a fragrant herb, simmer in water for about 15 mins max. If using a non-fragrant herb, consider making a 24 hour infusion from the Nourishing Herbal Infusion chapter and warm it up in a pot.

2.) Strain out the plant matter with a tightly woven mesh strainer.

3.) Place back into the pot. Warm back up if the temperature has dropped to lukewarm.

4.) Warm only to about bath water temperature. Don': burn yourself, but you want this to be pretty warm.

5.) Soak a clean towel in the herbal infused water.

6.) Gently ring out the towel. We still want a good amount of liquid in it, but there's no need for it to be overly dripping everywhere.

7.) Apply this warm wet towel to whatever area you are needing it for at least 30 minutes.

8.) If there is enough liquid left in the pot, stash it in the fridge **so long as you did not put the now used towel back into it**. You'll need to make fresh compressing brew every few days.

9.) Depending on what you've got going on once a day may do the trick, or you may need to do this 3-4 times a day. Watch how your individual body responds and go from there.

Poultice~

Dried plant option:

1.) Put about an ounce (28 grams) into a little soup pot with about 4 cups of water.

2.) Bring to a gentle simmer and hold for about 10 minutes.

3.) Allow to cool to a comfortable temp.

4.) Strain warm plant matter out of the water.

5.) Try to kinda mush it into a ball or patty.

6.) Smoosh this over top of whatever you are trying to heal.

7.) Wrap it with a cloth or saran wrap.

8.) Keep this in place for 30 minutes. You can place a heating pad over the top during this time too, to help it soak in a bit deeper.

Fresh plant option:

1.) Gather about a cup or two of the fresh plant you are wanting to use.

2.) You'll need to smash the plant in some way to break her cellular membranes some. A mortar and pestle is ideal, but you can also cut it up and then roll over it all clumped up with a rolling pin.

3.) Apply this to the area needing help, and use a cloth or plastic wrap to hold it in place for 2-5 hours.

Additional fresh plant option:

1.) Gather about a cup or two of the fresh plant you are wanting to use.

2.) Cut up the plant some.

3.) Place into a little pot.

4.) Add about ¼-½ cup water.

5.) Bring to a very gentle simmer for 5 minutes.

6.) Allow to cool a bit so you don't burn yourself.

7.) Remove the plant matter and apply it to the area that's giving you grief.

8.) Wrap in cloth or plastic wrap, and keep this in place for about an hour.

No matter which method you choose, you'll need new plant matter each time.

Sitz Bath~

1.) You will need to have about 2 gallons of water and about ½ pound of herbs to do this in a potent way. You can use more than one herb to make up the 8 ounces in half a pound.

2.) With such a large amount of water, it is best to use a clean white, cotton pillowcase - like a big tea bag for all of the herbs. You can also use a nut milk bag.

3.) Place this tied bag of herbs into the cold water and bring to a simmer.

4.) If there is a fragrant plant in the bag, like Yarrow, only simmer for about 15-20 minutes - up to an hour for non-fragrant herbs.

5.) Carefully pull out the bag of herbs.

6.) Allow the water to cool to a safe enough temperature for your sensitive bits to handle - but we still want it to be really warm!

7.) Pour the water into the bowl or tub that you will be sticking your ass into. It's best to make sure that you can fit into what you choose before pouring the water in, and only fill it up about halfway, so when you sit down it does not overflow.

8.) Make sure that the water covers the part you are wanting to soak fully.

9.) Relax, and sit there until the water cools off below lukewarm. Repeat as needed!

This infused water can only be used once, but you may get a second brew out of the herbs you used - so pop them in the fridge and rebrew within 1-2 days!

These really are an easy way to treat many different things we have going on with our skin or otherwise, and some of the plant allies in this book are great used in one or more of these ways!

Yarrow is fantastic for helping heal up wounds, and can be used as a compress, poultice, or in a sitz bath. As a sitz bath, she is really great for hemorrhoids and healing after birth. Any wound in these areas, really - especially since it's hard to keep things super clean down below when it comes to wound healing. Her antibacterial nature is a great match!

Just a quick story of a Yarrow compress to share: My father has type two diabetes, and this means he has a hard time healing wounds. Not to long ago he fell and ripped his knee up really badly. By the time my mom reached out to me it had become dangerously infected. Now, as a diabetic with a raging infection, going to the doctor was the prime choice - if he was not so stubborn . Stubbornness and a cultural distrust of doctors run deeply in his veins, and who am I kidding - mine too. So my mom has this huge Yarrow patch just outside of her door, and we started doing 8 hour compresses at night as he slept. Every day in between the compresses we applied Yarrow tincture to keep it from getting too moist. Within 7 days what was once an infection so bad that it had a very strong odor and clearly decaying flesh was healed to the point that when the huge scab fell off, it gave way to new skin!

Comfrey is a great choice as a compress, poultice, or sitz bath for any type of wound, including broken and sprained bones. Just read my personal story about healing with Comfrey for a pretty legit example of her ability to heal bones! She is also really ideal for skin issues like psoriasis and eczema.

Plantain is just like the rest, in the way that she shines being used in any of the options given above. Although, I will say she has a real affinity for skin issues and bringing boils to a head. In fact, one time (in a different trauma-filled section of my life) I woke up on top of a remote mountain in my shitty little cabin - just me and two young kids - with a Bartholin's cyst the size of a golf ball. These cysts are on the vagina, just to put the pain and awkwardness level into perspective. I could barely walk, let alone get into my jeep and drive the 14 miles of rutted out logging roads to the nearest pavement. My kids followed their hobbling mother way down the "road", looking for Plantain. In about 8 hours of direct warm water poulticing (and after sending the kids to bed), I was able to horrendously drain this thing and - no fucking joke - by the next morning I could not even tell it had happened!

Yep, I'm just gana end this chapter on a vagina cyst story.

.26.

This will have to do.

It's so funny to think about the pressure most writers likely feel to end a story with something that takes your breath away, or delivers one last punch to the gut. Something that gives the reader some sort of closure, or even makes them feel vindicated. I don't know, throw any phrasing in there that fits what you were hoping for in an end.

Whatever was expected is something that I can't likely give you, because my life did not end once I turned 18, 21, 25, now 34 and counting. I am still living this shit. It can be beautiful, but it is more likely brutal. It is flush with abundance, and it can be starved from needs unmet. At any given moment is all of these things, and I don't expect this will ever truly change.

The only thing I can really say that might give you some sort of something is the only thing I have yet to learn from all of this is how to let pain stop me from trying my damnedest to survive.

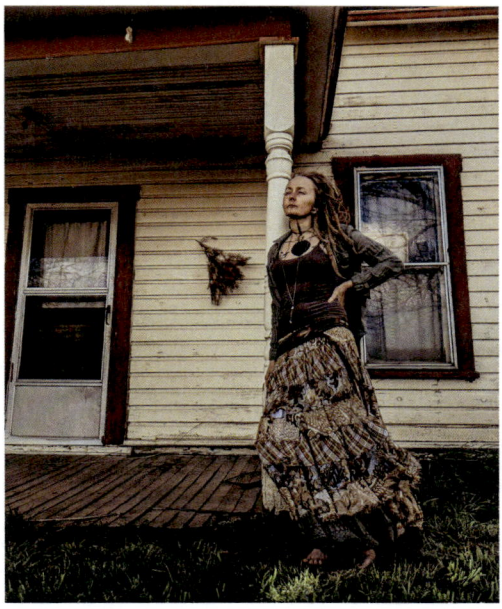

She keeps walking anyways.

References

Akkol EK, Koca U, Pesin I, Yilmazer D. Evaluation of the Wound Healing Potential of Achillea biebersteinii Afan. (Asteraceae) by in vivo Excision and Incision Models. Evid Based Complement Alternat Med. 2011;2011:474026.

Boswell-Ruys CL, Ritchie HE, Brown-Woodman PD. Preliminary screening study of reproductive outcomes after exposure to yarrow in the pregnant rat. Birth Defects Res B Dev Reprod Toxicol. 2003;68(5):416-420.

Cavalcanti AM, Baggio CH, Freitas CS, et al. Safety and antiulcer efficacy studies of Achillea millefolium L. after chronic treatment in Wistar rats. J Ethnopharmacol. 2006;107(2):277-284.

Dalsenter PR, Cavalcanti AM, Andrade AJ, Araujo SL, Marques MC. Reproductive evaluation of aqueous crude extract of Achillea millefolium L. (Asteraceae) in Wistar rats. Reprod Toxicol. 2004;18(6):819-823.

Ebrahimi M. Inter- and intra-specific genetic diversity of Iranian yarrow species Achillea santolina and Achillea tenuifolia based on ISSR and RAPD markers. Genet Mol Res. 2012;11(3):2855-2861.

Final report on the safety assessment of Yarrow (Achillea millefolium) Extract. Int J Toxicol. 2001;20 Suppl 2:79-84. Review.

Hausen BM. A 6-year experience with compositae mix. Am J Contact Dermat. 1996;7(2):94-99.

Karamenderes C, Apaydin S. Antispasmodic effect of Achillea nobilis L. subsp. sipylea (O. Schwarz) Bassler on the rat isolated duodenum. J Ethnopharmacol. 2003;84(2-3):175-179.

Kazemi M, Rostami H. Chemical composition and biological activities of Iranian Achillea wilhelmsii L. essential oil: a high effectiveness against Candida spp. and Escherichia strains. Nat Prod Res. 2015;29(3):286-288.

Khan AU, Gilani AH. Blood pressure lowering, cardiovascular inhibitory and bronchodilatory actions of Achillea millefolium. Phytother Res. 2011;25(4):577-583.

Nemeth E, Bernath J. Biological activities of yarrow species (Achillea spp.). Curr Pharm Des. 2008;14(29):3151-3167.

Rakel D, ed. Integrative Medicine. 3rd ed. Philadelphia, PA; Elsevier Saunders; 2012.

Rohloff J, Skagen EB, Steen AH, Iversen TH. Production of yarrow (Achillea millefolium L.) in Norway: essential oil content and quality. Agric Food Chem. 2000;48(12):6205-6209.

Rotblatt M, Ziment I. Evidence-Based Herbal Medicine. Philadelphia, PA: Hanley & Belfus, Inc.; 2002:369-371.

Stojanovic G, Radulovic N, Hashimoto T, Palic R. In vitro antimicrobial activity of extracts of four Achillea species: the composition of Achillea clavennae L. (Asteraceae) extract. J Ethnopharmacol. 2005;101(1-3):185-190.

Van der Weijden GA, Timmer CJ, Timmerman MF, Reijerse E, Mantel MS, Van der Velden U. The effect of herbal extracts in an experimental mouthrinse on established plaque and gingivitis. J Clin Periodontol. 1998;25(5):3099-3410.

Yaeesh S, Jamal Q, Khan AU, Gilani AH. Studies on hepatoprotective, antispasmodic and calcium antagonist activities of the aqueous-methanol extract of Achillea millefolium. Phytother Res. 2006;20:(7)546-551.

Nemeth E1, Bernath J. Biological activities of yarrow species (Achillea spp.). Corvinus University of Budapest, Department of Medicinal and Aromatic Plants, H-1118 Budapest, Villányi str. 29-35, Hungary.

Tiwari M1, Kakkar P. Plant derived antioxidants - Geraniol and camphene protect rat alveolar macrophages against t-BHP induced oxidative stress. Herbal Research Section, Indian Institute of Toxicology Research (CSIR), Mahatma Gandhi Marg, P.O. Box No. 80, Lucknow 226 001, Uttar Pradesh, India.

S. Saeidnia,1 AR. Gohari,1,* N. Mokhber-Dezfuli,1 and F. Kiuchi2. A review on phytochemistry and medicinal properties of the genus Achillea. Medicinal Plants Research Center, Faculty of Pharmacy, Tehran University of Medical Sciences, Tehran, Iran 2Faculty of Pharmacy, Keio University, 1-5-30 Shibakoen, Minato-ku, Tokyo 105-8512, Japan

Cheeke PR. 1988. Toxicity and Metabolism of Pyrrolizidine Alkaloids. Journal of Animal Science 66.

Macel M. 2010. Attract and deter: a dual role for pyrrolizidine alkaloids in plant-insect interactions. Phytochemistry Reviews 10:75–82.

Miller FM, Chow LM. 1954 Mar 5. Isolation and Characterization of Achilleine. Department of Chemistry and Pharmaceutical Chemistry of the University of Maryland.

Lucindo Quintans-Júnior, 1 José C. F. Moreira, 2 Matheus A. B. Pasquali, 2 Soheyla M. S. Rabie, 2 André S. Pires, 2 Rafael Schröder, 2 Thallita K. Rabelo, 2 João P. A. Santos, 2 Pollyana S. S. Lima, 3 Sócrates C. H. Cavalcanti, 1 Adriano A. S. Araújo, 1 Jullyana S. S. Quintans, 1 and Daniel P. Gelain 2 ,* Antinociceptive Activity and Redox Profile of the Monoterpenes (+)-Camphene, p-Cymene, and Geranyl Acetate in Experimental Models. 1Departamento de Bioquímica, Instituto de Ciências Básicas da Saúde, UFRGS, 90035-003 Porto Alegre, RS, Brazil 2Departamento de Fisiologia, Universidade Federal de Sergipe (DFS/UFS), Aracaju, 49100-000 São Cristovão, SE, Brazil 3Universidade Estadual de Feira de Santana (UEFS), 44031-460 Feira de Santana, BA, Brazil *Daniel P. Gelain

Martin Chadwick,1 Harriet Trewin,2,† Frances Gawthrop,2 and Carol Wagstaff1,*Sesquiterpenoids Lactones: Benefits to Plants and People. 1Food and Nutritional Sciences, University of Reading, PO Box 226, Whiteknights, RG6 6AP, UK; E-Mail: 2Tozer Seeds, Pyports, Downside Bridge Road, Cobham, Surrey, KT11 3EH, UK;

Mahtab Amiri, Jafar Navabi, Yalda Shokoohinia, Fatemeh Heydarpour, Gholamreza Bahrami, Leila Behbood, Padide Derakhshandeh, Saeideh Momtaz and Mohammad Hosein Farzaei, Efficacy and safety of a standardized extract from Achillea wilhelmsii C. Koch in patients with ulcerative colitis: A randomized double blind placebo-controlled clinical trial, Complementary Therapies in Medicine, 10.1016/j.ctim.2019.05.001, (2019).

Mikael M. Egebjerg, Pelle T. Olesen, Folmer D. Eriksen, Gitte Ravn-Haren, Lea Bredsdorff and Kirsten Pilegaard, Are wild and cultivated flowers served in restaurants or sold by local producers in Denmark safe for the consumer?, Food and Chemical Toxicology, 10.1016/j.fct.2018.07.007, 120, (129-142), (2018).

Sofi Imtiyaz Ali, B. Gopalakrishnan and V. Venkatesalu, Pharmacognosy, Phytochemistry and Pharmacological Properties of L.: A Review, Phytotherapy Research, 31, 8, (1140-1161), (2017).

Paola L. Minciullo, Gioacchino Calapai, Marco Miroddi, Carmen Mannucci, Ioanna Chinou, Sebastiano Gangemi and Richard J. Schmidt, Contact dermatitis as an adverse reaction to some topically used European herbal medicinal products – part 4: olidago virgaurea–itis vinifera, Contact Dermatitis, 77, 2, (67-87), (2017).

Lillian C. Becker, Wilma F. Bergfeld, Donald V. Belsito, Ronald A. Hill, Curtis D. Klaassen, Daniel C. Liebler, James G. Marks, Ronald C. Shank, Thomas J. Slaga, Paul W. Snyder and F. Alan Andersen, Safety Assessment of Achillea millefolium as Used in Cosmetics , International Journal of Toxicology, 10.1177/1091581816677717, 35, 3_suppl, (5S-15S), (2016).

Gioacchino Calapai, Marco Miroddi, Paola L. Minciullo, Achille P. Caputi, Sebastiano Gangemi and Richard J. Schmidt, Contact dermatitis as an adverse reaction to some topically used European herbal medicinal products – part 1: Achillea millefolium–Curcuma longa, Contact Dermatitis, 71, 1, (1-12), (2014).

Yusuke Watanabe, Paula Novaes, Rosa M. Varela, José M. G. Molinillo, Hisashi Kato-Noguchi and Francisco A. Macías, Phytotoxic Potential of Onopordum acanthium L. (Asteraceae), Chemistry & Biodiversity, 11, 8, (1247-1255), (2014).

T. K. Lim, Achillea millefolium, Edible Medicinal And Non-Medicinal Plants, 10.1007/978-94-007-7395-0_10, (138-162), (2013).

Chang-Hong Huo, Yong Li, Man-Li Zhang, Yu-Fang Wang, Qing Zhang, Fang Qin, Qing-Wen Shi and Hiromasa Kiyota, Cytotoxic flavonoids from the flowers of Achillea millefolium, Chemistry of Natural Compounds, 10.1007/s10600-013-0438-y, 48, 6, (958-962), (2013).

George E. Burrows and Ronald J. Tyrl, Asteraceae Martinov, Toxic Plants of North America, (150-256), (2012).

Farnood Shokouhi Sabet Jalali, Hossein Tajik and Mojtaba Hadian, Efficacy of topical application of alcoholic extract of yarrow in the healing process of experimental burn wounds in rabbit, Comparative Clinical Pathology, 10.1007/s00580-010-1081-7, 21, 2, (177-181), (2010).

Evy Paulsen and Klaus E. Andersen, Patch testing with constituents of Compositae mixes, Contact Dermatitis, 66, 5, (241-246), (2012).

Wendy L. Applequist and Daniel E. Moerman, Yarrow (Achillea millefolium L.): A Neglected Panacea? A Review of Ethnobotany, Bioactivity, and Biomedical Research1, Economic Botany, 10.1007/s12231-011-9154-3, 65, 2, (209-225), (2011).

Juliane Rocha de Sant'Anna, Claudinéia Conationi da Silva Franco, Claudia Tiemi Miyamoto, Miriam Machado Cunico, Obdulio Gomes Miguel, Lílian Cristina Cêcco, Carlos Itsuo Yamamoto, Cirino Corrêa Junior and Marialba Avezum Alves de Castro-Prado, Genotoxicity of Achillea millefolium essential oil in diploid cells of Aspergillus nidulans, Phytotherapy Research, 23, 2, (231-235), (2008).

Ch. Franz Vienna, R. Bauer Graz, R. Carle Hohenheim, D. Tedesco Milano, A. Tubaro Trieste and K. Zitterl-Eglseer Wien, Study on the assessment of plants/herbs, plant/herb extracts and their naturally or synthetically produced components as 'additives' for use in animal production, EFSA Supporting Publications, 4, 4, (2007).

O. Sticher, Isoprenoide als Inhaltsstoffe, Pharmakognosie — Phytopharmazie, 10.1007/978-3-540-34281-6_23, (809-914), (2007).

Ana Maria Cavalcanti, Cristiane Hatsuko Baggio, Cristina Setim Freitas, Lia Rieck, Renato Silva de Sousa, José Eduardo Da Silva-Santos, Sonia Mesia-Vela and Maria Consuelo Andrade Marques, Safety and antiulcer efficacy studies of Achillea millefolium L. after chronic treatment in Wistar rats, Journal of Ethnopharmacology, 10.1016/j.jep.2006.03.011, 107, 2, (277-284), (2006).

Edward Mills, Jean-Jacques Duguoa, Dan Perri and Gideon Koren, Herbal medicines, Herbal Medicines in Pregnancy and Lactation, 10.1201/b13984-5, (23-299), (2013).

Elke Marchart and Brigitte Kopp, Capillary electrophoretic separation and quantification of flavone-O- and C-glycosides in Achillea setacea W. et K., Journal of Chromatography B, 10.1016/S1570-0232(03)00262-9, 792, 2, (363-368), (2003).

Evy Paulsen, Contact sensitization from Compositae-containing herbal remedies and cosmetics, Contact Dermatitis, 47, 4, (189-198), (2002).

Sesquiterpenlactone [MAK Value Documentation in German language, 2006], The MAK-Collection for Occupational Health and Safety, (1-26), (2012).

Sabine Glasl, Disan Gunbilig, Samdan Narantuya, Ingrid Werner and Johann Jurenitsch, Combination of chromatographic and spectroscopic methods for the isolation and characterization of polar guaianolides from Achillea asiatica, Journal of Chromatography A, 10.1016/S0021-9673(01)00947-5, 936, 1-2, (193-200), (2001)

J. D. Guin, Occupational Contact Dermatitis to Plants, Handbook of Occupational Dermatology, 10.1007/978-3-662-07677-4_89, (730-766), (2000).

Sabine Glasl, Ulrike Kastner, Johann Jurenitsch and Wolfgang Kubelka, Qualitative and quantitative determination of sesquiterpenoids in Achillea species by reversed-phase high-performance liquid chromatography, mass-spectrometry and thin-layer chromatography, Journal of Chromatography B: Biomedical Sciences and Applications, 10.1016/S0378-4347(99)00134-6, 729, 1-2, (361-368), (1999).

Arnon Goldberg, Ronit Confino-Cohen and Yoav Waisel, Allergic responses to pollen of ornamental plants: High incidence in the general atopic population and especially among flower growers, Journal of Allergy and Clinical Immunology, 10.1016/S0091-6749(98)70088-0, 102, 2, (210-214), (1998).

Christiane Bayerl and E.G. Jung, Allergic contact stomatitis from Arislochol® a phytotherapeutic cholagogue, Contact Dermatitis, 34, 3, (222-223), (2006).

Karin Wrangsjö and Anne Marie Ros, Compsitae allergy, Seminars in Dermatology, 10.1016/S1085-5629(96)80027-7, 15, 2, (87-94), (1996).

A. C. Figueiredo, M. S. S. Pais and J. J. C. Scheffer, Achillea millefolium L. ssp. millefolium (Yarrow): In Vitro Culture and Production of Essential Oils, Medicinal and Aromatic Plants VIII, 10.1007/978-3-662-08612-4_1, (1-20), (1995).

H. Tunón, W. Thorsell and L. Bohlin, Mosquito repelling activity of compounds occurring inAchillea millefolium L. (asteraceae)Mückenabschreckende aktivität von substanzen ausachillea millefolium L., Economic Botany, 10.1007/BF02908196, 48, 2, (111-120), (1994).

Laurent Machet, Loïc Vaillant, Annick Callens, Maryvonne Demasure, Kossi Barruet and Gérard Lorette, Allergic contact dermatitis from sunflower (Helianthus annum) with cross-sensitivity to arnica, Contact Dermatitis, 28, 3, (184-185), (2006).

Gerhard Rücker, Detlef Manns and Judith Breuer, Peroxides as Constituents of Plants, XIV: On Further Guaianolide Peroxides from Yarrow, Achillea millefolium L., Archiv der Pharmazie, 326, 11, (901-905), (2006).

Baldassarre Santucci and Mauro Picardo, Occupational contact dermatitis to plants, Clinics in Dermatology, 10.1016/0738-081X(92)90100-D, 10, 2, (157-165), (1992).

Gerhard Rücker, Detlef Manns and Judith Breuer, , Archiv der Pharmazie, 324, 12, (979-981), (2010).

V. Lobo, A. Patil, A. Phatak, and N. Chandra. Free radicals, antioxidants and functional foods: Impact on human health. Department of Botany, Birla College, Kalyan – 421 304, Maharastra, India.

Bjelakovic, G., Nikolova, D., & Gluud, C. (2013, September 6). Meta-regression analyses, meta-analyses, and trial sequential analyses of the effects of supplementation with beta-carotene, vitamin A, and vitamin E singly or in different combinations on all-cause mortality: Do we have evidence for lack of harm? PLoS ONE, 8(9), e74558.

Cortés-Jofré, M., Rueda, J.-R., Corsini-Muñoz, G., Fonseca-Cortés, C., Caraballoso, M., & Cosp, X. B. (2012, October 17). Drugs for preventing lung cancer in healthy people. Cochrane Database of Systematic Reviews.

Grodstein, F., Kang, J. H., Glynn, R. J., Cook, N. R., & Gaziano, M. J. (2007, November 12). A randomized trial of beta-carotene supplementation and cognitive function in men: the physicians' health study II [Abstract]. Archives of Internal Medicine, 167(20), 2184-90.

Harman, D. (n.d.). Aging: A theory based on free radical and radiation chemistry.

Jang, Y. C., & Van Remmen, H. (2009, April). The mitochondrial theory of aging: Insight from transgenic and knockout mouse models [Abstract]. Experimental Gerontology, 44(4), 256-260.

Jiang, L., Yang, K. H., Tian, J. H., Guan, Q. L., Yao, N., Cao, N., . . . Yang, S. H. (2010). Efficacy of antioxidant vitamins and selenium supplement in prostate cancer prevention: A meta-analysis of randomized controlled trials [Abstract]. Nutrition and Cancer, 62(6), 719-727.

Knight, J. A. (1995, March-April). Diseases related to oxygen-derived free radicals [Abstract]. Annals of Clinical and Laboratory Science, 25(2), 111-21.

Labat-Robert, J., & Robert, L. (2014, April). Longevity and aging. Role of free radicals and xanthine oxidase. A review [Abstract]. Pathologie Biologie, 62(2), 61-66.

Liou, S. (2011, June 29). About free radical damage.

Pham-Huy, L. A., He, H., & Pham-Huy, C. (2008, June). Free radicals, antioxidants in disease and health. International Journal of Biomedical Science, 4(2), 89-96.

Sawada, M., & Carlson, J. C. (1987, November). Changes in superoxide radical and lipid peroxide formation in the brain, heart and liver during the lifetime of the rat [Abstract]. Mechanisms of Ageing and Development, 41(1-2), 125-137.

Singh, R., Devi, S., & Gollen, R. (2015, February 12). Role of free radical in atherosclerosis, diabetes and dyslipidaemia: Larger-than-life [Abstract]. Diabetes Metabolism Research and Reviews, 31(2), 113-126.

Vimal et al., "Eucalyptol, sabinene and cinnamaldehyde: potent inhibitors of salmonella target protein L-asparaginase", 3 Biotech, 2017, 7(4): 258.

Achotegui-Castells et al., "Strong Induction of Minor Terpenes in Italian Cypress, Cupressus sempervirens, in Response to Infection by the Fungus Seiridium cardinal", J ChemEcol, 2015, 41(3): 224.

Llena-Puy. The rôle of saliva in maintaining oral health and as an aid to diagnosis. Department 9, Valencian Health Service, CEU Cardenal Herrera University.

Brinker Francis (1997) Herbal Contraindications and Drug Interactions: Plus Herbal Adjuncts With Medicines, 4th Edition Eclectic Medical Publications.

Budd A.C. and J.B. Campbell. 1959. Flowering sequence of a local flora. Journal of Range Management 12: 127-132.

Callan, N. (December) 2002. Personal communication. Montana State University. Western Agricultural Research Station, Corvallis, MT. Clausen, J., D.D. Keck, and W.M. Hiesey. 1958.

Experimental studies on the nature of species: III. Environmental responses of climatic races of Achillea. Carnegie Institution of Washington Publication 581, Washington D.C. Cronquist, A., A.H. Holmgren, N.H. Holmgren, and J.L. Reveal. 2002.

Intermountain Flora, vascular plants of the intermountain west, Vol. 5: The Asterales. The New York Botanical Garden, NY. Hiesey, W.M. and M.A. Nobs. 1970.

Genetic and transplant studies on contrasting species and ecological races of the Achillea milllefolium complex. Botanical Gazette 131(3):245-259. Higgins, S.S. and R.N. Mack. 1987.

Comparative responses of Achillea millefolium ecotypes to competition and soil type. Oecologia 73:591-597 Hitchcock, C.L., A. Cronquist, M. Ownbey, and J.W. Thompson. 1955.

Vascular plants of the Pacific Northwest. University of Washington Press, Seattle and London. Hitchcock, C.L. and A. Cronquist. 1973. Flora of the Pacific Northwest: an illustrated manual. University of Washington Press, Seattle and London. Kannangara, H.W. and R.J. Field. 1985.

 Environmental and physiological factors affecting the fate of seeds of yarrow (Achillea millefolium) in arable land in New Zealand. Weed Research. 25:87- 92. Johnson, J.R. and G.E. Larson. 1999.

Grassland Plants of South Dakota and the Northern Great Plains. South Dakota State University. College of Agriculture and Biological Sciences. South Dakota Agricultural Experiment Station, Bulletin 566 (revised). Lavin, M. (November) 2002.

Personal communication. Montana State University, Bozeman. Lesica, P. (June) 2001. Personal communication. Conservation Biology Research. Missoula, MT.

Bianca Ivanescu,1 Anca Miron,2 and Andreia Corciova3. Sesquiterpene Lactones from Artemisia Genus: Biological Activities and Methods of Analysis. 1Department of Pharmaceutical Botany, Faculty of Pharmacy, University of Medicine and Pharmacy "Grigore T. Popa", 16 Universitatii Street, 700150 Iasi, Romani 2Department of Pharmacognosy, Faculty of Pharmacy, University of Medicine and Pharmacy "Grigore T. Popa", 16 Universitatii Street, 700150 Iasi, Romania 3Department of Drug Analysis, Faculty of Pharmacy, University of Medicine and Pharmacy "Grigore T. Popa", 16 Universitatii Street, 700150 Iasi, Romania

Imtiyaz, Sofi & Gopalakrishnan, Baskaran & Venkatesalu, Venugopalan. (2017). Pharmacognosy, Phytochemistry and Pharmacological Properties of Achillea millefolium L.: A Review. Phytotherapy research : PTR. 31. 10.1002/ptr.5840.

Yuan Feng,1,5,¶ Xiaozhou He,2,¶ Yilin Yang,2 Dongman Chao,1,3 Lawrence H. Lazarus,4 and Ying Xia1,3,*. Current Research on Opioid Receptor Function. 1Yale University School of Medicine, New Haven, CT, USA 2The Third Clinical College of Soochow University, Changzhou, Jiangsu, China 3The University of Texas Medical School at Houston, Houston, TX, USA 4National Institute of Environmental Health Sciences, Research Triangle Park, NC, USA 5The First Affiliated Hospital with Nanjing Medical University, Nanjing, Jiangsu, China *Address correspondence to this author at the The University of Texas Medical School at Houston, 6431 Fannin Street, Houston, TX 77030, USA;

Ali Esmail , Al-Snafi. ESCHSCHOLZIA CALIFORNICA: A PHYTOCHEMICAL AND PHARMACOLOGICAL - REVIEW. Department of Pharmacology, College of Medicine, Thi qar University, Iraq.

Chandler, R F., S. N. Hooper, and M. J. Harvey. 1982. Ethnobotany and phytochemistry of yarrow, Achillea millefoliurn, Compositae. Econ. Bot 36-203-223.

Dioscorides. 1933. The Greek Herbal of Dioscorides. R. T. Gunther, ed. Hafner Publ. Co., Inc., New York.

Solecki R., 1971: Shanidar: The First Flower People, Knopf, New York (1971).

Trinkaus E., 1983: The Shanidar Neanderthals, Academic Press, Inc.

Gerhard P. Shipley 1 , * and Kelly Kindscher 2. Evidence for the Paleoethnobotany of the Neanderthal: A Review of the Literature. 1Indigenous Studies Department, University of Kansas, Lippincott Hall, 1410 Jayhawk Boulevard, Lawrence, KS 66045, USA 2Kansas Biological Survey, University of Kansas, 2101 Constant Ave., Lawrence, KS 66047, USA *Gerhard P. Shipley

Karin M. Höld,* Nilantha S. Sirisoma,* Tomoko Ikeda,[†] Toshio Narahashi,[†] and John E. Casida*[‡]. α-Thujone (the active component of absinthe): γ-Aminobutyric acid type A receptor modulation and metabolic detoxification. *Environmental Chemistry and Toxicology Laboratory, Department of Environmental Science, Policy and Management, 114 Wellman Hall, University of California, Berkeley, CA 94720-3112; and †Department of Molecular Pharmacology and Biological Chemistry, Northwestern University Medical School, Chicago, IL 60611-3008

Shashank Kumar and Abhay K. Pandey* Chemistry and Biological Activities of Flavonoids: An Overview. Department of Biochemistry, University of Allahabad, Allahabad 211002, India *Abhay K. Pandey

Schafer H. L., Schafer H., Schneider W., Elstner E. F. Sedative action of extract combinations of Eschscholtzia californica and Corydalis cava . Arzneimittel-Forschung. 1995;45(2):124–126.

Rolland A., Fleurentin J., Lanhers M.-C., et al. Behavioural effects of the American traditional plant Eschscholzia californica: sedative and anxiolytic properties. Planta Medica. 1991;57(3):212–216. doi: 10.1055/s-2006-960076.

Rolland A., Fleurentin J., Lanhers M. C., Misslin R., Mortier F. Neurophysiological effects of an extract of Eschscholzia californica Cham. (Papaveraceae) Phytotherapy Research. 2001;15(5):377–381. doi: 10.1002/ptr.884.

Hanus M., Lafon J., Mathieu M. Double-blind, randomised, placebo-controlled study to evaluate the efficacy and safety of a fixed combination containing two plant extracts (Crataegus oxyacantha and Eschscholtzia californica) and magnesium in mild-to-moderate anxiety disorders. Current Medical Research and Opinion. 2004;20(1):63–71. doi: 10.1185/030079903125002603.

Kardos J., Blaskó G., Simonyi M. Enhancement of gamma-aminobutyric acid receptor binding by protopine-type alkaloids. Arzneimittel-Forschung. 1986;36(6):939–940.

Häberlein H., Tschiersch K.-P., Boonen G., Hiller K.-O. Chelidonium majus L.: components with in vitro Affinity for the GABAA Receptor. Positive Cooperation of Alkaloids. Planta Medica. 1996;62(3):227–231. doi: 10.1055/s-2006-957865.

Vacek J., Walterová D., Vrublová E., Šimánek V. The chemical and biological properties of protopine and allocryptopine. Heterocycles. 2010;81(8):1773–1789. doi: 10.3987/REV-10-673.

Şener B., Orhan I. Discovery of drug candidates from some Turkish plants and conservation of biodiversity. Pure and Applied Chemistry. 2005;77(1):53–64. doi: 10.1351/pac200577010053.

Gafner S., Dietz B. M., McPhail K. L., et al. Alkaloids from Eschscholzia californica and their capacity to inhibit binding of [3H]8-hydroxy-2-(di-N-propylamino) tetralin to 5-HT1A receptors in vitro. Journal of Natural Products. 2006;69(3):432–435. doi: 10.1021/np058114h.

Xu L.-F., Chu W.-J., Qing X.-Y., et al. Protopine inhibits serotonin transporter and noradrenaline transporter and has the antidepressant-like effect in mice models. Neuropharmacology. 2006;50(8):934–940. doi: 10.1016/j.neuropharm.2006.01.003.

Bugatti C., Colombo M. L., Tomé F. A new method for alkaloid extraction from Chelidonium majus L. Phytochemical Analysis. 1991;2(2):65–67. doi: 10.1002/pca.2800020204.

Suchomelová J., Bochořáková H., Paulová H., Musil P., Táborská E. HPLC quantification of seven quaternary benzo[c]phenanthridine alkaloids in six species of the family Papaveraceae . Journal of Pharmaceutical and Biomedical Analysis. 2007;44(1):283–287. doi: 10.1016/j.jpba.2007.02.005.

Sigel E. Properties of single sodium channels translated by Xenopus oocytes after injection with messenger ribonucleic acid. Journal of Physiology. 1987;386:73–90. doi: 10.1113/jphysiol.1987.sp016523.

Fabre N., Claparols C., Richelme S., Angelin M.-L., Fourasté I., Moulis C. Direct characterization of isoquinoline alkaloids in a crude plant extract by ion-pair liquid chromatography-electrospray ionization tandem mass spectrometry: example of Eschscholtzia californica . Journal of Chromatography A. 2000;904(1):35–46. doi: 10.1016/s0021-9673(00)00919-5.

Rey J.-P., Levesque J., Pousset J.-L., Roblot F. Analytical and quantitative studies of californin and protopin in aerial part extracts of Eschscholtzia californica Cham. with high-performance liquid chromatography. Journal of Chromatography A. 1991;587(2):314–317. doi: 10.1016/0021-9673(91)85174-e.

Tomè F., Colombo M. L., Caldiroli L. A comparative investigation on alkaloid composition in different populations of Eschscholtzia californica Cham. Phytochemical Analysis. 1999;10(5):264–267. doi: 10.1002/(sici)1099-1565(199909/10)10:5lt;264::aid-pca469>3.0.co;2-4.

Verma S. K., Jain V., Verma D., Khamesra R. Cratageus oxycantha—a cardioprotective herb. Journal of Herbal Medicine and Toxicology. 2007;1:65–71.

Goutman J. D., Waxemberg M. D., Doñate-Oliver F., Pomata P. E., Calvo D. J. Flavonoid modulation of ionic currents mediated by GABA(A) and GABA(C) receptors. European Journal of Pharmacology. 2003;461(2-3):79–87.

Aguirre-Hernández E., Martínez A. L., González-Trujano M. E., Moreno J., Vibrans H., Soto-Hernández M. Pharmacological evaluation of the anxiolytic and sedative effects of Tilia americana L. var. mexicana in mice. Journal of Ethnopharmacology. 2007;109(1):140–145. doi: 10.1016/j.jep.2006.07.017.

Aguirre-Hernández E., González-Trujano M. E., Martínez A. L., et al. HPLC/MS analysis and anxiolytic-like effect of quercetin and kaempferol flavonoids from Tilia americana var. mexicana . Journal of Ethnopharmacology. 2010;127(1):91–97. doi: 10.1016/j.jep.2009.09.044.

Martínez A. L., González-Trujano M. E., Aguirre-Hernández E., Moreno J., Soto-Hernández M., López-Muñoz F. J. Antinociceptive activity of Tilia americana var. mexicana inflorescences and quercetin in the formalin test and in an arthritic pain model in rats. Neuropharmacology. 2009;56:564–571. doi: 10.1016/j.neuropharm.2008.10.010.

Beck M.-A., Häberlein H. Flavonol glycosides from Eschscholtzia californica . Phytochemistry. 1999;50(2):329–332. doi: 10.1016/s0031-9422(98)00503-2.

Boettcher C., Fellermeier M., Boettcher C., Dräger B., Zenk M. H. How human neuroblastoma cells make morphine. Proceedings of the National Academy of Sciences of the United States of America. 2005;102(24):8495–8500. doi: 10.1073/pnas.0503244102.

Morais L. C. S. L., Barbosa-Filho J. M., Almeida R. N. Central depressant effects of reticuline extracted from Ocotea duckei in rats and mice. Journal of Ethnopharmacology. 1998;62(1):57–61. doi: 10.1016/s0378-8741(98)00044-0.

Ziegler J., Facchini P. J., Geißler R., et al. Evolution of morphine biosynthesis in opium poppy. Phytochemistry. 2009;70(15-16):1696–1707. doi: 10.1016/j.phytochem.2009.07.006.

Nikolaev V. O., Boettcher C., Dees C., Bünemann M., Lohse M. J., Zenk M. H. Live cell monitoring of μ-opioid receptor-mediated G-protein activation reveals strong biological activity of close morphine biosynthetic precursors. Journal of Biological Chemistry. 2007;282(37):27126–27132. doi: 10.1074/jbc.m703272200.

Laux A., Muller A. H., Miehe M., et al. Mapping of endogenous morphine-like compounds in the adult mouse brain: evidence of their localization in astrocytes and GABAergic cells. Journal of Comparative Neurology. 2011;519(12):2390–2416. doi: 10.1002/cne.22633.

Freund T. F., Katona I. Perisomatic inhibition. Neuron. 2007;56(1):33–42. doi: 10.1016/j.neuron.2007.09.012.

Beneyto M., Lewis D. A. Insights into the neurodevelopmental origin of schizophrenia from postmortem studies of prefrontal cortical circuitry. International Journal of Developmental Neuroscience. 2011;29(3):295–304. doi: 10.1016/j.ijdevneu.2010.08.003.

Zhu W., Ma Y., Cadet P., et al. Presence of reticuline in rat brain: a pathway for morphine biosynthesis. Molecular Brain Research. 2003;117(1):83–90. doi: 10.1016/s0169-328x(03)00323-1.

Laux-Biehlmann A., Mouheiche J., Vérièpe J., Goumon Y. Endogenous morphine and its metabolites in mammals: history, synthesis, localization and perspectives. Neuroscience. 2013;233:95–117. doi: 10.1016/j.neuroscience.2012.12.013.

Cahlíková L., Hulová L., Hrabinová M., et al. Isoquinoline alkaloids as prolyl oligopeptidase inhibitors. Fitoterapia. 2015;103:192–196. doi: 10.1016/j.fitote.2015.04.004.
Articles from Biochemistry Research International are provided here courtesy of Hindawi Limited

Modulation of CYPs, P-gp, and PXR by Eschscholzia californica (California Poppy) and Its Alkaloids.
[Planta Med. 2016]

Knockdown of berberine bridge enzyme by RNAi accumulates (S)-reticuline and activates a silent pathway in cultured California poppy cells.
[Transgenic Res. 2007]

Acetylcholinesterase and butyrylcholinesterase inhibitory compounds from Eschscholzia californica (Papaveraceae).
[Nat Prod Commun. 2010]

From ion currents to genomic analysis: recent advances in GABAA receptor research.
[Synapse. 1995]
Neuroactive steroid actions at the GABAA receptor.
[Horm Behav. 1994]

Salvador ÂC, Król E, Lemos VC, Santos SA, Bento FP, Costa CP, Almeida A, Szczepankiewicz D, Kulczyński B, Krejpcio Z, Silvestre AJ, Rocha SM. Effect of Elderberry (Sambucus nigra L.) Extract Supplementation in STZ-Induced Diabetic Rats Fed with a High-Fat Diet. Int J Mol Sci. 2016 Dec 22;18(1):13. doi: 10.3390/ijms18010013. PMID: 28025494; PMCID: PMC5297648.

Strugała P, Loi S, Bażanów B, Kuropka P, Kucharska AZ, Włoch A, Gabrielska J. A Comprehensive Study on the Biological Activity of Elderberry Extract and Cyanidin 3-O-Glucoside and Their Interactions with Membranes and Human Serum Albumin. Molecules. 2018 Oct 8;23(10):2566. doi: 10.3390/molecules23102566. PMID: 30297646; PMCID: PMC6222845.

.Loi M.C., Poli F., Sacchetti G., Selenu M.B., Ballero M. Ethnopharmacology of Ogliastra (Villagrande Strisaili, Sardinia, Italy) Fitoterapia. 2004;75:277–295. doi: 10.1016/j.fitote.2004.01.008. [PubMed] [CrossRef] [Google Scholar]

Uncini Manganelli R.E., Zaccaro L., Tomei P.E. Antiviral activity in vitro of Urtica dioica L., Parietaria diffusa M. et K. and Sambucus nigra L. J. Ethnopharmacol. 2005;98:323–327. doi: 10.1016/j.jep.2005.01.021. [PubMed] [CrossRef] [Google Scholar]

Konczak I., Zhang W. Anthocyanins-more than nature's colours. J. Biomed. Biotechnol. 2004;5:239–240. doi: 10.1155/S1110724304407013. [PMC free article] [PubMed] [CrossRef] [Google Scholar]

Olivas-Aguirre F.J., Rodrigo-García J., Martínez-Ruiz N.D., Cárdenas-Robles A.I., Mendoza-Díaz S.O., Álvarez-Parrilla E., González-Aguilar G.A., de la Rosa L.A., Ramos-Jiménez A., Wall-Medrano A. Cyanidin-3-O-glucoside: Physical-Chemistry. Foodomics and Health Effects. Molecules. 2016;21:1264. doi: 10.3390/molecules21091264. [PubMed] [CrossRef] [Google Scholar]

Vlachojannis J.E., Cameron M., Chrubasik S. A Systematic Review on the Sambuci fructus effect and efficacy profiles. Phytother. Res. 2010;24:1–8. doi: 10.1002/ptr.2729. [PubMed] [CrossRef] [Google Scholar]

Hendrich A.B. Flavonoid-membrane interactions: Possible consequences for biological effects of some polyphenolic compounds. Acta Pharmacol. Sin. 2006;27:27–40. doi: 10.1111/j.1745-7254.2006.00238.x. [PubMed] [CrossRef] [Google Scholar]

Pawlikowska-Pawlęga B., Dziubińska H., Krol E., Trębacz K., Jarosz-Wilkołazka A., Paduch R., Gawron A., Gruszecki W.I. Characteristics of quercetin interactions with liposomal and vacuolar membranes. Biochim. Biophys. Acta Biomembr. 2014;1838:254–265. doi: 10.1016/j.bbamem.2013.08.014. [PubMed] [CrossRef] [Google Scholar]

Cayahana Y., Gordon M.H. Interaction of anthocyanins with human albumin: Influence of pH and chemical structure on binding. Food Chem. 2013;141:2278–2285. doi: 10.1016/j.foodchem.2013.05.026. [PubMed] [CrossRef] [Google Scholar]

Muellera D., Junga K., Wintera M., Rogollb D., Melcherb R., Kulozikc U., Schwarzd K., Richling E. Encapsulation of anthocyanins from bilberries—Effects on bioavailability and intestinal accessibility in humans. Food Chem. 2018;15:217–224. doi: 10.1016/j.foodchem.2017.12.058. [PubMed] [CrossRef] [Google Scholar]

Patrasa A., Bruntona N.P., O'Donnell C.O., Tiwari B.K. Effect of thermal processing on anthocyanin stability in foods; mechanisms and kinetics of degradation. Trends Food Sci. Technol. 2010;21:3–11. doi: 10.1016/j.tifs.2009.07.004. [CrossRef] [Google Scholar]

Mahdavi S.A., Jafari S., Ghorbani M.M., Assadpoor E. Spray-Drying Microencapsulation of Anthocyanins by Natural Biopolymers: A Review. Drying Technol. 2014;32:509–518. doi: 10.1080/07373937.2013.839562. [CrossRef] [Google Scholar]

Duymuş H.G., Göger F., Başer K.H. In vitro antioxidant properties and anthocyanin compositions of elderberry extracts. Food Chem. 2014;15:112–119. doi: 10.1016/j.foodchem.2014.01.028. [PubMed] [CrossRef] [Google Scholar]

Dawidowicz A.L., Wianowska D., Baraniak B. The antioxidant properties of alcoholic extracts from Sambucus nigra L. (antioxidative properties of extracts) LWT-Food Sci. Technol. 2006;39:308–315. doi: 10.1016/j.lwt.2005.01.005. [CrossRef] [Google Scholar]

Olejnik A., Olkowicz M., Kowalska K., Rychlik J., Dembczyński R., Myszka K., Juzwa W., Białas W., Moyer M.P. Gastrointestinal digested Sambucus nigra L. fruit extract protects in vitro cultured human colon cells against oxidative stress. Food Chem. 2016;197:648–657. doi: 10.1016/j.foodchem.2015.11.017. [PubMed] [CrossRef] [Google Scholar]

Sidor A., Gramza-Michałowska A. Advanced research on the antioxidant and health benefit of elderberry (Sambucus nigra) in food—A review. J. Funct. Foods. 2015;18:941–958. doi: 10.1016/j.jff.2014.07.012. [CrossRef] [Google Scholar]

Kšonžeková P., Mariychuk R., Eliašová A., Mudroňová D., Csank T., Király J., Marcinčáková D., Pistl J., Tkáčiková L. In vitro study of biological activities of anthocyanin-rich berry extracts on porcineintestinal epithelial cells. J. Sci. Food Agric. 2015;96:1093–1100. doi: 10.1002/jsfa.7181. [PubMed] [CrossRef] [Google Scholar]

Kaack K., Frett X.C., Christensen L.P., Landbo A.-K., Meyer A.S. Selection of elderberry (Sambucus nigra L.) genotypes best suited for the preparation of juice. Eur. Food Res. Technol. 2008;226:843–855. doi: 10.1007/s00217-007-0605-0. [CrossRef] [Google Scholar]

Wu X., Gu L., Prior R.L., McKay S. Characterization of anthocyanins and proanthocyanidins in some cultivars of ribes, aronia, and sambucus and their antioxidant capacity. J. Agric. Food Chem. 2004;52:7846–7856. doi: 10.1021/jf0486850. [PubMed] [CrossRef] [Google Scholar]

Miculic-Petkovsek M., Schmitzer V., Slatnar A., Todorovic B., Veberic R., Stampar F., Ivancic A. Investigation of anthocyanin profile of four elderberry species and interspecific hybrids. J. Agric. Food Chem. 2014;62:5573–5580. doi: 10.1021/jf5011947. [PubMed] [CrossRef] [Google Scholar]

Strugała P., Dudra A., Gabrielska J. Interaction between mimic lipid membranes and acylated and nonacylated cyanidin and its bioactivity. J. Agric. Food Chem. 2016;64:7414–7422. doi: 10.1021/acs.jafc.6b03066. [PubMed] [CrossRef] [Google Scholar]

Williamson P., Mattocksa K., Schlegelb R.A. Merocyanine 540, a fluorescent probe sensitive to lipid packing. Biochim. Biophys. Acta. 1983;732:387–393. doi: 10.1016/0005-2736(83)90055-X. [PubMed] [CrossRef] [Google Scholar]

Manrique-Moreno M., Londoño-Londoño J., Jemioła-Rzemińska M., Strzałka K., Villena F., Avello M., Suwalsky M. Structural effects of the Solanum steroids solasodine, diosgenin and solanine on human erythrocytes and molecular models of eukaryotic membranes. Biochim. Biophys. Acta. 2014;1838:266–277. doi: 10.1016/j.bbamem.2013.08.003. [PubMed] [CrossRef] [Google Scholar]

Strugała P., Dudra A., Gabrielska J. Activity of blackcurrant and chokeberry extracts and two major cyanidin glycosides against lipid membrane oxidation and their binding properties to albumin. Acta Pol. Pharm. 2017;74:676–687. [PubMed] [Google Scholar]

Kaiser R.D., London E. Location of diphenylhexatriene (DPH) and its derivatives within membranes: Comparison of different fluorescence quenching analyses of membrane depth. Biochemistry. 1998;37:8180–8190. doi: 10.1021/bi980064a. [PubMed] [CrossRef] [Google Scholar]

Tammela P., Laitinen L., Galkin A., Wennberg T., Heczko R., Vuorela H., Slotte J.P., Vuorela P. Permeability characteristics and membrane affinity of flavonoids and alkyl gallates in Caco-2 cells and in phospholipid vesicles. Arch. Biochem. Biophys. 2004;425:193–199. doi: 10.1016/j.abb.2004.03.023. [PubMed] [CrossRef] [Google Scholar]

Inbar M. Fluidity of membrane lipids: A single cell analysis of mouse normal lymphocytes and malignant lymphoma cells. FEBS Lett. 1976;67:180–185. doi: 10.1016/0014-5793(76)80361-4. [PubMed] [CrossRef] [Google Scholar]

Kojima K. Molecular aspects of the plasma membrane in tumor cells. Nagoya J. Med. Sci. 1993;56:1–18. [PubMed] [Google Scholar]

Sok M., Šentjurc M., Schara M. Membrane fluidity characteristics of human lung cancer. Cancer Lett. 1999;139:215–220. doi: 10.1016/S0304-3835(99)00044-0. [PubMed] [CrossRef] [Google Scholar]

Inbar M., Shinitzky M. Cholesterol as a bioregulator in the development and inhibition of leukemia. Proc. Natl. Acad. Sci. USA. 1974;71:4229–4231. doi: 10.1073/pnas.71.10.4229. [PMC free article] [PubMed] [CrossRef] [Google Scholar]

Nakazawa I., Iwaizumi M. A role of the cancer cell membrane fluidity in the cancer metastases: An ESR study. Tohoku J. Exp. Med. 1989;157:193–198. doi: 10.1620/tjem.157.193. [PubMed] [CrossRef] [Google Scholar]

Rybczynska M., Spitaler M., Knebel N.G., Boeck G., Grunicke H., Hofmann J. Effects of miltefosine on various biochemical parameters in a panel of tumor cell lines with different sensitivities. Biochem. Pharmacol. 2001;62:765–772. doi: 10.1016/S0006-2952(01)00715-8. [PubMed] [CrossRef] [Google Scholar]

Berra B., Bordoni A., Rapelli S., Biagi P.L., Pezzotta S., Malgrassi L., Montorfano G., Hrelia S. Altered membrane lipid composition in a human meningosarcoma. Int. J. Clin. Lab. Res. 1994;24:54–57. doi: 10.1007/BF02592411. [PubMed] [CrossRef] [Google Scholar]

Tsuchiya H. Structure-dependent membrane interaction of flavonoids associated with their bioactivity. Food Chem. 2010;120:1089–1096. doi: 10.1016/j.foodchem.2009.11.057. [CrossRef] [Google Scholar]

Strugała P., Tronina T., Huszcza E., Gabrielska J. Bioactivity in vitro of quercetin glycoside obtained in beauveria bassiana culture and its interaction with liposome membranes. Molecules. 2017;22:1520. doi: 10.3390/molecules22091520. [PMC free article] [PubMed] [CrossRef] [Google Scholar]

Strugała P., Cyboran-Mikołajczyk S., Dudra A., Mizgier P., Kucharska A.Z., Olejniczak T., Gabrielska J. Biological activity of Japanese quince extract and its interaction with lipids, erythrocyte membrane and human albumin. J. Membr. Biol. 2016;249:393–410. doi: 10.1007/s00232-016-9877-2. [PMC free article] [PubMed] [CrossRef] [Google Scholar]

Strugała P., Gładkowski W., Kucharska A.Z., Sokół-Łętowska A., Gabrielska J. Antioxidant activity and anti-inflammatory effect of fruit extracts from blackcurrant, chokeberry, hawthorn, and rosehip, and their mixture with linseed oil on a model lipid membrane. Eur. J. Lipid Sci. Technol. 2016;118:461–474. doi: 10.1002/ejlt.201500001. [CrossRef] [Google Scholar]

Bratu M.M., Doroftei E., Negreanu-Pirjol T.A., Hostina C.A., Porta S. Determination of antioxidant activity and toxicity of Sambucus nigra fruit extract using alternative methods. Food Technol. Biotechnol. 2012;50:177–182. [Google Scholar]

Barak V., Birkenfeld S., Halperin T., Kalickman I. The effect of herbal remedies on the production of human inflammatory and anti-inflammatory cytokines. Isr. Med. Assoc. J. 2002;4:919–922. [PubMed] [Google Scholar]

. Farrell N.J., Norris G.H., Ryan J., Porter C.M., Jiang C., Blesso C.N. Black elderberry extract attenuates inflammation and metabolic dysfunction in diet-induced obese mice. Br. J. Nutr. 2015;114:1123–1131. doi: 10.1017/S0007114515002962. [PubMed] [CrossRef] [Google Scholar]

Fang Z., Bhandari B. Encapsulation of polyphenols—A review. Trends Food Sci. Technol. 2010;21:510–523. doi: 10.1016/j.tifs.2010.08.003. [CrossRef] [Google Scholar]

Patil Y.P., Jadhav S. Novel methods for liposome preparation. Chem. Phys. Lipids. 2014;177:8–18. doi: 10.1016/j.chemphyslip.2013.10.011. [PubMed] [CrossRef] [Google Scholar]

Robert P., Fredes C. The encapsulation of anthocyanins from berry-type fruits trends in foods. Molecules. 2015;20:5875–5888. doi: 10.3390/molecules20045875. [PMC free article] [PubMed] [CrossRef] [Google Scholar]

Cavalcanti R.N., Santos D.T., Meireles M.A.A. Non-thermal stabilization mechanisms of anthocyanins in model and food systems—An overview. Food Res. Int. 2011;44:499–509. doi: 10.1016/j.foodres.2010.12.007. [CrossRef] [Google Scholar]

Oehme A., Valotis A., Krammer G., Zimmermann I., Schreier P. Preparation and characterization of shellac-coated anthocyanin pectin beads as dietary colonic delivery system. Mol. Nutr. Food Res. 2011;55:S75–S85. doi: 10.1002/mnfr.201000467. [PubMed] [CrossRef] [Google Scholar]

Sharma A., Sharma U.S. Liposomes in drug delivery: Progress and limitations. Int. J. Pharm. 1997;154:123–140. doi: 10.1016/S0378-5173(97)00135-X. [CrossRef] [Google Scholar]

Nii T., Ishii F. Encapsulation efficiency of water-soluble and insoluble drugs in liposomes prepared by the microencapsulation vesicle method. Int. J. Pharm. 2005;14:198–205. doi: 10.1016/j.ijpharm.2005.04.029. [PubMed] [CrossRef] [Google Scholar]

Bryła A., Lewandowicz G., Juzwa W. Encapsulation of elderberry extract into phospholipid nanoparticles. J. Food Eng. 2015;167:189–195. doi: 10.1016/j.jfoodeng.2015.07.025. [CrossRef] [Google Scholar]

Yang S., Liu W., Liu C., Liu W., Tong G., Zenh H., Zhou W. Characterization and bioavailability of vitamin C nanparticles prepared by film evaporation—Dynamic high pressure microfluidization. J. Disper. Sci. Technol. 2011;33:1608–1614. doi: 10.1080/01932691.2011.629511. [CrossRef] [Google Scholar]

Siddiqi M., Nusrat S., Alam P., Malik S., Chaturvedi S.K., Ajmal M.R., Abdelhameed A.S., Khan R.H. Investigating the site selective binding of busulfan to human serum albumin: Biophysical and molecular docking approaches. Int. J. Biol. Macromol. 2018;107:1414–1421. doi: 10.1016/j.ijbiomac.2017.10.006. [PubMed] [CrossRef] [Google Scholar]

Lakowicz J.R. Quenching of fluorescence. In: Lakowicz J.R., editor. Principles of Fluorescence Spectroscopy. 3rd ed. Springer; New York, NY, USA: 2006. pp. 278–285. [Google Scholar]

Trnková L., Boušová I., Staňková V., Dršata J. Study on the interaction of catechins with human serum albumin using spectroscopic and electrophoretic techniques. J. Mol. Struct. 2011;985:243–250. doi: 10.1016/j.molstruc.2010.11.001. [CrossRef] [Google Scholar]

Dai J., Zou T., Wang L., Zhang Y., Liu Y. Investigation of the interaction between quercetin and human serum albumin by multiple spectra, electrochemical impedance spectra and molecular modeling. Luminescence. 2014;29:1154–1161. doi: 10.1002/bio.2676. [PubMed] [CrossRef] [Google Scholar]

Feroz S.R., Mohamad S.B., Bakri Z.S.D., Malek S.N.A., Tayyab S. Probing the interaction of a therapeutic flavonoid, pinostrobin with human serum albumin: Multiple spectroscopic and molecular modeling investigations. PLoS ONE. 2013;8:e76067. doi: 10.1371/journal.pone.0076067. [PMC free article] [PubMed] [CrossRef] [Google Scholar]

Klotz I.M. Physiochemical aspects of drug-protein interactions: A general perspective. Ann. N. Y. Acad. Sci. 1973;226:18–35. doi: 10.1111/j.1749-6632.1973.tb20465.x. [PubMed] [CrossRef] [Google Scholar]

. Xi J., Guo R. Interactions between flavonoids and hemoglobin in lecithin liposomes. Int. J. Biol. Macromol. 2007;40:305–311. doi: 10.1016/j.ijbiomac.2006.08.011. [PubMed] [CrossRef] [Google Scholar]

Ross P.D., Subramanian S. Thermodynamics of protein association reactions: Forces contributing to stability. Biochemistry. 1981;20:3096–3102. doi: 10.1021/bi00514a017. [PubMed] [CrossRef] [Google Scholar]

Remila S., Atmani-Kilani D., Delemasure S., Connat J.-L., Azib L., Richard T., Atmani D. Antioxidant, cytoprotective, anti-inflammatory and anticancer activities of Pistacia lentiscus (Anacardiaceae) leaf and fruit extracts. Eur. J. Integr. Med. 2015;7:274–286. doi: 10.1016/j.eujim.2015.03.009. [CrossRef] [Google Scholar]

Olsson M.E., Gustavsson K.E., Andersson S., Nilsson A., Duan R.D. Inhibition of cancer cell proliferation in vitro by fruit and berry extracts and correlations with antioxidant levels. J. Agric. Food Chem. 2004;52:7264–7271. doi: 10.1021/jf030479p. [PubMed] [CrossRef] [Google Scholar]

Chen P.N., Chu S.C., Chiou H.L., Chiang C.L., Yang S.F., Hsieh Y.S. Cyanidin 3-glucoside and peonidin 3-glucoside inhibit tumor cell growth and induce apoptosis in vitro and suppress tumor growth in vivo. Nutr. Cancer. 2005;53:232–243. doi: 10.1207/s15327914nc5302_12. [PubMed] [CrossRef] [Google Scholar]

Lee Y.K., Lee W.S., Kim G.S., Park O.J. Anthocyanins are novel AMPKα1 stimulators that suppress tumor growth by inhibiting mTOR phosphorylation. Oncol. Rep. 2010;24:1471–1477. doi: 10.3892/or_00001007. [PubMed] [CrossRef] [Google Scholar]

Li X., Xu J., Tang X., Liu Y., Yu X., Wang Z., Liu W. Anthocyanins inhibit trastuzumab-resistant breast cancer in vitro and in vivo. Mol. Med. Rep. 2016;13:4007–4013. doi: 10.3892/mmr.2016.4990. [PubMed] [CrossRef] [Google Scholar]

Malik M., Zhao C., Schoene N., Guisti M.M., Moyer M.P., Magnuson B.A. Anthocyanin-rich extract from Aronia meloncarpa E induces a cell cycle block in colon cancer but not normal colonic cells. Nutr. Cancer. 2003;46:186–196. doi: 10.1207/S15327914NC4602_12. [PubMed] [CrossRef] [Google Scholar]

Hakimuddin F., Paliyath G., Meckling K. Selective cytotoxicity of a red grape wine flavonoid fraction against MCF-7 cells. Breast Cancer Res. Treat. 2004;85:65–79. doi: 10.1023/B:BREA.0000021048.52430.c0. [PubMed] [CrossRef] [Google Scholar]

Thole J.M., Kraft T.F., Sueiro L.A., Kang Y.H., Gills J.J., Cuendet M., Pezzuto J.M., Seigler D.S., Lila M.A. A comparative evaluation of the anticancer properties of European and American elderberry fruits. J. Med. Food. 2006;9:498–504. doi: 10.1089/jmf.2006.9.498. [PubMed] [CrossRef] [Google Scholar]

Kucharska A.Z., Szumny A., Sokół-Łętowska A., Piórecki N., Klymenko S.V. Iridoids and anthocyanins in cornelian cherry (Cornus mas L.) cultivars. J. Food Compos. Anal. 2015;40:95–102. doi: 10.1016/j.jfca.2014.12.016. [CrossRef] [Google Scholar]

Sokół-Łętowska A., Kucharska A.Z., Wińska K., Szumny A., Nawirska-Olszańska A., Mizgier P., Wyspiańska D. Composition and antioxidant activity of red fruit liqueurs. Food Chem. 2014;157:533–539. doi: 10.1016/j.foodchem.2014.02.083. [PubMed] [CrossRef] [Google Scholar]

Brand-Williams B., Cuvelier M.E., Berset C. Use of free radical method to evaluate antioxidant activity. LWT-Food Sci. Technol. 1995;28:25–30. doi: 10.1016/S0023-6438(95)80008-5. [CrossRef] [Google Scholar]

Jang M.S., Pezzuto J.M. Assessment of cyclooxygenase inhibitors using in vitro assay systems. Method Cell Sci. 1997;19:25–31. doi: 10.1023/A:1009742504152. [CrossRef] [Google Scholar]

Bykowska A., Starosta R., Brzuszkiewicz A., Bażanów B., Florek M., Jackulak N., Król J., Grzesiak J., Kaliński K., Jeżowska-Bojczuk M. Synthesis, properties and biological activity of a novel phosphines ligand derived from ciprofloxacin. Polyhedron. 2013;60:23–29. doi: 10.1016/j.poly.2013.04.059. [CrossRef] [Google Scholar]

Rubin H. Chick embryo cells. In: Kruse P.F., Patterson M.K., editors. Tissue Culture Methods and Application. Academic Press; New York, NY, USA: 1973. pp. 119–123. [Google Scholar]

Tiralongo E, Wee SS, Lea RA. Elderberry Supplementation Reduces Cold Duration and Symptoms in Air-Travellers: A Randomized, Double-Blind Placebo-Controlled Clinical Trial. Nutrients. 2016 Mar 24;8(4):182. doi: 10.3390/nu8040182. PMID: 27023596; PMCID: PMC4848651.

Roxas M., Jurenka J. Colds and influenza: A review of diagnosis and conventional, botanical, and nutritional considerations. Altern. Med. Rev. 2007;12:25–48. [PubMed] [Google Scholar]

Raus K., Pleschka S., Klein P., Schoop R., Fisher P. Effect of an Echinacea-Based Hot Drink versus Oseltamivir in Influenza Treatment: A Randomized, Double-Blind, Double-Dummy, Multicenter, Noninferiority Clinical Trial. Curr. Ther. Res. Clin. Exp. 2015;77:66–72. doi: 10.1016/j.curtheres.2015.04.001. [PMC free article] [PubMed] [CrossRef] [Google Scholar]

Krawitz C., Mraheil M.A., Stein M., Imirzalioglu C., Domann E., Pleschka S., Hain T. Inhibitory activity of a standardized elderberry liquid extract against clinically-relevant human respiratory bacterial pathogens and influenza A and B viruses. BMC Complement. Altern. Med. 2011;11:182. doi: 10.1186/1472-6882-11-16. [PMC free article] [PubMed] [CrossRef] [Google Scholar]

Roschek B., Jr., Fink R.C., McMichael M.D., Li D., Alberte R.S. Elderberry flavonoids bind to and prevent H1N1 infection in vitro. Phytochemistry. 2009;70:1255–1261. doi: 10.1016/j.phytochem.2009.06.003. [PubMed] [CrossRef] [Google Scholar]

Vlachojannis J.E., Cameron M., Chrubasik S. A systematic review on the sambuci fructus effect and efficacy profiles. Phytother. Res. 2010;24:1–8. doi: 10.1002/ptr.2729. [PubMed] [CrossRef] [Google Scholar]

Kong F. Pilot clinical study on a proprietary elderberry extract: Efficacy in addressing influenza symptoms. Online J. Pharmacol. Pharmacokinet. 2009;5:32–43. [Google Scholar]

Netzel M., Strass G., Herbst M., Dietrich H., Bitsch R., Bitsch I., Frank T. The excretion and biological antioxidant activity of elderberry antioxidants in healthy humans. Food Res. Int. 2005;38:905–910. doi: 10.1016/j.foodres.2005.03.010. [CrossRef] [Google Scholar]

Gray A.M., Abdel-Wahab Y.H., Flatt P.R. The traditional plant treatment, Sambucus nigra (elder), exhibits insulin-like and insulin-releasing actions in vitro. J. Nutr. 2000;130:15–20. [PubMed] [Google Scholar]

Staiger C. Comfrey: a clinical overview. Phytother Res. 2012 Oct;26(10):1441-8. doi: 10.1002/ptr.4612. Epub 2012 Feb 23. PMID: 22359388; PMCID: PMC3491633.

Staiger C. Comfrey root: from tradition to modern clinical trials. Wien Med Wochenschr. 2013 Feb;163(3-4):58-64. doi: 10.1007/s10354-012-0162-4. Epub 2012 Dec 7. PMID: 23224633; PMCID: PMC3580139.

Schmelzer G., Gurib-Fakim A. Plant Resources of Tropical Africa: Medicinal Plants 1. Backhuys Publishers CTA; Kerkwerve, The Netherlands: 2008. [Google Scholar]

Horinouchi C.D., Otuki M.F. Botanical briefs: comfrey (Symphytum officinale) Cutis. 2013;91:225–228. [PubMed] [Google Scholar]

Frost R., MacPherson H., O'Meara S.M. A critical scoping review of external uses of comfrey (Symphytum spp.) Complementary Ther. Med. 2013;21:724–745. doi: 10.1016/j.ctim.2013.09.009. [PubMed] [CrossRef] [Google Scholar]

Staiger C. Comfrey: A clinical overview. Phytother. Res. 2012;26:1441–1448. doi: 10.1002/ptr.4612. [PMC free article] [PubMed] [CrossRef] [Google Scholar]

Riet-Correa F., Medeiros R., Tokarnia C., Dobereiner J. Toxic plants for livestock in Brazil: Economic impact, toxic species, control measures and public health implications. In: Panter K.E., Wierenga T.L., Pfister J.A., editors. Poisonous Plants: Global Research and Solutions. CABI Press; Wallingford, UK: 2007. pp. 2–14. [Google Scholar]

Cameron M., Chrubasik S. Topical herbal therapies for treating osteoarthritis. Cochrane Database Syst. Rev. 2013:Cd010538. doi: 10.1002/14651858.CD010538. [PMC free article] [PubMed] [CrossRef] [Google Scholar]

MacKay D., Miller A.L. Nutritional support for wound healing. Altern. Med. Rev. 2003;8:359–377. [PubMed] [Google Scholar]

Neagu E., Paun G., Radu G. Antioxidant capacity of some Symphytum officinalis extracts processed by ultrafiltration. Rom. Biotechnol. Lett. 2010;15:5505–5511. [Google Scholar]

Sowa I., Paduch R., Strzemski M., Zielińska S., Rydzik-Strzemska E., Sawicki J., Kocjan R., Polkowski J., Matkowski A., Latalski M., et al. Proliferative and antioxidant activity of Symphytum officinale root extract. Nat. Prod. Res. 2018;32:605–609. doi: 10.1080/14786419.2017.1326492. [PubMed] [CrossRef] [Google Scholar]

Barbakadze V., Mulkijanyan K., Merlani M.M., Gogilashvili L., Amiranashvili L., K. Shaburishvili E. Extraction, composition and the antioxidant and anticomplement activities of high molecular weight fractions from the leaves of Symphytum asperum and S. caucasicum. Pharm. Chem. J. 2011;44:604–607. doi: 10.1007/s11094-011-0527-9. [CrossRef] [Google Scholar]

Chen S., Shang H., Yang J., Li R., Wu H. Effects of different extraction techniques on physicochemical properties and activities of polysaccharides from comfrey (Symphytum officinale L.) root. Ind. Crop. Prod. 2018;121:18–25. doi: 10.1016/j.indcrop.2018.04.063. [CrossRef] [Google Scholar]

Brown A.W., Stegelmeier B.L., Colegate S.M., Gardner D.R., Panter K.E., Knoppel E.L., Hall J.O. The comparative toxicity of a reduced, crude comfrey (Symphytum officinale) alkaloid extract and the pure, comfrey-derived pyrrolizidine alkaloids, lycopsamine and intermedine in chicks (Gallus gallus domesticus) J. Appl. Toxicol. 2016;36:716–725. doi: 10.1002/jat.3205. [PubMed] [CrossRef] [Google Scholar]

Kurucu S., Kartal M., Choudary M.I., Topcu G. Pyrrolizidine Alkaloids from Symphytum sylvaticum Boiss. subsp. sepulcrale. (Boiss. & Bal.) Greuter & Burdet var. sepulcrale and Symphytum aintabicum Hub. - Mor. & Wickens. Turk. J. Chem. 2002;26:195–199. [Google Scholar]

Mei N., Guo L., Fu P.P., Fuscoe J.C., Luan Y., Chen T. Metabolism, Genotoxicity, annd Carcinogenicity of Comfrey. J. Toxicol. Environ. Health Part B. 2010;13:509–526. doi: 10.1080/10937404.2010.509013. [PMC free article] [PubMed] [CrossRef] [Google Scholar]

Adeneye A.A. 6 - Subchronic and Chronic Toxicities of African Medicinal Plants. In: Kuete V., editor. Toxicological Survey of African Medicinal Plants. Elsevier; Amsterdam, The Netherlands: 2014. [CrossRef] [Google Scholar]

Kruse L.H., Stegemann T., Sievert C., Ober D. Identification of a Second Site of Pyrrolizidine Alkaloid Biosynthesis in Comfrey to Boost Plant Defense in Floral Stage() Plant Physiol. 2017;174:47–55. doi: 10.1104/pp.17.00265. [PMC free article] [PubMed] [CrossRef] [Google Scholar]

Mazzocchi A., Montanaro F. Observational study of the use of Symphytum 5CH in the management of pain and swelling after dental implant surgery. Homeopathy. 2012;101:211–216. doi: 10.1016/j.homp.2012.07.002. [PubMed] [CrossRef] [Google Scholar]

. Colegate S.M., Stegelmeier B.L., Edgar J.A. 14 - Dietary exposure of livestock and humans to hepatotoxic natural products. In: Fink-Gremmels J., editor. Animal Feed Contamination. Woodhead Publishing; Amsterdam, The Netherlands: 2012. [CrossRef] [Google Scholar]

Singh H., Du J., Singh P., Yi T.H. Role of green silver nanoparticles synthesized from Symphytum officinale leaf extract in protection against UVB-induced photoaging. J. Nanostructure Chem. 2018;8:359–368. doi: 10.1007/s40097-018-0281-6. [CrossRef] [Google Scholar]

Karavaev V.A., Solntsev M.K., Iurina T.P., Iurina E.V., Poliakova I.B., Kuznetsov A.M. Antifungal activity of aqueous extracts from the leaf of cowparsnip and comfrey. Izv. Akad. Nauk. Seriia Biol. 2001;4:435–441. [PubMed] [Google Scholar]

Pileggi M., Raiman P.M., Micheli A., Beatriz S., Bobalto V. Antimicrobial Action and Endophytic interaction in Symphytum officinale L. Publ. Uepg. 2002;8:47–55. [Google Scholar]

Avancini C., Wiest J.M., Dall'Agnol R., Haas J.S., von POSER G.L. Antimicrobial activity of plants used in the prevention and control of bovine mastitis in Southern Brazil. Lat. Am. J. Pharm. 2008;27:894–899. [Google Scholar]

Rodrigues Oliveira P., Ramos Santos F., Ferreira Duarte E., Silva Guimarães G., Sartori Carvalho Mattos N., Minafra C. Symbiotics and Aloe vera and Symphytum officinale extracts in broiler feed. Semin.: Ciências Agrárias. 2016;37:2677. doi: 10.5433/1679-0359.2016v37n4Supl1p2677. [CrossRef] [Google Scholar]

Pawlowski B. Symphytum L. and Procopiania Gusul. In: Tutin T., Heywood V., Burges H., Moore N.A., Valentine D.M., Walters D.H., Webb S.M., editors. Flora of Europea. Volume 3. Cambridge University Press; Cambridge, UK: 1972. pp. 103–106. [Google Scholar]

Peruzzi L., Garbari F., Bottega S. Symphytum tanaicense (Boraginaceae) new for the Italian flora. Willdenowia. 2001;31:33–41. doi: 10.3372/wi.31.31102. [CrossRef] [Google Scholar]

Tarıkahya B. The Revision of Turkish Symphytum L. (Boraginaceae) Genus. Hacettepe University; Ankara, Turkey: 2010. [Google Scholar]

Hacıoğlu B.T., Erik S. Phylogeny of Symphytum L.(Boraginaceae) with special emphasis on Turkish species. Afr. J. Biotechnol. 2011;10:15483–15493. doi: 10.5897/AJB11.1094. [CrossRef] [Google Scholar]

Teynor T.M., Putnam D.H., Doll J.D., Kelling K.A., Oelke E.A., Undersander D.J., Oplinger E.S. Comfrey - Alternative Field Crops Manual. Minnesota Extension Service, University of Minnesota; Minneapolis, MN, USA: 1992. [Google Scholar]

Chittendon F. RHS Dictionary of Plants Plus Supplement. Oxford University Press; Oxford, UK: 1956. [Google Scholar]

Grieve B. A Modern Herbal. Penguin; London, UK: 1984. [Google Scholar]

Huxley A. The New RHS Dictionary of Gardening. MacMillan Press; London, UK: 1992. [Google Scholar]

Bogert L.J., Briggs G.M., Calloway D.H. Nutrition and physical fitness. W.B. Saunders Co.; Philadelphia, PA, USA: 1973. [Google Scholar]

Harris P.J.C., Grove C.G., Havard A.J. In vitro propagation of Symphytum species. Sci. Hortic. 1989;40:275–281. doi: 10.1016/0304-4238(89)90101-5. [CrossRef] [Google Scholar]

Robinson R.G. Comfrey—A Controversial Crop. University of Minnesota. Agricultural Experiment Station; St. Paul, MN, USA: 1983. [Google Scholar]

Thoresen E.M. Symphytum officinale Common comfrey. Szent Istvan University; Budapest, Hungary: 2013. [Google Scholar]

Bellardi M.G., Benni A. The occurrence of alfalfa mosaic virus in Symphytum tuberosum L. J. Plant Pathol. 2005;87:75. [Google Scholar]

Juhl V.M. Liste over vaertplanter for blad nematoden Aphelenchoides ritzemabosi. Ugeskr. Agron. HortonomerForstkandidater Og Licent. 1978;123:183–186. [Google Scholar]

Knight K.W., Barber C.J., Page G.D. Plant-parasitic Nematodes of New Zealand Recorded by Host Association. J. Nematol. 1997;29:640–656. [PMC free article] [PubMed] [Google Scholar]

Neagu E., PĂun G., Radu L.G. Phytochemical study of some Symphytum officinalis extracts concentrated by membranous procedures. Sci. Bull. -Univ. Politeh. Buchacharest. 2011:3–7. [Google Scholar]

Stickel F., Seitz H.K. The efficacy and safety of comfrey. Public Health Nutr. 2000;3:501–508. doi: 10.1017/S1368980000000586. [PubMed] [CrossRef] [Google Scholar]

Trifan A., Opitz S.E.W., Josuran R., Grubelnik A., Esslinger N., Peter S., Bräm S., Meier N., Wolfram E. Is comfrey root more than toxic pyrrolizidine alkaloids? Salvianolic acids among antioxidant polyphenols in comfrey (Symphytum officinale L.) roots. Food Chem. Toxicol. 2018;112:178–187. doi: 10.1016/j.fct.2017.12.051. [PubMed] [CrossRef] [Google Scholar]

Mulkijanyan K., Barbakadze V., Novikova Z., Sulakvelidze M., Gogilashvili L., Amiranashvili L., Merlani M. Burn healing compositions from Caucasian species of comfrey (Symphytum L.) Bull. Georg. Natl. Acad. Sci. 2009;3:114–117. [Google Scholar]

Roeder I.E., Bourauel T., Neuberger V. Symviridine, a new pyrrolizidine alkaloid from Symphytum species. Phytochemistry. 1992;31:4041–4042. doi: 10.1016/S0031-9422(00)97585-X. [CrossRef] [Google Scholar]

Roeder E. Medicinal plants in Europe containing pyrrolizidine alkaloids. Pharmazie. 1995;50:83–98. [PubMed] [Google Scholar]

Onduso S.O. Determination of levels of pyrrolizidine alkaloids in Symphytum asperum Lepech growing in selected parts of Keniya. Kenyatta University; Nairobi, Kenia: 2014. [Google Scholar]

Barbakadze V.V., Kemertelidze E.P., Shashkov A.S., Usov A.I. Structure of a new anticomplementary dihydroxycinnamate-derived polymer from Symphytum asperum (Boraginaceae) Mendeleev Commun. 2000;10:148–149. doi: 10.1070/MC2000v010n04ABEH001295. [CrossRef] [Google Scholar]

Barbakadze V., Kemertelidze E., Targamadze I., Mulkijanyan K., Shashkov A.S., Usov A.I. Poly[3-(3,4-dihydroxyphenyl)glyceric acid], a new biologically active polymer from Symphytum asperum Lepech. and S. caucasicum Bieb. (Boraginaceae) Molecules. 2005;10:1135–1144. doi: 10.3390/10091135. [PMC free article] [PubMed] [CrossRef] [Google Scholar]

Barbakadze V.V., Kemertelidze E.P., Mulkijanyan K.G., Van Den Berg A.J.J., Beukelman C.J., Van Den Worm E., Quarles Van Ufford H.C., Usov A.I. Antioxidant and anticomplement activity of poly[3-(3,4-dihydroxyphenyl) glyceric acid] from Symphytum asperum and Symphytum caucasicum plants. Pharm. Chem. J. 2007;41:14–16. doi: 10.1007/s11094-007-0004-7. [CrossRef] [Google Scholar]

Melkumova Z.V., Telezhenetskaya M.V., Yunusov S.Y., Manko I.V. Refinement of the structure of asperumine. Chem. Nat. Compd. 1974;10:483–485. doi: 10.1007/BF00563814. [CrossRef] [Google Scholar]

Mroczek T., Ndjoko-Ioset K., Głowniak K., Mietkiewicz-Capała A., Hostettmann K. Investigation of Symphytum cordatum alkaloids by liquid–liquid partitioning, thin-layer chromatography and liquid chromatography–ion-trap mass spectrometry. Anal. Chim. Acta. 2006;566:157–166. doi: 10.1016/j.aca.2006.03.016. [CrossRef] [Google Scholar]

Avula B., Sagi S., Wang Y.H., Zweigenbaum J., Wang M., Khan I.A. Characterization and screening of pyrrolizidine alkaloids and N-oxides from botanicals and dietary supplements using UHPLC-high resolution mass spectrometry. Food Chem. 2015;178:136–148. doi: 10.1016/j.foodchem.2015.01.053. [PubMed] [CrossRef] [Google Scholar]

. Liu F., Wan S.Y., Jiang Z., Li S.F.Y., Ong E.S., Osorio J.C.C. Determination of pyrrolizidine alkaloids in comfrey by liquid chromatography–electrospray ionization mass spectrometry. Talanta. 2009;80:916–923. doi: 10.1016/j.talanta.2009.08.020. [PubMed] [CrossRef] [Google Scholar]

Kim N.C., Oberlies N.H., Brine D.R., Handy R.W., Wani M.C., Wall M.E. Isolation of symlandine from the roots of common comfrey (Symphytum officinale) using countercurrent chromatography. J. Nat. Prod. 2001;64:251–253. doi: 10.1021/np0004653. [PubMed] [CrossRef] [Google Scholar]

Janeš D., Kreft S. TLC densitometric method for screening of lycopsamine in comfrey root (Symphytum officinale L.) extracts using retrorsine as a reference compound. Acta. Pharm. 2014;64:503–508. doi: 10.2478/acph-2014-0031. [PubMed] [CrossRef] [Google Scholar]

Janes D., Kalamar B., Kreft S. Improved method for isolation of lycopsamine from roots of comfrey (Symphytum officinale) Nat. Prod. Commun. 2012;7:861–862. [PubMed] [Google Scholar]

Brauchli J., Lüthy J., Zweifel U., Schlatter C. Pyrrolizidine alkaloids from Symphytum officinale L. and their percutaneous absorption in rats. Experientia. 1982;38:1085–1087. doi: 10.1007/BF01955382. [PubMed] [CrossRef] [Google Scholar]

Altamirano J.C., Gratz S.R., Wolnik K.A. Investigation of pyrrolizidine alkaloids and their N-oxides in commercial comfrey-containing products and botanical materials by liquid chromatography electrospray ionization mass spectrometry. J. Aoac Int. 2005;88:406–412. [PubMed] [Google Scholar]

Tsutomu F., Hikich M. Alkaloids and triterpenoids of Symphytum officinale. Phytochemistry. 1971;10:2217–2220. doi: 10.1016/S0031-9422(00)97225-X. [CrossRef] [Google Scholar]

Dresler S., Szymczak G., Wojcik M. Comparison of some secondary metabolite content in the seventeen species of the Boraginaceae family. Pharm. Biol. 2017;55:691–695. doi: 10.1080/13880209.2016.1265986. [PMC free article] [PubMed] [CrossRef] [Google Scholar]

Ahmad V.U., Noorwala M., Mohammad F.V., Sener B., Aftab K. Symphytoxide A, a triterpenoid saponin from the roots of Symphytum officinale. Phytochemistry. 1993;32:1003–1006. doi: 10.1016/0031-9422(93)85244-L. [PubMed] [CrossRef] [Google Scholar]

Haaß D., Abou-Mandour A.A., Blaschek W., Franz G., Czygan F.C. he influence of phytohormones on growth, organ differentiation and fructan production in callus of Symphytum officinale L. Plant Cell Rep. 1991;10:421–424. [PubMed] [Google Scholar]

Abou-Mandour A.A., Czygan F.C., Haaß D., Franz G. Fructan synthesis in tissue cultures of Symphytum officinale L.: initiation, differentiation, and metabolic activity. Planta Med. 1987;53:482–487. doi: 10.1055/s-2006-962778. [PubMed] [CrossRef] [Google Scholar]

Mohammad F.V., Noorwala M., Ahmad V.U., Sener B. A bidesmosidic hederagenin hexasaccharide from the roots of Symphytum officinale. Phytochemistry. 1995;40:213–218. doi: 10.1016/0031-9422(95)00246-4. [PubMed] [CrossRef] [Google Scholar]

Yunusova S.G., Lyashenko S.S., Fedorov N.I., Fedorov N.I., Denisenko O.N. Lipids and lipophilic constituents of comfrey (Symphytum officinale L.) seeds. Pharm. Chem. J. 2017;50:728–731. doi: 10.1007/s11094-017-1521-7. [CrossRef] [Google Scholar]

Grabias B., Swiatek L. Phenolic acids in Symphytum officinale L. Pharmaceutical and Pharmacological Letters. 1998;8:81–83. [Google Scholar]

Ulubelen A., Öcal F. Alkaloids and other compounds of Symphytum tuberosum. Phytochemistry. 1977;16:499–500. doi: 10.1016/S0031-9422(00)94343-7. [CrossRef] [Google Scholar]

Culvenor C.C.J., Edgar J.A., Frahn J.L., Smith L.W. The alkaloids of Symphytum × uplandicum (Russian comfrey) Aust. J. Chem. 1980;33:1105–1113. doi: 10.1071/CH9801105. [CrossRef] [Google Scholar]

Tamariz J., Burgueño-Tapia E., Vázquez M.A., Delgado F. Pyrrolizidine Alkaloids. In The Alkaloids. Chem. Biol. 2018;80:1–314. [PubMed] [Google Scholar]

Chou M.W., Fu P.P. Formation of DHP-derived DNA adducts in vivo from dietary supplements and Chinese herbal plant extracts containing carcinogenic pyrrolizidine alkaloids. Toxicol Ind Health. 2006;22:321–327. doi: 10.1177/0748233706071765. [PubMed] [CrossRef] [Google Scholar]

Gomes M.F.P.L., Massoco C.O., Xavier J.G., Bonamin L.V. Comfrey (Symphytum officinale L.) and experimental hepatic carcinogenesis: a short-term carcinogenesis model study. eCAM. 2010;7:197–202. doi: 10.1093/ecam/nem172. [PMC free article] [PubMed] [CrossRef] [Google Scholar]

Mutterlein R., Arnorld C.G. Investigations concerning the content and the pattern of pyrrolizidine alkaloids in Symphytum officinale L. (comfrey) Pharm Ztg Wiss. 1993;138:119–125. [Google Scholar]

Couet C.E., Crews C., Hanley A.B. Analysis, separation, and bioassay of pyrrolizidine alkaloids from comfrey (Symphytum officinale) Nat Toxins. 1996;4:163–167. doi: 10.1002/19960404NT3. [PubMed] [CrossRef] [Google Scholar]

Oberlies N.H., Kim N.C., Brine D.R., Collins B.J., Handy R.W., Sparacino C.M., Wani M.C., Wall M.E. Analysis of herbal teas made from the leaves of comfrey (Symphytum officinale): reduction of N-oxides results in order of magnitude increases in the measurable concentration of pyrrolizidine alkaloids. Public Health Nutr. 2004;7:919–924. doi: 10.1079/PHN2004624. [PubMed] [CrossRef] [Google Scholar]

Savić V.L., Nikolić V.D., Arsić I.A., Stanojević L.P., Najman S.J., Stojanović S., Mladenović-Ranisavljević I. Comparative Study of the Biological Activity of Allantoin and Aqueous Extract of the Comfrey Root. Phytother. Res. 2015;29:1117–1122. doi: 10.1002/ptr.5356. [PubMed] [CrossRef] [Google Scholar]

Al-Nimer M.S., Wahbee Z. Ultraviolet light assisted extraction of flavonoids and allantoin from aqueous and alcoholic extracts of Symphytum officinale. J. Intercult. Ethnopharmacol. 2017;6:280–285. doi: 10.5455/jice.20170630092831. [PMC free article] [PubMed] [CrossRef] [Google Scholar]

. Becker L.C., Bergfeld W.F., Belsito D.V., Klaassen C.D., Marks J.G., Shank R.C., Slaga T.J., Snyder P.W., Andersen F.A. Final report of the safety assessment of allantoin and its related complexes. Int. J. Toxicol. 2010;29:84S–97S. doi: 10.1177/1091581810362805. [PubMed] [CrossRef] [Google Scholar]

Alkan F.U., Anlas C., Ustuner O., Bakırel T., Sari A.B. Antioxidant and proliferative effects of aqueous and ethanolic extracts of Symphytum officinale on 3T3 Swiss albino mouse fibroblast cell line. Asian J. Plant Sci. Res. 2014;4:62–68. [Google Scholar]

. Rode D. Comfrey toxicity revisited. Trends Pharmacol. Sci. 2002;23:497–499. doi: 10.1016/S0165-6147(02)02106-5. [PubMed] [CrossRef] [Google Scholar]

. Merlani M., Barbakadze V., Amiranashvili L., Gogilashvili L., Yannakopoulou E., Papadopoulos K., Chankvetadze B. Enantioselective synthesis and antioxidant activity of 3-(3,4-dihydroxyphenyl)-glyceric acid--basic monomeric moiety of a biologically active polyether from Symphytum asperum and S. caucasicum. Chirality. 2010;22:717–725. doi: 10.1002/chir.20823. [PubMed] [CrossRef] [Google Scholar]

Kucera M., Kálal J., Polesna Z. Effects ofSymphytum ointment on muscular symptoms and functional locomotor disturbances. Adv. Ther. 2000;17:204–211. doi: 10.1007/BF02850297. [PubMed] [CrossRef] [Google Scholar]

Schmid K., Ivemeyer S., Vogl C., Klarer F., Meier B., Hamburger M., Walkenhorst M. Traditional use of herbal remedies in livestock by farmers in 3 Swiss cantons (Aargau, Zurich, Schaffhausen) Forschende Komplementarmedizin (2006) 2012;19:125–136. doi: 10.1159/000339336. [PubMed] [CrossRef] [Google Scholar]

Neagu E., Moroeanu V., Radu G. Concentration of Symphytum officinale extracts with cytostatic activity by tangential flow ultrafiltration. Roum. Biotechnol. Lett. 2008;13:4008–4013. [Google Scholar]

Staiger C. Comfrey root: from tradition to modern clinical trials. Wien Med Wochenschr. 2013;163:58–64. doi: 10.1007/s10354-012-0162-4. [PMC free article] [PubMed] [CrossRef] [Google Scholar]

De Albuquerque U.P., Monteiro J.M., Ramos M.A., de Amorim E.L. Medicinal and magic plants from a public market in northeastern Brazil. J. Ethnopharmacol. 2007;110:76–91. doi: 10.1016/j.jep.2006.09.010. [PubMed] [CrossRef] [Google Scholar]

Aceves-Avila F.J., Medina F., Fraga A. Herbal therapies in rheumatology: the persistence of ancient medical practices. Clin. Exp. Rheumatol. 2001;19:177–183. [PubMed] [Google Scholar]

. Smith N., Shin D.B., Brauer J.A., Mao J., Gelfand J.M. Use of complementary and alternative medicine among adults with skin disease: results from a national survey. J. Am. Acad. Dermatol. 2009;60:419–425. doi: 10.1016/j.jaad.2008.11.905. [PubMed] [CrossRef] [Google Scholar]

Petkeviciute Z., Savickiene N., Savickas A., Bernatoniene J., Simaitiene Z., Kalveniene Z., Lazauskas R., Mekas T.A. Urban ethnobotany study in Samogitia region, Lithuania. J. Med. Plants Res. 2010;4:064–071. [Google Scholar]

Cavero R.Y., Akerreta S., Calvo M.I. Pharmaceutical ethnobotany in Northern Navarra (Iberian Peninsula) J. Ethnopharmacol. 2011;133:138–146. doi: 10.1016/j.jep.2010.09.019. [PubMed] [CrossRef] [Google Scholar]

Cavero R.Y., Calvo M.I. Medicinal plants used for musculoskeletal disorders in Navarra and their pharmacological validation. J. Ethnopharmacol. 2015;168:255–259. doi: 10.1016/j.jep.2015.03.078. [PubMed] [CrossRef] [Google Scholar]

Sharifi-Rad M., Nazaruk J., Polito L., Morais-Braga M., Rocha J., Coutinho H., Salehi B., Tabanelli G., Montanari C., Del M.M.C. Matricaria genus as a source of antimicrobial agents: From farm to pharmacy and food applications. Microbiol. Res. 2018;215:76–88. doi: 10.1016/j.micres.2018.06.010. [PubMed] [CrossRef] [Google Scholar]

Kapil A.J.I.J.M.R. The challenge of antibiotic resistance: need to contemplate. Ind. J. Med. Res. 2005;121:83–91. [PubMed] [Google Scholar]

Lewis K., Ausubel F.M.J.N.B. Prospects for plant-derived antibacterials. Nature Biotechnol. 2006;24:1504. doi: 10.1038/nbt1206-1504. [PubMed] [CrossRef] [Google Scholar]

Leach M. A critical review of natural therapies in wound management. Ostomy/Wound Manag. 2004;50:36–40. [PubMed] [Google Scholar]

Sharifi-Rad J., Sharifi-Rad M., Salehi B., Iriti M., Roointan A., Mnayer D., Soltani-Nejad A., Afshari A. In vitro and in vivo assessment of free radical scavenging and antioxidant activities of Veronica persica Poir. Cell. Mol. Biol. (Noisy-Le-GrandFr.) 2018;64:57–64. doi: 10.14715/cmb/2018.64.8.9. [PubMed] [CrossRef] [Google Scholar]

Koll R., Buhr M., Dieter R., Pabst H., Predel H.-G., Petrowicz O., Giannetti B., Klingenburg S., Staiger C. Efficacy and tolerance of a comfrey root extract (Extr. Rad. Symphyti) in the treatment of ankle distorsions: results of a multicenter, randomized, placebo-controlled, double-blind study. Phytomedicine. 2004;11:470–477. doi: 10.1016/j.phymed.2004.02.001. [PubMed] [CrossRef] [Google Scholar]

Salehi B., Valussi M., Jugran A.K., Martorell M., Ramírez-Alarcón K., Stojanović-Radić Z.Z., Antolak H., Kręgiel D., Mileski K.S., Sharifi-Rad M. Nepeta Species: From Farm to Food applications and Phytotherapy. Trends Food Sci. Technol. 2018;80:104–122. doi: 10.1016/j.tifs.2018.07.030. [CrossRef] [Google Scholar]

EFSA Scientific Opinion on the re-evaluation of ascorbic acid (E 300), sodium ascorbate (E 301) and calcium ascorbate (E 302) as food additives. Efsa J. 2015;13:4087. doi: 10.2903/j.efsa.2015.4087. [CrossRef] [Google Scholar]

EFSA, T.r.-E.v.o.E.s.f.a.A.i.S., 2018. The re-'E'valuation of Europe's food additives. [(accessed on 1 September 2018)]; Available online: https://www.efsa.europa.eu/en/press/news/120130b. 100. Lee N.K., Paik H.D. Status, Antimicrobial Mechanism, and Regulation of Natural Preservatives in Livestock Food Systems. Korean J. Food Sci. Anim. Resour. 2016;36:547–557. doi: 10.5851/kosfa.2016.36.4.547. [PMC free article] [PubMed] [CrossRef] [Google Scholar]

Settanni L., Corsetti A. Application of bacteriocins in vegetable food biopreservation. Int. J. Food Microbiol. 2008;121:123–138. doi: 10.1016/j.ijfoodmicro.2007.09.001. [PubMed] [CrossRef] [Google Scholar]

MacDonald R., Reitmeier C. Understanding Food Systems: Agriculture, Food Science, and Nutrition in the United States. Academic Press; Cambridge, MA, USA: 2017. [Google Scholar]

Carocho M., Morales P., Ferreira I.C.F.R. Antioxidants: Reviewing the chemistry, food applications, legislation and role as preservatives. Trends Food Sci. Technol. 2018;71:107–120. doi: 10.1016/j.tifs.2017.11.008. [CrossRef] [Google Scholar]

Wedzicha B.L. PRESERVATIVES | Classifications and Properties. 2013 doi: 10.1016/B0-12-227055-X/00969-X. [CrossRef] [Google Scholar]

Sharifi-Rad J., Soufi L., Ayatollahi S., Iriti M., Sharifi-Rad M., Varoni E.M., Shahri F., Esposito S., Kuhestani K. Anti-bacterial effect of essential oil from Xanthium strumarium against shiga toxin-producing Escherichia coli. Cell. Mol. Biol. 2016;62:69–74. [PubMed] [Google Scholar]

Erdemoglu N., Ozkan S., Tosun F. Alkaloid profile and antimicrobial activity of Lupinus angustifolius L. alkaloid extract. Phytochem. Rev. 2007;6:197–201. doi: 10.1007/s11101-006-9055-8. [CrossRef] [Google Scholar]

Morteza-Semnani K., Amin G., Shidfar M., Hadizadeh H., Shafiee A. Antifungal activity of the methanolic extract and alkaloids of Glaucium oxylobum. Fitoterapia. 2003;74:493–496. doi: 10.1016/S0367-326X(03)00113-8. [PubMed] [CrossRef] [Google Scholar]

Slobodníková L., KoSt'álová D., Labudová D., Kotulová D., Kettmann V. Antimicrobial activity of Mahonia aquifolium crude extract and its major isolated alkaloids. Phytother. Res.: Int. J. Devoted Pharmacol. Toxicol. Eval. Nat. Prod. Deriv. 2004;18:674–676. doi: 10.1002/ptr.1517. [PubMed] [CrossRef] [Google Scholar]

Wuilloud J.C., Gratz S.R., Gamble B.M., Wolnik K.A. Simultaneous analysis of hepatotoxic pyrrolizidine alkaloids and N-oxides in comfrey root by LC-ion trap mass spectrometry. Analyst. 2004;129:150–156. doi: 10.1039/b311030c. [PubMed] [CrossRef] [Google Scholar]

Ma C., Liu Y., Zhu L., Ji H., Song X., Guo H., Yi T. Determination and regulation of hepatotoxic pyrrolizidine alkaloids in food: A critical review of recent research. Food and Chemical Toxicology. Food Chem. Toxicol. 2018;119:50–60. doi: 10.1016/j.fct.2018.05.037. [PubMed] [CrossRef] [Google Scholar]

. Neuman M.G., Cohen L., Opris M., Nanau R.M., Jeong H. Hepatotoxicity of pyrrolizidine alkaloids. J. Pharm. Pharm. Sci. 2015;18:825–843. doi: 10.18433/J3BG7J. [PubMed] [CrossRef] [Google Scholar]

Kartal M., Kurucu S., Choudary M.I. Antifungal activities of different extracts and echimidine-N-oxide from Symphytum sylvaticum Boiss subsp. sepulcrale (Boiss. & Bal.) Greuter & Burdet var. Sepulcrale. Turk. J. Med Sci. 2001;31:487–492. [Google Scholar]

Savić V.L., Savić S.R., Nikolić V.D., Nikolić L.B., Najman S.J., Lazarević J.S., Đorđević A.S. The identification and quantification of bioactive compounds from the aqueous extract of comfrey root by UHPLC-DAD-HESI-MS method and its microbial activity. Hem. Ind. 2015;69:1–8. doi: 10.2298/HEMIND131202013S. [CrossRef] [Google Scholar]

Sumathi S., Kumar S.S., Bai A., Glory L. Evaluation of Phytochemical Constituents and Antibacterial Activities of Symphytum officinale L. J. Pure Appl. Microbiol. 2011;5:323–328. [Google Scholar]

. Sumathi S. Antibacterial Activity of the plant extract of Symphytum officinale L. against selected pathogenic bacteria. Int. J. Res. Pharm. Sci. 2016;2:92–94. [Google Scholar]

Woods-Panzaru S., Nelson D., McCollum G., Ballard L.M., Millar B.C., Maeda Y., Goldsmith C.E., Rooney P.J., Loughrey A., Rao J.R., et al. An examination of antibacterial and antifungal properties of constituents described in traditional Ulster cures and remedies. Ulst. Med J. 2009;78:13–15. [PMC free article] [PubMed] [Google Scholar]

Barbakadze V., Van Den Berg A., Beukelman C., Kemmink J., van Ufford H.Q. Poly [3-(3, 4-dihydroxyphenyl) glyceric acid] from Symphytum officinale roots and its biological activity. Chem. Nat. Compd. 2009;45:6–10. doi: 10.1007/s10600-009-9221-5. [CrossRef] [Google Scholar]
118. Sharifi-Rad M., Fokou P., Sharopov F., Martorell M., Ademiluyi A., Rajkovic J., Salehi B., Martins N., Iriti M., Sharifi-Rad J.J.M. Antiulcer agents: From plant extracts to phytochemicals in healing promotion. Molecules. 2018;23:1751. doi: 10.3390/molecules23071751. [PMC free article] [PubMed] [CrossRef] [Google Scholar]

Prakash A.M., Sharifi-Rad M., Shariati M., Mabkhot Y., Al-Showiman S., Rauf A., Salehi B., Župunski M., Gusain P., Sharifi-Rad J. Bioactive compounds and health benefits of edible Rumex species-A review. Cell. Mol. Biol. (Noisy-Le-GrandFr.) 2018;64:27–34. doi: 10.14715/cmb/2018.64.8.5. [PubMed] [CrossRef] [Google Scholar]

Prakash Mishra A., Saklani S., Salehi B., Parcha V., Sharifi-Rad M., Milella L., Iriti M., Sharifi-Rad J., Srivastava M. Satyrium nepalense, a high altitude medicinal orchid of Indian Himalayan region: chemical profile and biological activities of tuber extracts. Cell. Mol. Biol. (Noisy-Le-GrandFr.) 2018;64:35–43. doi: 10.14715/cmb/2018.64.8.6. [PubMed] [CrossRef] [Google Scholar]

. Abdolshahi A., Naybandi-Atashi S., Heydari-Majd M., Salehi B., Kobarfard F., Ayatollahi S., Ata A., Tabanelli G., Sharifi-Rad M., Montanari C. Antibacterial activity of some Lamiaceae species against Staphylococcus aureus in yoghurt-based drink (Doogh) Cell. Mol. Biol. (Noisy-Le-GrandFr.) 2018;64:71–77. doi: 10.14715/cmb/2018.64.8.11. [PubMed] [CrossRef] [Google Scholar]

WHO WHO Traditional Medicine Strategy 2014-2023. World Health Organization: 2014. [(accessed on 18 June 2019)]; Available online: http:llapps.who.int7irislbitstream710665l92455l1l9789241506090eng.pdf?ua.
123. Knaak N., Dias da Silva L., Finger Andreis T., Mariana Fiuza L. Chemical characterization and anti-fungal activity of plant extracts and essential oils on the Bipolaris oryzae and Gerlachia oryzae phytopathogens. Australas. Plant Pathol. 2013;42:469–475. doi: 10.1007/s13313-013-0220-4. [CrossRef] [Google Scholar]

Rocha R., Eleutério da Luz D., Engels C., Pileggi S., de Souza Jaccoud Filho D., Matiello R., Pileggi M. Selection of endophytic fungi from comfrey (Symphytum officinale L.) for in vitro biological control of the phytopathogen Sclerotinia sclerotiorum (Lib.) Braz. J. Microbiol. 2009;40:73–78. doi: 10.1590/S1517-83822009000100011. [PMC free article] [PubMed] [CrossRef] [Google Scholar]

Cvetkovic D., Stanojević L., Kundaković T., Zlatkovic S., Nikolić G. Antioxidant and antimicrobial activity of a new generation phyto-gel. Adv. Technol. 2015;4:11–18. doi: 10.5937/savteh1502011C. [CrossRef] [Google Scholar]

Bouzada M.L.M., Fabri R.L., Nogueira M., Konno T.U.P., Duarte G.G., Scio E. Antibacterial, cytotoxic and phytochemical screening of some traditional medicinal plants in Brazil. Pharm. Biol. 2009;47:44–52. doi: 10.1080/13880200802411771. [CrossRef] [Google Scholar]

Borchardt J.R., Wyse D.L., Sheaffer C.C., Kauppi K.L., Ehlke R.G.F.N.J., Biesboer D.D., Bey R.F. Antimicrobial activity of native and naturalized plants of Minnesota and Wisconsin. J. Med. Plants Res. 2008;2:098–110. [Google Scholar]

Onofre N.A., Magalhães L.P.M., Amaral J.P.D., Yara R., Lima C.S.A., Sena K.X.F.R. Antimicrobial activity of plants used in manufacture of traditional phytotherapics in community centres of Recife metropolitan region. Exp. Pathol. Health Sci. 2016;8:23–24. [Google Scholar]

Savic V., Nikolic V., Stanojevic L., Ilic D., Stankovic B. Extraction kinetics and antioxidant activity of an aqueous extract from comfrey root (Symphytum officinale L.) Adv. Technol. 2012;1:41–47. [Google Scholar]

Dolganiuc A., Radu L., Olinescu A. The effect of products of plant and microbial origin on phagocytic function and on the release of oxygen free radicals by mouse peritoneal macrophages. Bacteriol Virusol Parazitol Epidemiol. 1997;42:65–69. [PubMed] [Google Scholar]

Repetto M., Llesuy S. Antioxidant properties of natural compounds used in popular medicine for gastric ulcers. Braz. J. Med Biol. Res. 2002;35:523–534. doi: 10.1590/S0100-879X2002000500003. [PubMed] [CrossRef] [Google Scholar]

Barthomeuf C., Debiton E., Barbakadze V., Kemertelidze E. Evaluation of the dietetic and therapeutic potential of a high molecular weight hydroxycinnamate-derived polymer from Symphytum asperum Lepech. Regarding its antioxidant, antilipoperoxidant, antiinflammatory, and cytotoxic properties. J. Agric. Food Chem. 2001;49:3942–3946. doi: 10.1021/jf010189d. [PubMed] [CrossRef] [Google Scholar]

Oktay M., Yildirim A., Bilaloglu V., Gülçin I. Antioxidant activity of different parts of isgin (Rheum ribes L.) Asian J. Chem. 2007;19:3047. [Google Scholar]

Paun G., Neagu E., Litescu S.C., Rotinberg P., Radu G.L. Application of membrane processes for the concentration of Symphytum officinale and Geranium robertianum extracts to obtain compounds with high anti-oxidative activity. J. Serb. Chem. Soc. 2012:77. [Google Scholar]

Thring T.S., Hili P., Naughton D.P. Anti-collagenase, anti-elastase and anti-oxidant activities of extracts from 21 plants. Bmc Complementary Altern. Med. 2009;9:27. doi: 10.1186/1472-6882-9-27. [PMC free article] [PubMed] [CrossRef] [Google Scholar]

Nossa González D.L., Pérez T., Verónica Y., Núñez R., Elías W. Determination of polyphenols and antioxidant activity of polar extracts of comfrey (Symphytum officinale L) Rev. Cuba. De Plantas Med. 2016;21:125–132. [Google Scholar]

adridze G., Kacharava N., Chkhubianishvili E., Rapava L., Kikvidze M., Chigladze L., Chanishvili S. Content of antioxidants in leaves of some plants of Tbilisi environs. Bull. Georg. Natl. Acad. Sci. 2013:7. [Google Scholar]

Smith D.B., Jacobson B.H. Effect of a blend of comfrey root extract (Symphytum officinale L.) and tannic acid creams in the treatment of osteoarthritis of the knee: randomized, placebo-controlled, double-blind, multiclinical trials. J. Chiropr. Med. 2011;10:147–156. doi: 10.1016/j.jcm.2011.01.003. [PMC free article] [PubMed] [CrossRef] [Google Scholar]

. Liu C., Chang J., Zhang L., Zhang J., Li S. Purification and antioxidant activity of a polysaccharide from bulbs of Fritillaria ussuriensis Maxim. Int. J. Biol. Macromol. 2012;50:1075–1080. doi: 10.1016/j.ijbiomac.2012.03.006. [PubMed] [CrossRef] [Google Scholar]

Pielesz A. Vibrational spectroscopy and electrophoresis as a "golden means" in monitoring of polysaccharides in medical plant and gels. Spectrochim. Acta-Part A: Mol. Biomol. Spectrosc. 2012;93:63–69. doi: 10.1016/j.saa.2012.03.003. [PubMed] [CrossRef] [Google Scholar]

Duan M., Shang H., Chen S., Li R., Wu H. Physicochemical properties and activities of comfrey polysaccharides extracted by different techniques. Int. J. Biol. Macromol. 2018;115:876–882. doi: 10.1016/j.ijbiomac.2018.04.188. [PubMed] [CrossRef] [Google Scholar]

Barbakadze V.V., Kemertelidze E.P., Targamadze I.L., Shashkov A.S., Usov A.I. Poly[3-(3,4-dihydroxyphenyl)glyceric acid]: A new biologically active polymer from two comfrey species Symphytum asperum and S. caucasicum (Boraginaceae) Russ. J. Bioorganic Chem. 2002;28:326–330. doi: 10.1023/A:1019552110312. [PMC free article] [PubMed] [CrossRef] [Google Scholar]

Matcovschi C., Calistru Z., Cojocaru M., Vaˆlcu S. Symphytum officinale (L) gaertn — A prospective hepatoprotective and hepatoregenerative plant. Pharmacol. Res. 1995;31:91. doi: 10.1016/1043-6618(95)86625-6. [CrossRef] [Google Scholar]

Oberbaum M., Yakovlev E., Kaufman D., Shoshan S. Effect of Arnica montana and Symphytum officinalis on bone healing in guinea pigs. Br. Homeopath. J. 1994;83:90. doi: 10.1016/S0007-0785(94)80017-0. [CrossRef] [Google Scholar]

Araujo L.U., Reis P.G., Barbosa L.C., Saude-Guimaraes D.A., Grabe-Guimaraes A., Mosqueira V.C., Carneiro C.M., Silva-Barcellos N.M. In vivo wound healing effects of Symphytum officinale L. leaves extract in different topical formulations. Pharmazie. 2012;67:355–360. [PubMed] [Google Scholar]

. Kommission E. Monographie Symphyti radix (Beinwellwurzel) Bundesanzeiger. 1990:318. [Google Scholar]

Vostinaru O., Conea S., Mogosan C., Toma C., Borza C., Vlase L. Anti-inflammatory and antinociceptive effect of Symphytum officinale root. Rom. Biotechnol. Lett. 2017 [Google Scholar]

Hiermann A., Writzel M. Antiphlogistic glycopeptide from the roots of Symphytum officinale. Pharm. Pharmacol. Lett. 1998;8:154–157. [Google Scholar]

Grigore A., Pirvu L., Bubueanu C., Minerva P., Rasit I. Influence of chemical composition on the antioxidant and anti-inflammatory activity of Rosmarinus officinalis extracts. Rom. Biotechnol. Lett. 2015;20:10047–10054. [Google Scholar]

Schmidtke-Schrezenmeier G. The efficacy of a phytotherapeutic agent in the treatment of non-activated osteoarthritis of the knee [Behandlung der nichtaktivierten Gonarthrose: Besserung durch ein Phytotherapeutikum] Therapiewoche. 1992;42:1322–1325. [Google Scholar]

Grube B., Grünwald J., Krug L., Staiger C. Efficacy of a comfrey root (Symphyti offic. radix) extract ointment in the treatment of patients with painful osteoarthritis of the knee: results of a double-blind, randomised, bicenter, placebo-controlled trial. Phytomedicine. 2007;14:2–10. doi: 10.1016/j.phymed.2006.11.006. [PubMed] [CrossRef] [Google Scholar]

Laslett L., Quinn S., Darian-Smith E., Kwok M., Fedorova T., Körner H., Steels E., March L., Jones G. Treatment with 4Jointz reduces knee pain over 12 weeks of treatment in patients with clinical knee osteoarthritis: a randomised controlled trial. Osteoarthr. Cartil. 2012;20:1209–1216. doi: 10.1016/j.joca.2012.07.019. [PubMed] [CrossRef] [Google Scholar]

Giannetti B.M., Staiger C., Bulitta M., Predel H.-G. Efficacy and safety of comfrey root extract ointment in the treatment of acute upper or lower back pain: Results of a double-blind, randomised, placebo controlled, multicentre trial. Br. J. Sports Med. 2009;44:637–641. doi: 10.1136/bjsm.2009.058677. [PubMed] [CrossRef] [Google Scholar]

Pabst H., Schaefer A., Staiger C., Junker-Samek M., Predel H.G. Combination of comfrey root extract plus methyl nicotinate in patients with conditions of acute upper or low back pain: a multicentre randomised controlled trial. Phytother. Res. 2013;27:811–817. doi: 10.1002/ptr.4790. [PMC free article] [PubMed] [CrossRef] [Google Scholar]

. Petersen G., Lorkowski G., Kasper F., Gottwald R., Lücker P. Anti-inflammatory activity of a pyrrolizidine alkaloid-free extract of roots of Symphytum officinale in humans. Planta Med. 1993;59:A703–A704. doi: 10.1055/s-2006-960000. [CrossRef] [Google Scholar]

Predel H.-G., Giannetti B., Koll R., Bulitta M., Staiger C. Efficacy of a Comfrey root extract ointment in comparison to a Diclo-fenac gel in the treatment of ankle distortions: Results of an observer-blind, randomized, multicenter study. Phytomedicine. 2005;12:707–714. doi: 10.1016/j.phymed.2005.06.001. [PubMed] [CrossRef] [Google Scholar]

. Kučera M., Barna M., Horáček O., Kováriková J., Kučera A. Efficacy and safety of topically applied Symphytum herb extract cream in the treatment of ankle distortion: Results of a randomized controlled clinical double-blind study. Wien. Med. Wochenschr. 2004;154:498–507. doi: 10.1007/s10354-004-0114-8. [PubMed] [CrossRef] [Google Scholar]

Kucera M., Barna M., Horácek O., Kálal J., Kucera A., Hladíkova M. TopicalSymphytum herb concentrate cream against myalgia: A randomized controlled double-blind clinical study. Adv. Ther. 2005;22:681–692. doi: 10.1007/BF02849961. [PubMed] [CrossRef] [Google Scholar]

Barna M., Kucera A., Hladícova M., Kucera M. Der wundheilende Effekt einer Symphytum-Herba-Extrakt-Creme (Symphytum× uplandicum Nyman): Ergebnisse einer randomisierten, kontrollierten Doppelblindstudie. Wien. Med. Wochenschr. 2007;157:569–574. doi: 10.1007/s10354-007-0474-y. [PubMed] [CrossRef] [Google Scholar]

Grünwald J., Bitterlich N., Nauert C., Schmidt M. Anwendung und Verträglichkeit von Beinwellcreme (Symphyti herba) bei Kindern mit akuten stumpfen Traumen. Z. Für Phytother. 2010;31:61–66. doi: 10.1055/s-0030-1247646. [CrossRef] [Google Scholar]

Barna M., Kucera A., Hladikova M., Kucera M. Randomized double-blind study: Wound-healing effects of a Symphytum herb extract cream (Symphytum× uplandicum Nyman) in children. Arzneimittelforschung. 2012;62:285–289. doi: 10.1055/s-0032-1308981. [PubMed] [CrossRef] [Google Scholar]

Andreas P., Brenneisen R., Clerc J. Relating antiphlogistic efficacy of dermatics containing extracts of Symphytum officinale to chemical profiles. Planta Med. 1989;7:55–66. [Google Scholar]

Štepán J., Ehrlichova J., Hladikova M. Therapieergebnisse und Anwendungssicherheit von Symphytum-Herba-Extrakt-Creme in der Behandlung von Dekubitus. Z. Für Gerontol. Und Geriatr. 2014;47:228–235. doi: 10.1007/s00391-013-0522-8. [PubMed] [CrossRef] [Google Scholar]

Gafar M., Dumitriu H., Dumitriu S., Guti L. Apiphytotherapeutic original preparations in the treatment of chronic marginal parodontopathies. A clinical and microbiological study. Rev. De Chir. Oncol. Radiol. O.R.L., Oftalmol. Stomatol. Ser.: Stomatol. 1989;36:91–98. [PubMed] [Google Scholar]

Orescanin V. Treatment of atopic dermatitis in children with Bioapifit® anti-inflammatory herbal ointment - a preliminary study. Ijrdo-J. Biol. Sci. 2016;2:1–17. [Google Scholar]

166. Binić I., Janković A., Janković D., Janković I., Vručinić Z. Evaluation of healing and antimicrobiological effects of herbal therapy on venous leg ulcer: pilot study. Phytother. Res. 2010;2010 [PubMed] [Google Scholar]

Orescanin V., Guštek Štefica F., Krivak Bolanca I. Development and Aplication of New Herbal Pessaries for the Treatment of Squamous Endocervical Metaplasia. Indian J. Appl. Res. 2015;5:176–182. [Google Scholar]

Bhatia D., Bejarano T., Novo M. Current interventions in the management of knee osteoarthritis. J. Pharm. Bioallied Sci. 2013;5:30. doi: 10.4103/0975-7406.106561. [PMC free article] [PubMed] [CrossRef] [Google Scholar]

Assandri A., Canali S., Giachetti C. Local tolerability and pharmacokinetic profile of a new transdermal delivery system, diclofenac hydroxyethylpyrrolidine plaster. Drugs Under Exp. Clin. Res. 1993;19:89–95. [PubMed] [Google Scholar]

Radermacher J., Jentsch D., Scholl M., Lustinetz T., Frolich J. Diclofenac concentrations in synovial fluid and plasma after cutaneous application in inflammatory and degenerative joint disease. Br. J. Clin. Pharmacol. 1991;31:537–541. doi: 10.1111/j.1365-2125.1991.tb05576.x. [PMC free article] [PubMed] [CrossRef] [Google Scholar]

Riess W., Schmid K., Botta L., Kobayashi K., Moppert J., Schneider W., Sioufi A., Strusberg A., Tomasi M. The percutaneous absorption of diclofenac. Arzneim. Forsch. 1986;36:1092–1096. [PubMed] [Google Scholar]

EMA Committee for Proprietary Medicinal Products (CPMP). Points to consider on switching between superiority and non-inferiority. Br. J. Clin. Pharmacol. 2000;52:223–228. [PMC free article] [PubMed] [Google Scholar]

. Barnes J., Anderson L.A., Phillipson J.D. Herbal Medicines. Pharmaceutical Press; London, UK: 2007. [Google Scholar]

. Coulombe R.A., Jr. Pyrrolizidine Alkaloids in Foods. Centre for Food Safety; Hong Kong, China: 2003. [Google Scholar]

Prakash A.S., Pereira T.N., Reilly P.E., Seawright A.A. Pyrrolizidine alkaloids in human diet. Mutat. Res. /Genet. Toxicol. Environ. Mutagenesis. 1999;443:53–67. doi: 10.1016/S1383-5742(99)00010-1. [PubMed] [CrossRef] [Google Scholar]

. EMA . Assessment report on Symphytum officinale L., radix. EMA; Amsterdam, The Netherlands: 2005. Committee on Herbal Medicinal Products. EMA/HMPC/572844/2009. [Google Scholar]

Blumenthal M., Busse W. American Botanical Council. Integr. Med. Commun. Ger. 1998 [Google Scholar]

Najafian Y, Hamedi SS, Farshchi MK, Feyzabadi Z. Plantago major in Traditional Persian Medicine and modern phytotherapy: a narrative review. Electron Physician. 2018 Feb 25;10(2):6390-6399. doi: 10.19082/6390. PMID: 29629064; PMCID: PMC5878035.

Wang H, Zhao C, Huang Y, Wang F, Li Y, Chung HY. Chemical Constituents and Bioactivities of Plantaginis Herba. Hong Kong Med J. 2015;22:29–35. [Google Scholar]

Aghili M. Makhzan-O-L Advieh. Tehran: Tehran University of Medical Science Press; 2008. [Google Scholar]

Mozaffarian V. Identification of medicinal and aromatic plants of Iran. Tehran: Farhang moaser; 2012. [Google Scholar]

Shahabi S, Hassan ZM, Mahdavi M, Dezfouli M, Torabi Rahvar M, Naseri M, et al. Hot and Cold natures and some parameters of neuroendocrine and immune systems in traditional Iranian medicine: a preliminary study. J Altern Complement Med. 2008;14:147–56. doi: 10.1089/acm.2007.0693. [PubMed] [CrossRef] [Google Scholar]

. Samuelsen AB. The traditional uses, chemical constituents and biological activities of Plantago major L. A review. J Ethnopharmacol. 2000;71:1–21. [PubMed] [Google Scholar]

. Al-Nafis I. Al-Shamil fi al-Tibb. Abu Dhabi: United Arab Emirates Pub; 2000. [Google Scholar]

Avicenna. The Canon of medicine. Beirut: Dar Maktab Al-Helal; 2009. [Google Scholar]

Aghili M. Qarabadin Kabir. Tehran: Tehran University of Medical Science Press; 1999. [Google Scholar]

. Meteria Medica. Tehran: Tehran University of Medical Siences; 2005. Dioscorides's. [Google Scholar]

Osbaldeston T. Dioscorides. Johannesburg: IBIDIS Press; 2000. [Google Scholar]

. Biruni A. Al-saydanah Fi-elteb. Tehran: Asar publisher; 2004. [Google Scholar]

Razi M. Al-havi (Arabic) Beirut: Lebanon: Dar Al -EHIA Al-Tourath Al-Arabi; 2002. [Google Scholar]

Arzani M. Tebb-E-Akbari Qom. Institute of Medical History, Islamic and Complementary Medicine, Iran University of Medical Sciences publisher; 2007. [Google Scholar]

Yavari M, Khodabandeh F, Tansaz M, Rouholamin S. A neuropsychiatric complication of oligomenorrhea according to iranian traditional medicine. Iran J Reprod Med. 2014;12(7):453–8. [PMC free article] [PubMed] [Google Scholar]

Jorjani S. Zakhireh Kharazmshahi. [Treasure of Kharazmshahi]. Tehran: Iranian Culture Foundation; 1976. (Original work published 1206 AD Tehran) [Google Scholar]

Nemereshina ON, Tinkov AA, Gritsenko VA, Nikonorov AA. Influence of Plantaginaceae species on E. coli K12 growth in vitro: Possible relation to phytochemical properties. Pharm Biol. 2015;53:715–24. doi: 10.3109/13880209.2014.940426. [PubMed] [CrossRef] [Google Scholar]

Mazzutti S, Ferreira S, Herrero M, Ibañez E. Intensified aqueous-based processes to obtain bioactive extracts from Plantago major and Plantago lanceolata. J Supercrit Fluids. 2017;119:64–71. doi: 10.1016/j.supflu.2016.09.008. [CrossRef] [Google Scholar]

El-Gawad AMA, Mashaly IA, Ziada MEA, Deweeb MR. Phytotoxicity of three Plantago species on germination and seedling growth of hairy beggarticks (Bidens pilosa L.) J Basic Appl Sci. 2015;2:303–9. doi: 10.1016/j.ejbas.2015.07.003. [CrossRef] [Google Scholar]

. Gonçalves S, Romano A. The medicinal potential of plants from the genus Plantago (Plantaginaceae) Ind Crops Prod. 2016;83:213–26. doi: 10.1016/j.indcrop.2015.12.038. [CrossRef] [Google Scholar]

Akram M, Hamid A, Khalil A, Ghaffar A, Tayyaba N, Saeed A, et al. Review on medicinal uses, pharmacological, phytochemistry and immunomodulatory activity of plants. Int J Immunopathol Pharmacol. 2014;27:313–9. [PubMed] [Google Scholar]

Fons F, Gargadennec A, Rapior S. Culture of Plantago species as bioactive components resources: a 20-year review and recent applications. Acta Bot Gall. 2008;155:277–300. doi: 10.1080/12538078.2008.10516109. [CrossRef] [Google Scholar]

Kuhn MA, Winston D. Herbal therapy and supplements: a scientific and traditional approach. Lippincott Williams & Wilkins; 2000. [Google Scholar]

Jamilah J, Sharifa A, Sharifah N. GC-MS analysis of various extracts from leaf of Plantago major used as traditional medicine. World Appl Sci J. 2012;17:67–70. [Google Scholar]

Gomez-Flores R, Calderon C, Scheibel L, Tamez-Guerra P, Rodriguez-Padilla C, Tamez-Guerra R, et al. Immunoenhancing properties of Plantago major leaf extract. Phytother Res. 2000;14:617–22. [PubMed] [Google Scholar]

Chiang LC, Chiang W, Chang MY, Lin CC. In vitro cytotoxic, antiviral and immunomodulatory effects of Plantago major and Plantago asiatica. Am J Chin Med. 2003;31:225–34. [PubMed] [Google Scholar]

Türel I, Özbek H, Erten R, Öner AC, Cengiz N, Yilmaz O. Hepatoprotective and anti-inflammatory activities of Plantago major L. Indian J Pharmacol. 2009;41:120–4. doi: 10.4103/0253-7613.55211. [PMC free article] [PubMed] [CrossRef] [Google Scholar]

. Atta AH, Nasr SM, Mouneir SM. Potential protective effect of some plant extracts against carbon tetrachloride–induced hepatotoxicity. Afr J Tradit Complement Altern Med. 2006;3:1–9. doi: 10.4314/ajtcam.v3i3.114. [CrossRef] [Google Scholar]

. Gómez-Estrada H, Díaz-Castillo F, Franco-Ospina L, Mercado-Camargo J, Guzmán-Ledezma J, Medina J, et al. Folk medicine in the northern coast of Colombia: an overview. J Ethnobiol Ethnomed. 2011;7:27. doi: 10.1186/1746-4269-7-27. [PMC free article] [PubMed] [CrossRef] [Google Scholar]

Hriscu A, Stănescu U, Ionescu A, Verbuţă A. A pharmacodynamic investigation of the effect of polyholozidic substances extracted from Plantago sp. on the digestive tract. Rev Med Chir Soc Med Nat Iasi. 1989;94:165–170. [PubMed] [Google Scholar]

Lans C, Turner N, Khan T, Brauer G. Ethnoveterinary medicines used to treat endoparasites and stomach problems in pigs and pets in British Columbia, Canada. Vet Parasitol. 2007;148:325–340. doi: 10.1016/j.vetpar.2007.06.014. [PubMed] [CrossRef] [Google Scholar]

Atta A, Nasr SM, Mouneir SM. Antiulcerogenic effect of some plants extracts. Nat Prod Rad. 2005;4:258–63. [Google Scholar]

Lima GR, Montenegro CD, Almeida CL, Athayde-Filho PF, Barbosa-Filho JM, Batista LM. Database Survey of Anti-Inflammatory Plants in South America. Int J Mol Sci. 2011;12:2692–749. doi: 10.3390/ijms12042692. [PMC free article] [PubMed] [CrossRef] [Google Scholar]

Atta AH, Mouneir SM. Evaluation of some medicinal plant extracts for antidiarrhoeal activity. Phytother Res. 2005;19:481–5. doi: 10.1002/ptr.1639. [PubMed] [CrossRef] [Google Scholar]

Ikawati Z, Wahyuono S, Maeyama K. Screening of several Indonesian medicinal plants for their inhibitory effect on histamine release from RBL-2H3 cells. J Ethnopharmacol. 2001;75:249–56. doi: 10.1016/S0378-8741(01)00201-X. [PubMed] [CrossRef] [Google Scholar]

. Hetland G, Samuelsen A, Loslash V, Paulsen B, Aaberge I, Groeng E, et al. Protective effect of Plantago major L. pectin polysaccharide against systemic Streptococcus pneumoniae infection in mice. Scand J Immunol. 2000;52:348–55. doi: 10.1046/j.1365-3083.2000.00793.x. [PubMed] [CrossRef] [Google Scholar]

. Matev M, Angelova I, Koĭchev A, Leseva M, Stefanov G. Clinical trial of a Plantago major preparation in the treatment of chronic bronchitis. Vutr Boles. 1981;21:133–7. [PubMed] [Google Scholar]

 Doan DD, Nguyen N, Doan H, Nguyen T, Phan T, Van Dau N, et al. Studies on the individual and combined diuretic effects of four Vietnamese traditional herbal remedies (Zea mays, Imperata cylindrica, Plantago major and Orthosiphon stamineus) J Ethnopharmacol. 1992;36:225–31. doi: 10.1016/0378-8741(92)90048-V. [PubMed] [CrossRef] [Google Scholar]

Nhiem NX, Tai BH, Van Kiem P, Van Minh C, Cuong NX, Tung NH, et al. Inhibitory activity of Plantago major L. on angiotensin I-converting enzyme. Arch Pharm Res. 2011;34:419–23. [PubMed] [Google Scholar]

. Aziz SA, See TL, Khuay LY, Osman K, Bakar MAA. In vitro effects of plantago major extract on urolithiasis. Malays J Med Sci. 2005;12:22–6. [PMC free article] [PubMed] [Google Scholar]

. Yazdian MA, Gheisari M, Khodadoost M, Barikbin B, Yazdian M, Askarfarashah M, et al. Evaluation of Plantago major aqueous extract in treatment of acute urticaria. Int J Biosci. 2014;5:182–8. [Google Scholar]

Yazdian MA, Khodadoost M, Gheisari M, Kamalinejad M, Ehsani AH, Barikbin B. A Hypothesis on the Possible Potential of Plantago Major in the Treatment of Urticaria. Hong Kong Med J. 2014;3:123–6. [Google Scholar]
Angarskaya M, Sokolova V. The effect of plantain (Plantago major) on the course of experimental atherosclerosis in rabbits. Bull Exp Biol Med. 1963;53:410–2. doi: 10.1007/BF00783859. [CrossRef] [Google Scholar]

Alarcon-Aguilar F, Vega-Avila E, Almanza-Perez J, Velasco-Lezama R, Vazquez-Carrillo L, Roman-Ramos R. Hypoglycemic effect of Plantago major seeds in healthy and alloxan-diabetic mice. Proc West Pharmacol Soc. 1998;2006:51. [Google Scholar]

Matsuura N, Aradate T, Kurosaka C, Ubukata M, Kittaka S, Nakaminami Y, et al. Potent protein glycation inhibition of plantagoside in Plantago major seeds. Biomed Res Int. 2014;2014:208539. doi: 10.1155/2014/208539. [PMC free article] [PubMed] [CrossRef] [Google Scholar]

Atta A, El-Sooud KA. The antinociceptive effect of some Egyptian medicinal plant extracts. J Ethnopharmacol. 2004;95:235–8. doi: 10.1016/j.jep.2004.07.006. [PubMed] [CrossRef] [Google Scholar]

Mazzutti S, Riehl CA, Ibañez E, Ferreira SR. Green-based methods to obtain bioactive extracts from Plantago major and Plantago lanceolata. J Supercrit Fluids. 2017;119:211–20. doi: 10.1016/j.supflu.2016.09.018. [CrossRef] [Google Scholar]

Mello JC, Gonzalez MV, Moraes VW, Prieto T, Nascimento OR, Rodrigues T. Protective Effect of Plantago major Extract against t-BOOH-Induced Mitochondrial Oxidative Damage and Cytotoxicity. Molecules. 2015;20:17747–59. doi: 10.3390/molecules201017747. [PMC free article] [PubMed] [CrossRef] [Google Scholar]

Mello JC, Guimaraes NS, Gonzalez MV, Paiva JS, Prieto T, Nascimento OR, et al. Hydroxyl scavenging activity accounts for differential antioxidant protection of Plantago major against oxidative toxicity in isolated rat liver mitochondria. J Pharm Pharmacol. 2012;64:1177–87. doi: 10.1111/j.2042-7158.2012.01496.x. [PubMed] [CrossRef] [Google Scholar]

Karima S, Farida S, Mihoub ZM. Antioxidant and antimicrobial activities of Plantago major. Int j pharm sci. 2015;7:58–64. [Google Scholar]

Stenholm A, Goransson U, Bohlin L. Bioassay-guided supercritical fluid extraction of cyclooxygenase-2 inhibiting substances in Plantago major L. Phytochem Anal. 2013;24:176–83. doi: 10.1002/pca.2398. [PubMed] [CrossRef] [Google Scholar]

Chiang L, Chiang W, Chang M, Ng L, Lin C. Antiviral activity of Plantago major extracts and related compounds in vitro. Antiviral Res. 2002;55:53–62. doi: 10.1016/S0166-3542(02)00007-4. [PubMed] [CrossRef] [Google Scholar]

Metiner K, Ozkan O, Ak S. Antibacterial effects of ethanol and acetone extract of Plantago major L. on Gram positive and Gram negative bacteria. Kafkas Univ Vet Fak Derg. 2012;18:503–5. doi: 10.9775/kvfd.2011.5824. [CrossRef] [Google Scholar]

Ponce-Macotela M, Navarro-Alegria I, Martinez-Gordillo M, Alvarez-Chacon R. In vitro effect against Giardia of 14 plant extracts. Rev Invest Clin. 1993;46:343–7. [PubMed] [Google Scholar]

Sharma H, Yunus G, Agrawal R, Kalra M, Verma S, Bhattar S. Antifungal efficacy of three medicinal plants Glycyrrhiza glabra, Ficus religiosa, and Plantago major against oral Candida albicans: A comparative analysis. Indian J Dent Res. 2016;27:433–6. doi: 10.4103/0970-9290.191895. [PubMed] [CrossRef] [Google Scholar]

Galvez M, Martí C, Lopez-Lazaro M, Cortes F, Ayuso J. Cytotoxic effect of Plantago spp. on cancer cell lines. J Ethnopharmacol. 2003;88:125–30. doi: 10.1016/S0378-8741(03)00192-2. [PubMed] [CrossRef] [Google Scholar]

Oto G, Ekin S, Ozdemir H, Levent A, Berber I. The effect of Plantago Major Linnaeus on serum total sialic acid, lipid-acibound sialic d, some trace elements and minerals after administration of 7, Dimethylbenz (a) anthracene in rats. Toxicol Ind Health. 2011;28:334–42. doi: 10.1177/0748233711412422. [PubMed] [CrossRef] [Google Scholar]

Velasco-Lezama R, Tapia-Aguilar R, Román-Ramos R, Vega-Avila E, Pérez-Gutiérrez MS. Effect of Plantagomajor on cell proliferation in vitro. J Ethnopharmacol. 2006;103:36–42. doi: 10.1016/j.jep.2005.05.050. [PubMed] [CrossRef] [Google Scholar]

Amini M, Kherad M, Mehrabani D, Azarpira N, Panjehshahin M, Tanideh N. Effect of Plantago major on burn wound healing in rat. J Appl Anim Res. 2010;37:53–6. doi: 10.1080/09712119.2010.9707093. [CrossRef] [Google Scholar]

. Zubair M, Ekholm A, Nybom H, Renvert S, Widen C, Rumpunen K. Effects of Plantago major L. leaf extracts on oral epithelial cells in a scratch assay. J Ethnopharmacol. 2012;141:825–30. doi: 10.1016/j.jep.2012.03.016. [PubMed] [CrossRef] [Google Scholar]

Nazarizadeh A, Mikaili P, Moloudizargari M, Aghajanshakeri S, Javaherypour S. Therapeutic uses and pharmacological properties of Plantago major L. and its active constituents. J Basic Appl Sci Res. 2013;3:212–21. [Google Scholar]

61. Guil J, Rodríguez-Garcí I, Torija E. Nutritional and toxic factors in selected wild edible plants. Plant Foods Hum Nutr. 1997;51:99–107. doi: 10.1023/A:1007988815888. [PubMed] [CrossRef] [Google Scholar]

Parra AL, Yhebra RS, Sardiñas IG, Buela LI. Comparative study of the assay of Artemia salina L. and the estimate of the medium lethal dose (LD50 value) in mice, to determine oral acute toxicity of plant extracts. Phytomedicine. 2001;8:395–400. doi: 10.1078/0944-7113-00044. [PubMed] [CrossRef] [Google Scholar]

Zubair M, Nybom H, Ahnlund M, Rumpunen K. Detection of genetic and phytochemical differences between and within populations of Plantago major L.(plantain) Sci Hortic. 2012;136:9–16. https://doi.org/10.1016/j.scienta.2012.01.002. [Google Scholar]

Balakhnina TI, Borkowska A, Nosalewicz M, Nosalewicz A, Włodarczyk TM, Kosobryukhov AA, et al. Effect of temperature on oxidative stress induced by lead in the leaves of Plantago major L. Int Agrophys. 2016;30:285–92. doi: 10.1515/intag-2015-0094. [CrossRef] [Google Scholar]

Doan DD, Nguyen NH, Doan HK, Nguyen TL, Phan TS, Van Dau N, et al. Studies on the individual and combined diuretic effects of four Vietnamese traditional herbal remedies (Zea mays, Imperata cylindrica, Plantago major and Orthosiphon stamineus) J Ethnopharmacol. 1992;36:225–31. [PubMed] [Google Scholar]

Doyle BJ, Frasor J, Bellows LE, Locklear TD, Perez A, Gomez-Laurito J, et al. Estrogenic effects of herbal medicines from Costa Rica used for the management of menopausal symptoms. Menopause. 2009;16:748–55. [PMC free article] [PubMed] [Google Scholar]

Kavyanifard S, Heidarieh N, Jamalo F, Alinejad G, Alinejad M, Mohammad EA. Effect of hydro alcoholic extract of Plantago major L. on pentilentetrazol-induced seizures in male mice. J Gorgan Uni Med Sci. 2016;18:41–5. [Google Scholar]

Shipochliev T. Uterotonic action of extracts from a group of medicinal plants. Vet Med Nauki. 1980;18:94–8. [PubMed] [Google Scholar]

Stewart A. Plantain (Plantago lanceolata)-a potential pasture species. Proceedings of the Conference-New Zealand Grassland Association; 1996. pp. 77–86. [Google Scholar]

. Tiwari A, Soni V, Londhe V, Bhandarkar A, Bandawane D, Nipate S. An overview on potent indigenous herbs for urinary tract infirmity: urolithiasis. Asian J Pharm Clin Res. 2012;5:7–12. [Google Scholar]

Hamedi S, Shams-Ardakani MR, Sadeghpour O, Amin G, Hajighasemali D, Orafai H. Designing mucoadhesive discs containing stem bark extract of Ziziphus jujuba based on Iranian traditional documents. Iran J Basic Med Sci. 2016;19:330–6. [PMC free article] [PubMed] [Google Scholar]

Hamedi S, Sadeghpour O, Shamsardekani MR, Amin G, Hajighasemali D, Feyzabadi Z. The Most Common Herbs to Cure the Most Common Oral Disease: Stomatitis Recurrent Aphthous Ulcer

(RAU) Iran Red Crescent Med J. 2016;18:e21694. doi: 10.5812/ircmj.21694. [PMC free article] [PubMed] [CrossRef] [Google Scholar]

Gautam R, Saklani A, Jachak SM. Indian medicinal plants as a source of antimycobacterial agents. J Ethnopharmacol. 2007;110:200–34. [PubMed] [Google Scholar]

Afsharypour S, Shafii K, Akbary ME, Zargarzadeh MR. Preparation and clinical evaluation of some anti-anorectal disease drugs obtained from medicineal. Med J Islam Repub Iran. 1996;10:73–7. [Google Scholar]

. Awaad AS, El-Meligy RM, Soliman GA. Natural products in treatment of ulcerative colitis and peptic ulcer. Saudi J Gastroenterol. 2013;17:101–24. doi: 10.1016/j.jscs.2012.03.002. [CrossRef] [Google Scholar]

Ozaslan M, Karagoz ID, Kiliç IH, Cengiz B, Kalender ME, Güldür ME, et al. Effect of Plantago major sap on Ehrlich ascites tumours in mice. Afr J Biotechnol. 2009;8:955–59. doi: 10.5897/AJB09.033. [CrossRef] [Google Scholar]

Ibn Beytar Z. Al-Jamee Le-Mofradaat al- Adwiah wal- Aghziyah (Comprehensive Book in Simple Drugs and Foods) Beirut: Dar-Al-Kotob Al-ilmiyah; 2001. [Google Scholar]

. Thomé RG, Santos HB, Santos FV, Oliveira RJ, De Camargos LF, Pereira MN, et al. Evaluation of healing wound and genotoxicity potentials from extracts hydroacoholic of Plantago major and Siparuna guianensis. Exp Biol Med (Maywood) 2012;237:1379–86. doi: 10.1258/ebm.2012.012139. [PubMed] [CrossRef] [Google Scholar]

Rahimi R, Shams-Ardekani MR, Abdollahi M. A review of the efficacy of traditional Iranian medicine for inflammatory bowel disease. World J Gastroenterol. 2010;16:4504–14. doi: 10.3748/wjg.v16.i36.4504. [PMC free article] [PubMed] [CrossRef] [Google Scholar]

Rotblatt M. Herbal medicine: expanded commission E monographs. Ann Intern Med. 2000;133:487. doi: 10.7326/0003-4819-133-6-200009190-00031. [CrossRef] [Google Scholar]

Haddadian K, Haddadian K, Zahmatkash M. A review of Plantago plant. Indian J Traditional Knowedlege. 2014;13:681–5. [Google Scholar]

Antal DS, Canciu CM, Dehelean CA, Anke M. How much selenium do medicinal plants contain? Results of a research on wild-growing species from Western Romania. An Univ Oradea Fasc Biol. 2010;17:23–8. [Google Scholar]

Balmus IM, Ciobica A, Antioch I, Dobrin R, Timofte D. Oxidative Stress Implications in the Affective Disorders: Main Biomarkers, Animal Models Relevance, Genetic Perspectives, and Antioxidant Approaches. Oxid Med Cell Longev. 2016;2016:3975101. doi: 10.1155/2016/3975101. Epub 2016 Aug 1. PMID: 27563374; PMCID: PMC4983669.

Chatgilialoglu C, Ferreri C, Masi A, Melchiorre M, Sansone A, Terzidis MA, Torreggiani A. Free radicals in chemical biology: from chemical behavior to biomarker development. J Vis Exp. 2013 Apr 15;(74):50379. doi: 10.3791/50379. PMID: 23629513; PMCID: PMC3664958.

Radulović NS1, Genčić MS2, Stojanović NM3, Randjelović PJ4, Stojanović-Radić ZZ5, Stojiljković NI4. Toxic essential oils. Part V: Behaviour modulating and toxic properties of thujones and thujone-containing essential oils of Salvia officinalis L., Artemisia absinthium L., Thuja occidentalis L. and Tanacetum vulgare L. 1Department of Chemistry, Faculty of Science and Mathematics, University of Niš, Višegradska 33, 18000 Niš, Serbia.
2Department of Chemistry, Faculty of Science and Mathematics, University of Niš, Višegradska 33, 18000 Niš, Serbia.3Faculty of Medicine, University of Niš, Bulevar Zorana Đinđića 81, 18000 Niš, Serbia.
4Department of Physiology, Faculty of Medicine, University of Niš, Bulevar Zorana Đinđića 81, 18000 Niš, Serbia.5Department of Biology and Ecology, Faculty of Science and Mathematics, University of Niš, Višegradska 33, 18000 Niš, Serbia.

Public statement on the use of herbal medicinal products containing thujone. 27 January 2011
EMA/HMPC/732886/2010
Committee on Herbal Medicinal Products (HMPC)

In vitro toxicological evaluation of essential oils and their main compounds used in active food packaging: A review.Llana-Ruiz-Cabello M, Pichardo S, Maisanaba S, Puerto M, Prieto AI, Gutiérrez-Praena D, Jos A, Cameán AM.Food Chem Toxicol. 2015 Jul; 81:9-27. Epub 2015 Apr 9.